Newer Trends in Management of Nursing Services and Education

Newer Trends in Management of Nursing Services and Education

Dr Alamelu Venketaraman PhD (N)
Director, Nursing Education and Research
Westfort College of Nursing
Westfort Academy for Higher Education
Thrissur, Kerala, India
Former Principal and Dean
Omayal Achi College of Nursing
Avadi, Chennai, Tamil Nadu, India

Foreword
SA Samuel

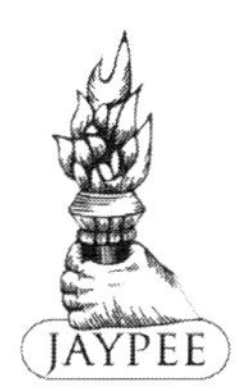

The Health Sciences Publisher
New Delhi | London | Panama

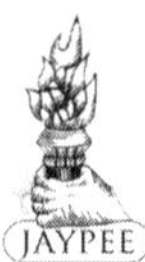

Jaypee Brothers Medical Publishers (P) Ltd

Headquarters

Jaypee Brothers Medical Publishers (P) Ltd
4838/24, Ansari Road, Daryaganj
New Delhi 110 002, India
Phone: +91-11-43574357
Fax: +91-11-43574314
Email: jaypee@jaypeebrothers.com

Overseas Offices

J.P. Medical Ltd
83 Victoria Street, London
SW1H 0HW (UK)
Phone: +44 20 3170 8910
Fax: +44 (0)20 3008 6180
Email: info@jpmedpub.com

Jaypee-Highlights Medical Publishers Inc
City of Knowledge, Bld. 235, 2nd Floor, Clayton
Panama City, Panama
Phone: +1 507-301-0496
Fax: +1 507-301-0499
Email: cservice@jphmedical.com

Jaypee Brothers Medical Publishers (P) Ltd
17/1-B Babar Road, Block-B, Shaymali
Mohammadpur, Dhaka-1207
Bangladesh
Mobile: +08801912003485
Email: jaypeedhaka@gmail.com

Jaypee Brothers Medical Publishers (P) Ltd
Bhotahity, Kathmandu, Nepal
Phone +977-9741283608
Email: kathmandu@jaypeebrothers.com

Website: www.jaypeebrothers.com
Website: www.jaypeedigital.com

Inquiries for bulk sales may be solicited at: jaypee@jaypeebrothers.com

Newer Trends in Management of Nursing Services and Education

First Edition: **2017,** Reprint: 2023

ISBN: 978-93-86261-59-5

Printed at: Sterling Graphics Pvt. Ltd.

DEDICATED TO

*My husband, Dr S Venketaraman who has supported me
in everything I have ever done or gone through and to my loving son,
Vasudevan, a writer who constantly amazes me
with his own work and his love for writing.
His inspiration and advice has been invaluable.*

Foreword

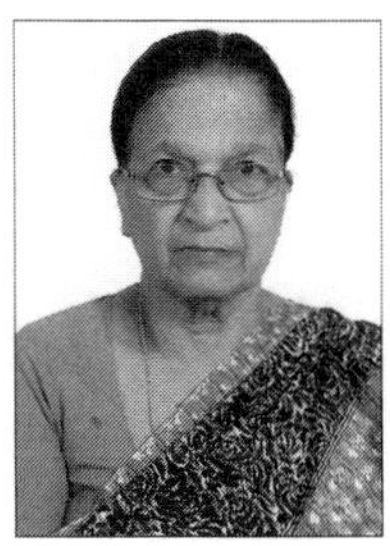

Newer Trends in Management of Nursing Services and Education authored by Dr Alamelu Venketaraman is a long felt need of nurses in India, both in the areas of nursing practice and education. This era, characterized by rapid change in medical and health system technology, knowledge explosion, consumerism and the complex health care demands, challenges the nurses' knowledge, technical competence, interpersonal skills and commitment today, more than ever before. Nurses are working in varied levels of health care system, shouldering responsibilities of contributing to *Health for All* are constantly in contact with people in health and sickness. Coping with this soaring demand and ensuring unlimited career opportunities for nurses, comparable to those in other disciplines, graduate and postgraduate nurses require knowledge and skill in managing nursing care. This textbook will ultimately prepare them to be nurse managers, hospital administrators and nurse leaders. Further, nurses with leadership skills and a clear vision for the future can motivate associates to work towards common goals of survival of the organization, strengthening the workforce and to thrive during rapid change.

It is a known fact that the development and use of Information Technology has revolutionized the world today. Thus, it has also influenced nursing service and educational administration. Significant developments are the use of management by objectives, program evalution review technique (PERT), critical path method, management information system in nursing and electronic health records.

I commend Dr Mrs Venketaraman is rising to the occasion to provide this invaluable book, designed with fifteen units containing twenty-eight chapters. The setting of the chapters with learning objectives, conceptualization of the contents, supportive figures, tables and examples in boxes, research highlights, summary points, review questions, selected readings, index and glossary are most useful to the students of BSc, post basic BSc and MSc nursing courses. Special care taken by the author to deal with application of principles of administration in nursing services and education, issues and challenges faced by nurse leaders and newer trends in management are a ready reckoner for students of management courses prescribed by the Indian Nursing Council.

This textbook, anchored on Dr Mrs Venketaraman's vast experience in varied levels of nursing services and education, focusing especially on the Indian settings, is a blessing in disguise to the learners. I have no doubt that our nursing students and faculty will enjoy learning and applying these principles in their professional practice and reach greater heights in their chosen career.

My heartiest congratulations to Dr Venketaraman, whom I have known for many years, for completing this book on management, which is very very close to my heart. She has met one of the unmet needs of nursing in India through this textbook. I eagerly look forward to the improvement in the quality of nursing services and education in the country to make nurses equal partners in health care with their medical counterparts to make India a healthier Nation.

Ms SA Samuel
Former Principal
College of Nursing
National Institute of Nursing Education (NINE)
PGIMER, Chandigarh, India

Preface

Nursing is a dynamic, progressive and developing profession which ensures unlimited career opportunities for graduate and postgraduate nurses. Clinical nurses, teaching nurses, unit management, departmental or hospital nursing service administrator or clinical nurse researcher are the major roles where nurses focus to take up in future. This denotes that nurses are not only health care providers, but also health care managers who exercise both clinical and administrative role.

Today, health care delivery system is more complex, chaotic and challenging. Medical and health-related technological advancements, global shortage of nurses, quality and patient safety as benchmark of nursing practice, increased diversified work force in work setting, greater accountability for nursing care practice, ethical and legal aspects of care, consumerism, accreditation preparedness, nursing standards, best practices evidence informed in administration and many other factors warrants effective nurse managers, administrators and educational administrators who demonstrate core competencies of nursing leadership at all levels of nursing service administration and education. The framework of nursing management and administration requires a conceptualization of various functions, roles and responsibilities of nurse manager and administrator in hospital and academic setting.

Though many textbooks on management are available in the country, yet this book on ***Newer Trends in Management of Nursing Services and Education*** reflects on application of principles of administration in ward units, hospital and nursing school, administrative theories, leadership, innovations in nursing service administration, nursing standards, quality control in nursing and other features for undergraduates, post basic BSc nursing and postgraduate nursing program in nursing in management of nursing services and education course.

This textbook is very comprehensive and can be used by hospital nursing administrators, ward sisters and academic administrators.

Dr Alamelu Venketaraman

Acknowledgments

With a deep sense of fulfillment and gratitude, first and foremost I thank the Omnipotent, Omnipresent Almighty God for enabling me to complete the First Edition of this textbook ***Newer Trends in Management of Nursing Services and Education.***

It was my long cherished desire to write a book on Nursing Administration and this was made possible when Mr Jayanandan, Senior Commissioning Editor, and Mr Senthil, Team Leader, Jaypee Brothers Medical Publishers, Chennai, encouraged me to write this textbook. I whole heartedly thank them for their constant support and guidance.

My special gratitude to Ms Ruby Sharma, Project Manager, Jaypee Brothers Medical Publishers, for her untiring support which kept me more engaged and updated. I also appreciate the production team for their cooperation in maintaining precision in completing this textbook. I appreciate the extraordinary patience of the team members that provided me a source of inspiration.

I wish to express my solemn sentiments and heartiest thanks to each of the authors of various textbooks, journal articles, and websites whose references are being cited in the textbook without which the scientific base for the facts would not be possible.

I wish to thank personally Mr K Mohan Das, our Managing Director of Westfort Hospital Group, a farsighted visionary leader and administrator to permit me to include in the mission, vision and philosophy of nursing service administration, performance appraisal format, and philosophy of staffing of Westfort College of Nursing as example in the related topics. I accord a special gratitude to Prof Shirley Prakash, Principal, Westfort College of Nursing for her sincere support.

I am grateful to Prof R Rekha, Principal, VNSS College of Nursing, Kollam (Kerala) for her constant encouragement and Library support.

I accord special gratitude to Dr Gayatri Vyas Mahindroo, Director, National Accreditation Board for Hospitals and Healthcare Providers (NABH) for granting permission to include the National Assessment and Accreditation Council (NAAC), India.

I owe deepest gratitude and huge thanks to Dr Annie Grace Kalaimathi, Registrar, Tamil Nadu Nurses and Midwives Council and Dr Latha R, Principal, Goverment College of Nursing, Thrissur Medical College, Kerala and former Registrar of Kerala Nurses and Midwives Council for providing information regarding State Nursing Council and excellent support.

It is a pleasure to thank those who made contributions by sharing their research findings related to the topic and expanded knowledge to this textbook.

- Dr Susan Armstrong, Faculty of Health Sciences, Johannesburg, South Africa.
- Dr Hemant Kumar, Commandant, Rajouri Hospital, Jammu and Kashmir, India.
- Dr Usha Marath, Prof-cum-Principal, Lisie College of Nursing, Ernakulum, Kerala, India.
- Dr Sunita Lawrence, Principal, Pragyan College of Nursing, Bhopal, Madhya Pradesh, India.
- Dr Usha Ukhande and Faculty Members, Choithram College of Nursing, Indore, Madhya Pradesh, India.
- Prof Shija Binoy and Prof Jaya Binoy, Faculty, Pragyan College of Nursing, Bhopal, Madhya Pradesh, India.
- Prof Rajani Bhagga and Viashali, Faculty (Through the kindness of Dr Usha Ukhande, NRSI) New Delhi, India.

I owe my special thanks to all principals, nursing faculties, and nursing students of colleges of nursing for their request to write this textbook and their encouragement and confidence showed on me.

The responsibility of completing this edition would have been impossible without the sacrifice made by Dr S Venketaraman, my dear husband and Vasudevan, my beloved son, allowing me to spare the family time in writing this humble textbook. I appreciate my heartiest appreciation and sentiments to them.

Finally, I thank all those who helped me directly or indirectly to complete this textbook.

Dr Alamelu Venketaraman

Contents

Unit I: Introduction to Health Administration

Introduction

This textbook on *Newer Trends in Management of Nursing Services and Education* comprising of fifteen units with twenty-eight chapters covering all the contents comprehensively, built on sequential order and presented systematically in a simple manner.

Unit I: Introduction to Health Administration

This unit consists of two chapters which are dealt with very important aspects of postgraduate nursing curriculum on management. **Chapter 1** focuses on overview of Indian health care system constitutes Indian constitution, and Indian administrative system. Special emphasis is given on health care delivery system at national, state, district and local level. It also includes India's five year plans and has taken special attention to present the impact of five year plans in development of nursing services in the country.

Chapter 2 highlights India's health care policies. Author has presented all the health committee reports from its inception till date and a meticulous care has been taken to present the impact of various health committee reports on nursing profession. It also depicts national health policies, national population policies and national policies on AYUSH and plans.

Unit II: Introduction to Nursing Service Administration

This unit consists of two chapters. **Chapter 3** concentrates on the basic and advanced concept of nursing administration and management with their differences in significance, principles and functions in an elaborate manner. It also describes various management theories in detail and its application in nursing service administration.

Chapter 4 presents the role of a nurse administrator and manager in a hospital. The role of nurse administrator in a hospital and a nurse manager in a unit (ward) describes, administrative, supervisory, educative, and research role in detail. Few nursing research highlights are presented in the end of chapter.

Unit III: Functions of Administration

This unit consists of two chapters. **Chapter 5** mainly focuses on planning, its concept, definition, principles, goals and objectives. In-depth description is given in various types of planning like operational plan, strategic planning, proactive planning, organizational Planning and managerial planning and each of their application in nursing service administration and management. In this chapter the philosophy, vision and mission of administration is dealt in detail with an example planning for change and planning a new venture is a special feature which is very beneficial for nurse managers and administrators in the current scenario.

Chapter 6 describes the concept and purposes of program evaluation review technique (PERT), critical path method (CPM), use of Gantt chart and management by objectives (MBO) that are current trends in management. It describes the topics in an elaborate manner and has furnished examples from nursing. It ends with a related research highlight.

Unit IV: Organization

Organization is the second function of administration This unit consists of five chapters. **Chapter 7** presents conceptualization of organization, organization structure of nursing service department and organization chart with diagram, advantages and disadvantages.

Chapter 8 focuses on organization process. It is built on the major principles of organization such as centralization *vs* decentralization, delegation of authority, span of control (supervision), division of service, and departmentalization. Attempt has been made to apply each principle in nursing service administration with their advantages and disadvantages.

Chapter 9 reviews organizational theories. Organizational effectiveness, organizational climate and organizational culture are explained in detail with greater emphasis on application of these concepts and the role of nurse administrator in their work setting.

Chapter 10 focuses on organizing nursing services and patient care deals with patient classification system, advantages and their disadvantages. Methods of patient assignment is dealt in detail with diagrammatic representation for easy understanding. Planning and organizing of hospital unit is dealt elaborately with ancillary services. Planning and establishing an intensive care unit is presented as an example in this chapter.

Chapter 11 focuses on power and politics in an organization. It includes the concept, types and factors influencing political behavior in nursing. It also presents the role of nurse administrator in power and politics in administration.

Unit V: Staffing

Staffing is one of the important functions of administration. This unit consists of two chapters. **Chapter 12** emphasizes the concept staffing and scheduling and staffing norms prescribed by various regulatory and government bodies. It highlights estimation of nursing staff requirement based on an activity analysis study.

Chapter 13 deals in detail the staffing process on personnel administration/human resource management. It focuses on recruitment: credentialing, selection, placement, promotion, retention, personnel policies, termination, staff development programme. Supervision, duties and responsibilities of various category of nursing personnel and their applications to nursing service and education. It ends with research highlights.

Unit VI: Directing

This unit consists of two chapters. **Chapter 14** conceptualizes leadership in nursing, theories of motivation and emphasizes in depth the role of nurse administrator as a leader in creating a motivational climate in work setting for quality care outcome. It emphasizes on communication skills and communication strategies which are important for smooth administration of hospital/unit.

Chapter 15 presents organizational behavior and human relations that are backbone strength in nursing administration. Role of nurse administrator in group dynamics, human relations, public relation in context of nursing, decision-making, delegation, conflict management, negotiation and collective bargaining are explained in detail and the chapter ends with research highlights in leadership.

Unit VII: Controlling

This unit consists of two chapters. **Chapter 16** presents quality assurance in detail. It describes the concepts and the role of nurse administrator in quality control, quality assurance, total quality improvement and nursing audit. It also highlights quality improvement models.

Chapter 17 presents performance appraisal as a managerial tool to control administration with example format. It also elaborately discusses coaching and mentoring to improve performance of nurses/employees, discipline and disciplinary strategies for smooth running of the nursing administration and employee's grievance procedure to rectify their problems.

Unit VIII: Material Management

Utilization of resources is an important function of nurse administrator. **Chapter 18** elaborately discusses concept, principles and procedures of material management. It also presents planning and procurement procedures and specifications, ABC analysis, and very important and essential daily use (VED) analysis. The essence of this chapter is the role of hospital nurse administrator and unit managers in planning equipments and supplies for nursing care: Unit and hospital, inventory control and condemnation.

Unit IX: Financial Administration

Like materials, finance is also essential to run a department. **Chapter 19** presents budget for nursing service department in detail. Apart from conceptualizing budget, it emphasizes plan and non-plan, zero budgeting, mid-term appraisal, capital and revenue. More focus is given on role of nurse administrator in budget estimate, revised estimate, performance budget and auditing. Cost effectiveness, cost accounting, critical pathways, health care reforms, health economics, and health insurance are other important features of this chapter. Example of nursing budget for nursing department is presented for easy understanding.

Unit X: Legal and Ethical Issues

Today, nurses are confronted with various legal issues and ethical dilemmas. **Chapter 20** presents conceptualization of law and ethics, legal system, legal issues in nursing, medicolegal issues and patient care issues. The role of regulatory bodies in nursing ethics, patients' rights, consumer protection act, professional responsibility and accountability, infection control, standard safety measures national accreditation boards for hospitals and ethical committee in an institution are special features in this chapter. It ends with research highlights.

Unit XI: Nursing Informatics

We are living in digital era today and the advances in information technology have created new roles for nurses, and stressed the need for all nursing personnel irrespective of their position to become more knowledgeable about health information concepts and the technology. **Chapter 21** present concepts, use of computers by health care professional in hospital and community, patient record system, nursing records and reports including electronic medical records, management information and evaluation system (MIES), e-nursing, telemedicine, and telenursing.

Unit XII: Nursing Unit Management

Chapter 22 presents introduction to ward management. It emphasizes the role of ward manger or head nurse in planning physical facilities, floor space, time planning daily/weekly plan, and maintaining therapeutic environment for patients. It also elaborates the factors influencing ward management and the role of a head nurse in student education specifically nursing rounds, nursing care conference, etc. to enhance their clinical knowledge.

Unit XIII: Educational Administration

Chapter 23 on applications of principles of administration in nursing education focuses on the role of academic administrator in application of principles of, planning, organizing, staffing, directing, controlling and budgeting in nursing school administration.

Unit XIV: Issues and Challenges

This unit consists of three chapters. **Chapter 24** presents issues and challenges in administration specific to nursing service and education.

Chapter 25 presents emergencies and disaster management specific to epidemiology of disasters, role of nurses in disaster management and rehabilitation.

Chapter 26 on nursing standards describe the concept, importance, characteristics and type of standards. The most important aspect of the chapter is, it describes the framework and steps in developing nursing standards.

Unit XV: Nursing as a Profession

This unit consists of two chapters. **Chapter 27** focuses on introduction to nursing as a profession, philosophy of nursing practice, aims and objectives of nursing, characteristics of professional nurse and regulatory bodies—NINC, SNC acts and functions for nursing.

Chapter 28 stresses on professional advancement for nurses that include, continuing education, career opportunities, membership in professional organization participation in research activities and publication of research findings in journals and newspapers.

I am sure that the students may enjoy studying this textbook. However, there is always a room for improvement of this textbook. Your comments and suggestions for improvement of this humble book shall be highly appreciated.

Dr Alamelu Venketaraman

UNIT I
INTRODUCTION TO HEALTH ADMINISTRATION

1. Overview of Indian Health Care System
2. India's Health Care Policies

1

Overview of Indian Health Care System

LEARNING OBJECTIVES

This chapter imparts learning about:

- Introduction to Constitution of India
- The Purpose, Functions and Provision of Health-Related Facilities to Indian Citizens as Per the Constitution
- Description of the Current Health Administration at Various Levels in India
- The Organizational Structure of Health System in the Country
- Introduction to Five Year Plans and their Impact on Health
- Current Five Year Plan and Health

INTRODUCTION

India is the largest populated democratic country in the world comprising 29 states, and 7 union territories. The states are administered by respective state Governments and Union Territories by Central government. The Indian Republic is controlled by her Constitution headed by the President of India. India became Republic on 26th of January in 1950, though the constitution was officially adopted on 26th November 1949.

THE CONSTITUTION OF INDIA

As per the constitution of India, the Indian Parliamentary system of administration, constitute the President and two houses. According to its Article 79, they are:

- The Rajya Sabha (The council of States) also called Upper House
- The Lok Sabha (The house of people) also called Lower House.

Apart from this, there is a provision in the constitution that there shall be council of ministers headed by the Prime Minister of India. This council and the prime minister advises the President of India in matters related to Indian administration and the President functions accordingly.

The prime minister is vested with all executive powers. The council of Ministers are responsible to the function of Lok Sabha.

Every state has a legislative assembly and legislative council. The Governor of the state is the administrative head of the legislative assembly. The Chief Minister of the State as the head of the Legislative council advises the Governor in execution of Governmental program.

The Indian Constitution is being the longest written document in the worldcountries, it comprises 448 articles in 22 parts, 12 schedules and 100 amendments as on 2015. The architect of Indian Constitution is believed to be Dr Bhimrao Ambedkar.

The major functions of the constitution is to ensure all citizens of the country protection and safeguard against their rights, define the characteristics of the government system and establish a strong government in the country.

The three component parts of Government are (Fig. 1.1):

1. **Executive Body:** The executive body consists of temporary and permanent executives. Prime Minister along with his council of ministers are the Temporary Executives. These officials are elected for every five years and hence called as Temporary Executives. These executives often are drawn from the legislature. The permanent executives are civil servants and other officials working under the government of India. They are assigned the task of policy implementation.
2. **Legislative Body:** According to the constitution, Legislature is the policy making body of India. Each and every Act/bill is initiated/proposed by the executive Body has to be discussed, reviewed, analyzed and amended and voted upon in the legislature for approval. So ultimately it is the legislature that decides which bills should be passed. The executive can bypass the legislature through ordinance. But the validity of this ordinance is six months only and it has to be ratified by the legislature.
3. **Judiciary Body:** Judiciary is the evaluation body. Supreme court is the head of the body and independent. Judiciary has the power to review any bill or law passed by the Parliament and can declare a law null and void if it violates the constitution of the country.

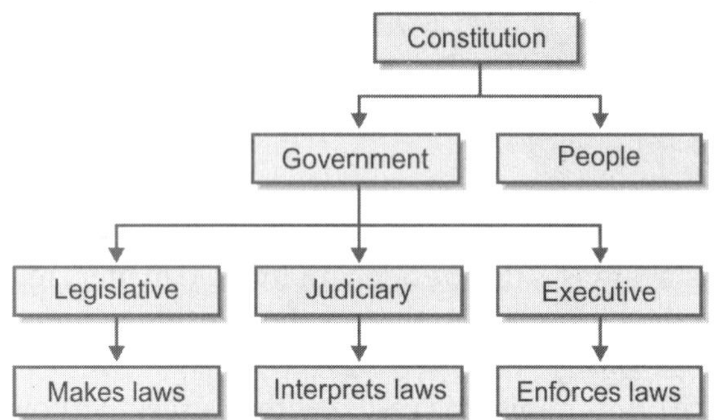

Fig. 1.1: Role of constitution in relationship between the government and people

Functions of the Constitution

- To provide a set of basic rules that permits for minimal coordination amongst citizen of a society to clarify the authority who has the power to make decisions in a society and the government constituted.
- To set a frame of reference on the rules that government can impose on its citizens.
- To help the government to fulfill and establish conditions for a society.

Preamble of Constitution

Preamble describes the philosophy, values, ideals, goals and objectives of the constitution. It forms as a preface to the constitution.

'We the people of India having solemnly resolved to constitute India into a sovereign socialist secular democratic republic and to secure to all its citizens:

Justice, social, economic and political; Liberty of thought, expression, belief, faith and worship; equality of status and of opportunity and to promote among them all; Fraternity: assuring the dignity of the individual and the unity and integrity of the nation; in our constituent assembly this twenty sixth day of November 1949, do hereby adopt, enact and give to ourselves this constitution.'

As of June 2015, there were 100 amendments since it was first enacted in 1950.

Structure of Constitution of India

The constitution of India (Fig. 1.2) in the current form consists of 1 preamble, 25 parts containing 450 articles, 12 schedules, 2 appendices and 100 Amendments (June 2015). The parts and articles describe fundamental rights, directive principles and fundamental duties.

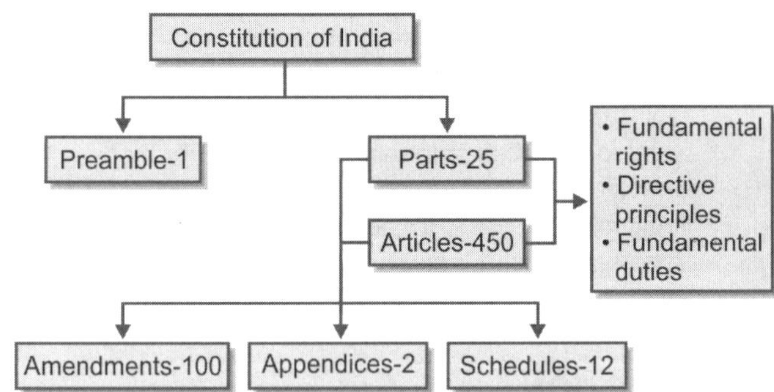

Fig. 1.2: Structure of constitution of India

It is every citizen's responsibility to safeguard our constitution apart from the responsibilities of the jurists and policy makers, that will enable each countrymen to work in harmony for the development of the nation. The first book of constitution of India is preserved in Parliament Library Building, New Delhi, India.

INDIAN ADMINISTRATIVE SYSTEM: HEALTH CARE DELIVERY SYSTEM–NATIONAL, STATE AND LOCAL LEVEL

Health care delivery system in India includes both facilities at state and central governments. The various form of health care delivery in India are three tier health care system include a system of Community Health Centers (CHC) Primary Health Centers (PHC) and Sub Health Centers (SHC) are available for people in rural areas, hospitals at state and district levels. Maternal and Child Health Service (MCH) and family welfare (FW) centre, family planning clinics, maternity homes are available in urban areas. Health insurance, national health programmes private hospitals and corporate/contributory hospitals indigenous systems of medicine NGO's and voluntary health organizations. are also delivering health care for the people at district and state levels.

HEALTH ADMINISTRATION AT NATIONAL LEVEL

It comprises of:

- Central ministry of Health and Family Welfare.
- Directorate General of Health Services (DGHS) headed by Director General of Health services. The Directorate is responsible to look into the matters affecting medical care and hospitals, public health and general administration.
- Central Council of Health (CCH).

Administration and organization of central ministry of health and family welfare has three departments:

- Department of Health that is helped by the Director General of Health services by supporting technical guidance and advice on medical and public health affairs including supervising and monitoring national health schemes.
- Department of Family Welfare supports family welfare program sponsored by the central government.
- Department of Indian Systems of Medicine and Homeopathy: This department is responsible for supporting Indian system of medicine (AYUSH).

NATIONAL LEVEL

Organization Structure of Union Ministry of Health and Family Welfare (Fig. 1.3)

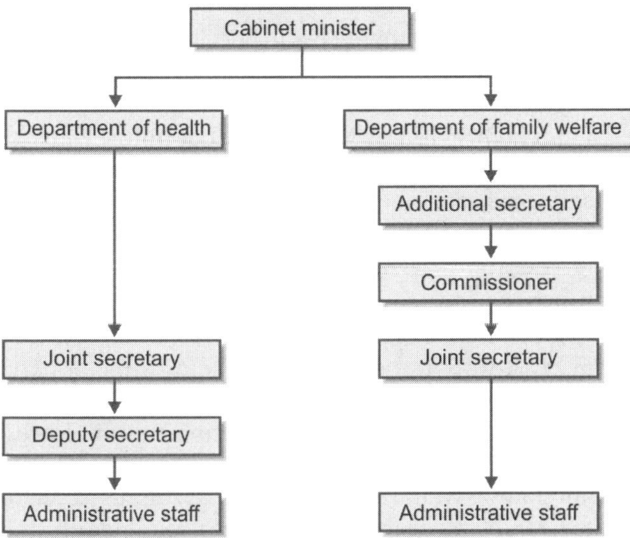

Fig. 1.3: Organization structure of union ministry of health and family welfare

Functions of Central Government under Union List

- Establishing international health relations and quarantine regulation.
- Monitor and control of drug standards in the country.
- Administration and supervision of centrally sponsored establishments.
- Enhancing research activities through research centers and institutions.
- Development of medical, dental, nursing and pharmacy as professions through proper regulation and control.
- Collection and publication of census data.
- For statistical data facilitating health intelligence publications.
- Monitoring immigration and emigration.
- Support and formulation of regulation of workers engaged in mines/coal fields.

Specific Functions according to the Concurrent List

The following listed functions are the responsibilities of both the central and state government:

- Prevention and control of communicable diseases
- Prevention of adulteration of food
- Control of drug and poisons
- Vital statistics
- Labor welfare
- Ports other than those declared by or under law made by Parliament
- Economic and social planning
- Population control and family planning
- Preparation of health education materials for creating awareness through Central Health Education Board
- Collection, compilation analysis, evaluation and dissemination of information through Central Bureau of Health Intelligence
- National Medical library.

Organization Structure of Directorate General of Health Services

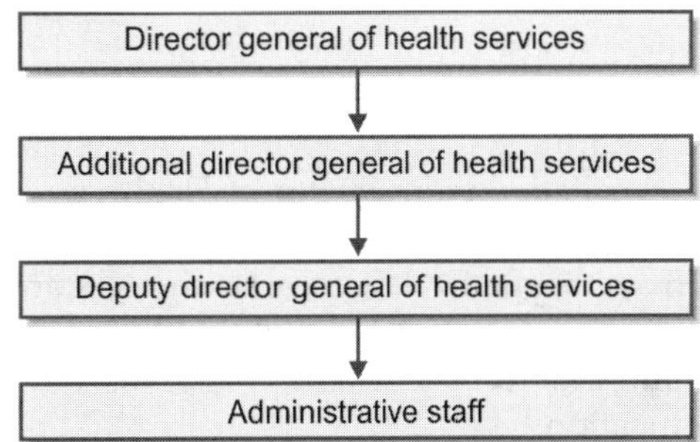

Fig. 1.4: Organization structure of directorate of health services

Functions of Directorate General of Health Services

- International health relations and quarantine of all major ports and international airports in India
- Control of drug standards
- Maintenance of medical store depots
- Administration of Postgraduate training program
- Administration of selected medical colleges in India
- Conduct of medical research through Indian Council of Medical Research
- Preparation of health education materials for creating awareness through Central Health Education Board
- Collection, compilation analysis, evaluation and dissemination of information through Central Bureau of Health Intelligence
- National medical library.

Organization Structure of Central Council of Health

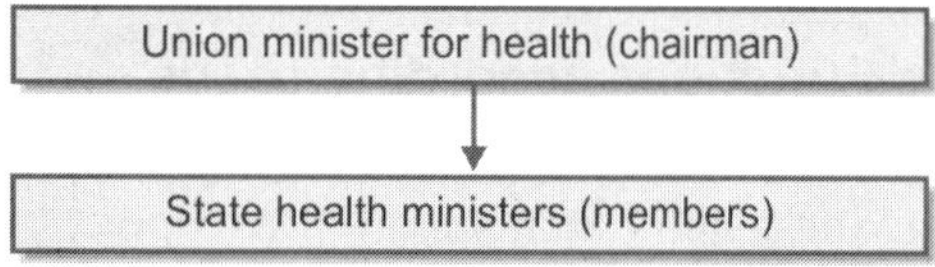

Fig. 1.5: Organization structure of central council of health

Functions of Central Council of Health

- To consider and recommend broad outlines of policies regarding health–environmental hygiene, nutrition and health education
- To make proposals for legislation relating to medical and public health matter
- To make recommendations to central government regarding distribution of grant-in-aid.

HEALTH ADMINISTRATION AT STATE LEVEL

India has 29 states and 7 union territories as per census 2011. Health is a state subject and state health ministry takes responsibility to take care the health of the people like union health ministry. The health ministry of the state is supported by the Health Secretariat headed by Health Secretary and the Health Directorate headed by the Director of health services. Director of health services is a technical advisor to matters affecting health and he is assisted by the deputy and additional directors of health. The additional director for the Family Welfare of the state is called Commissioner of Health and Family Welfare. In most of the states, medical education has been isolated from the medical directorate services and a post of Director of Medical Education has been introduced to support and monitor medical, nursing and other allied health education.

Organization Structure of State Ministry of Health and Family Welfare

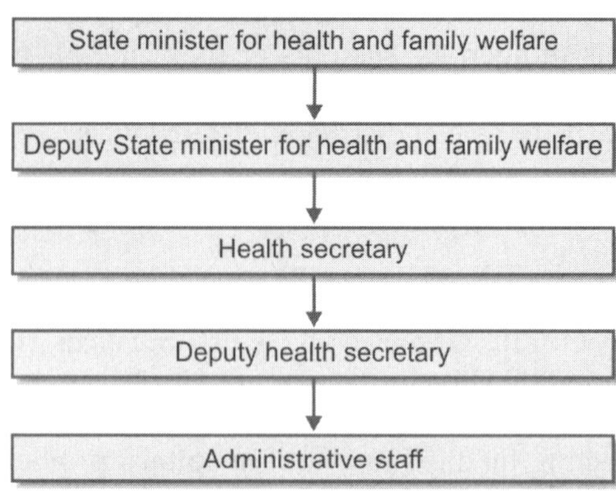

Fig. 1.6: Organization structure of state ministry of health and family welfare

Functions of the State Health Department

- Facilitate quality medical care in urban and rural population through hospitals, dispensaries and health centers
- Arrange and promote medical, nursing education and research
- Implementation of all the national health programmes.
- Facilitate for nutrition, industrial health, family planning services to population
- Monitor and control adulteration of drug
- Support, monitor, supervise and control of local bodies
- Establishment of laboratories
- Promotion of AYUSH care.

STATE DIRECTORATE FOR HEALTH

It is headed by Director of Health Services with a staffing pattern comprising of Joint Secretary, Special Secretary, Deputy Secretary and additional Directors.

- Under Director of Medical Education, Deans of medical colleges and deputy director of nursing services functions.
- Under deputy director of nursing services, colleges of nursing and nursing services of the hospitals functions.
- Under Director of Medical and Rural Health Services, many additional directors and joint directors and deputy directors are functioning such as additional directors for indigenous medicine, public health and preventive medicine, commissioner of Health and family welfare (H and FW), Additional Director for MCH. Research Statistics, Public Health and Preventive Medicine, Primary Health Centers.

- Joint directors holding responsibilities of PHC Department, Immunization. Prevention of Food Adulteration, Training, Health Education Bureau Epidemiology and Nutrition.
- Deputy director for school health program.

Functions of Directorate of Health Services

- Studies the health problems and needs of the state and plans for various schemes for addressing those problems identified
- Prevention and curative health services
- Provision for control of milk and food sanitation
- Prevention of outbreak of communicable diseases
- Promotion of health education
- Promotion of school health, family planning and occupational health
- Supervision of community health centers and primary health centers
- Establishing training for health personnel
- Coordination of all health services with other ministers of health.

ADMINISTRATION AND ORGANIZATION AT REGIONAL LEVEL

Some of the states like Bihar, Madhya Pradesh, Uttar Pradesh, Karnataka and other zonal/regional/divisional areas have the State Directorate of Health Services and District Health administration. There is a difference in zonal and regional administration headed by Additional/Joint/Deputy Directors of Health Services.

ADMINISTRATION AND ORGANIZATION AT DISTRICT LEVEL

As per census 2011, India has 640 districts, 5767 Tehsils, 7,933 Towns, 6,00,000 villages. District administration provides a link between state and the region and acts middle management on one end and peripheral level organization on the other end. The aim of the district level administration is collecting information from the state and communicates to the peripheral institutions. Each district, there are six types of administrative areas:

- Subdivision
- Tehsil (Taluka)
- Community Development Block
- Municipalities and Corporation
- Villages
- Panchayats.

Collector is the administrative head of the district and subdivision is administered by assistant collector or sub collector. Each district is divided into two or more subdivisions. Each subdivision is divided into Taluka with 200–600 villages. The administrative head of the Taluka is Tehsildar. Community development block is headed by Block Development Officer (BDO), each block comprising of 100 villages with a population of 20,000 to 1,20,000 population.

ADMINISTRATION AND ORGANIZATION AT SUBDIVISION LEVEL

For easy administration, each district is divided into two or more subdivisions, called Tehsils or Taluka having Taluka hospitals, dispensaries, nursing homes and general hospital or rural hospitals for the people, run by the Government. General physicians are responsible to take care of the patients.

Organization: Assistant District Health and Family Welfare Officer (ADHO) is responsible for Taluka hospitals or other government sponsored clinics who is assisted by medical officers of health and lady medical officers of general hospitals. these are now being converted in CHC for a population of 3,00,000.

ADMINISTRATION AND ORGANIZATION AT BLOCK LEVEL

In each Block a Community Health Center (CHC) is available to provide health care for 3, 00,000 population. Under each CHC, primary health centers (PHC) are established to cater health services for 10,000 population. Under each PHC, 5–6 sub health centers (SHCs) are available serving 5,000 population comprising of 5–6 villages with a population of each village 1000. Administratively the block comes under Panchayat Samiti headed by Block of Development officer and the village administration comes under Panchayat headed by Panchayat president.

Medical Services at Block Level in Rural Areas

Community Health Center is the First Referral Unit (FRU) that facilitates

- Emergency care, routine medical and surgical care for patients.
- Maternal and child health care for 24 × 7 days
- Family planning and abortion care services
- Essential newborn care and care of sick children
- Implementation of all national health program.

The community center is manned by 22–29 health personnel including Medical officer and Block Medical Officer (Civil Surgeon)-3, Staff Nurses-2, health supervisor-1, Community Health Nurse-1, Sector Health Nurse 3–5, Health Worker (Male/Female) 6–10, Female Nursing Assistant-1, Pharmacist-1.

Laboratory technician-1, Ophthalmic assistant-1, Radiographer-1, Hospital Worker-1.

Primary Health Center (PHC) comes under block.

The main functions of PHC are:

- Medical care MCH including Family Planning
- Safe water supply and basic sanitation
- Prevention and control of local endemic diseases
- Collection and reporting vital statistics
- Implementation of national programs
- Referral Services to CHC
- Training of health guides, health workers
- Basic laboratory services and education about health
- Collection of vital statistics.

The PHC is manned by (a total 15 persons headed by Medical officer-1 and the following health personnel:

- Pharmacist: 1
- Nurse Midwife: 1
- Health Worker (Female)/ANM/VHN: 1
- Health Educator: 1
- Health Assistant (Male): 1
- Health Assistant (Female): 1
- Apart from the above upper division clerk/store keeper/Superintendent-1, Laboratory Technician-1, Driver (Subject to availability of vehicle)-1 and Class IV workers are posted.
- Subcenter Level is manned by Health worker (Female)-1, HealthWorker (male)/HealthInspector-1 and Voluntary Paid worker.

VILLAGE LEVEL ADMINISTRATION

The village comprising of average 1000 population, the subcenter caters health services to the villages, it is manned by basic health worker: Anganwadi worker, Accredited Social Health Activist (ASHA) under National Rural Health Mission (NRHM).

DISTRICT ADMINISTRATION URBAN AREAS

The urban areas of District organized into Town areas with a population of 5,000–10,000 and Municipals Board with a population of 10,000–2,00,000 headed by a **chairman** elected by members.

Functions of Municipal Board

- Construction and maintenance of roads
- Sanitation and drainage
- Provision of street lights
- Safe water supply
- Maintenance of hospital and dispensaries
- Education
- Registration of Births and Deaths.

The Corporation is next higher level with a population of more than 2,00,000 population. It is headed by **Mayor** elected by Councillors. The executive agency of corporation include Commissioner, Secretary Engineer and health Officer.

OTHER AGENCIES FOR HEALTH CARE

- Employee's State Insurance Scheme (ESI hospitals).
- Defensive/railway/private hospitals.
- Voluntary agencies in India.

PLANNING PROCESS: FIVE YEAR PLANS

Since independence, the government of India focused on planning for economic developments. Five year plans were conceived by the government and implemented to achieve the economic aim. Five year plans are run by the central government and amalgamated in national economic program. The Government established Planning commission headed by the Prime minister of India as ex-officio chairman. A deputy chairman at the rank of Cabinet minister was nominated by the commission to help the chairman. The government has successfully completed 11 five year plans by 2012 and at present the 12th five year plan is running.

The concept of five year plans are originated from Soviet Union by Joseph Stalin in early 1920. Gradually many communist and capitalist countries adopted it in the world

The following presents the five year plans executed by the government of India year-wise:

- First Plan (1951–1956)
- Second Plan (1956–1961)
- Third Plan (1961 1966)
- Fourth Plan (1969–1974)
- Fifth Plan (1974–1979)
- Rolling plan (1979–1980)
- Sixth Plan (1980–1985)
- Seventh Plan (1985–1990)
- Annual Plans (1990–1992)
- Eighth Plan (1992–1997)

- Ninth Plan (1997–2002)
- Tenth Plan (2002–2007)
- Eleventh Plan (2007–2012)
- Twelfth Plan (2012–2017)

The following are the achievement of each five year plans in India.

First Five Year Plan (1951–1956)

In 1951 the first five year plan was commissioned in India focusing the development of primary sector which was based on modified Harrod–Domar Model. The budget allocated for the first plan was 2378 crore.

The budget distributed in the following areas (presented in percentage):

- Irrigation and energy (27.2%).
- Agriculture and community development (17.4%).
- Transport and communications (24%).
- Industry (8.4%).
- Social services (16.64%).
- Land rehabilitation (4.1%).
- Other sectors and services (2.5%).

All the states had taken responsibility for the economic development of the country.

Achievement of First Five Year Plans

- The target growth rate increased from 2.1%–3.6%
- Growth of domestic product increased to 15%
- Per capita income increased by 8%
- Because of rapid expansion of population growth the national income increased more than the per capita income
- For irrigation purpose Bhakra Nangal dam and Hirakud dam were launched
- In the education sector, five IITs (Indian Institutes of Technology) were established by 1956. University Grants Commission (UGC) was setup to plan, implement, monitor and strengthen the higher education in India
- To establish five steel plants for that planning and contract were signed. First five year plan was partially successful in achieving its aims.

First Five Year Plan: Impact on Health

- With the assistance from WHO, the government brought down the infant mortality.
- The National Malaria program launched in 1953 with the support from Technical Mission USA and WHO and DDT spraying program started.
- With the assistance of UNICEF, WHO and Rockefeller foundation, tuberculosis control program initiated with opening of more TB clinics, BCG vaccination, Domiciliary services and follow-up care of tuberculosis patients.
- Family planning program launched in 1951 and India was the first country to accept Family planning program.

Second Five Year Plan (1956–1961)

The Second Plan was aiming at maximal economic growth and focused on developing public sector. This plan was based on Mahalanobis model of economic development. It was initiated by an Indian statistician Prasanta Chandra Mahalanobis. The production sector was concentrated by allocating more budgets envisaging more economic growth. To achieve this aim novel methods of statistical application and operational research were used that was developed by Indian statistical Institute.

The budget allocated for second five year plan was ₹ 48 Billion to support power and irrigation, social services communication and transport and other miscellaneous factors. Though the target growth rate fixed was 4.5%, the actual rate achieved was 4.27% only.

Achievements of Second Five Year Plan

- Five steel plants in Bihar, Durgapur and Rourkela were established
- Hydroelectric power stations were launched
- Increased the amount of coal production
- In Northeast regions, Railway lines were increased
- In 1957 Tata Institute of Fundamental research was commissioned
- Scholarships were allocated for conducting research in nuclear power.

Second Five Year Plan: Impact on Health

- Rural health care was given special attention under community development program, more PHCs were established.
- Family planning programs were supported by nongovernmental agencies apart from the governmental program.

Third Five Year Plan (1961–1966)

After Sino-Indian war the Indian economy became weak and more attention was paid to defense industry. The Third Five-year plan focused on agriculture and improvement in the production of wheat, and prioritized to check inflation rate and stabilize prices of commodities.

Achievement of Third Five Year Plans

- For irrigation process and to enhance food production construction of dams were emphasized

- Many cement and fertilizer factories were established
- Wheat production was increased specially in Punjab state
- To strengthen educational program, more primary schools, and secondary and higher secondary education boards were formed. States were given responsibility to develop secondary and higher secondary education
- Panchayat election were started to strengthen grass root level administration
- States stated participating in development program.

State electricity boards, transportation, corporation and construction of roads were became a state responsibility. Though the target growth rate was 5.6%, but the actual growth rate was only 2.4%.

Annual Plans (1966–67, 1967–68, and 1968–69)

Because of the unsuccessful development observed due to war, lack of resources, and increase in inflation during third five year plans, the government was compelled to announce holidays (from 1966–67, 1967–68, and 1968–69). These years it was an annual plan not five-year plan.

Unfortunately, there was a drought during 1966–67. The plan prioritized to develop agriculture and industrial sector.

Annual Plans: Impact on Health

Problems observed by this plan in health sector:

- The problems affecting PHCs due to shortage of health care personnel
- Delay in construction of PHCs and staff residences
- Inadequate training facilities for health personnel required in rural areas
- Inadequate funding for training of personnel
- Proposal made to start new Medical Colleges
- Proposal made for the establishment of preventive and social medicine and psychiatric departments
- Priority were given for the completion of the All India Institute of Medical Sciences and schemes for upgrading departments in Medical Colleges for postgraduate training and research continued to be high (Batliwala, 1978)
- Unipurpose workers continued to give services
- The Chadha Committee had recommended the integration of health and family planning services and its delivery through one male and one female multipurpose worker per 10,000
- Camp approach was launched to implement family planning program and population control
- Family planning department became independent department in ministry of health
- This recommendation is reinforced the camp programme services (Banerjee, 1973)
- Mukherjee Committee recommended introduction of Intra-uterine Device (IUD) for family planning, target fixation, payments for motivation and incentives to acceptor
- It was proposed the reorganization of the family planning (FP) program into a vertical program like malaria
- Proposed to post addition of one more health visitor per PHC who would supervise the ANMs for achieving the targets of this program.
- Recommendation of retaining of private practitioners.

Fourth Five Year Plan (1969–1974)

During this plan period more concentration was on fertility reduction and given high priority. Though the target growth rate proposed was 5.6% and the achievement was only 3.3%.

Achievement of Fourth Five Year Plan

- To improve agriculture, the concept of green revolution was brought in
- 14 major Indian banks were nationalized.

Fourth Five Year Plans: Impact on Health

- Water supply and sanitation were separated and separate allocation of budget was made under housing and regional development.
- PHCs were given separate budget for their development, 42% of budget allocated for health and family planning.
- Subdivisional and district hospital were declared as referral centers.
- Prevention and control of communicable diseases were given due attention. Sudden increase of malaria rose from 100,000 cases annually between 1963–65.

Fifth Five Year Plan (1974–1979)

Fifth plan period is an important land mark in health care delivery system. The major emphasis were provision of employment, reduction of poverty and provision of justice to people. During this plan the government also stressed on self-reliance in agricultural production and defense materials. The target growth rate of the plan was 4.4% and the actual growth rate observed was 3.8%.

Achievements of Fifth Five Year Plan

- In 1975 the Electricity Supply Act was amended which helped the union government generate power and transmission of power supply

- To reduce traffic accidents, many roads were widened and expanded and the Indian National Highway system also introduced.

Fifth five Year Plan: Impact on Health

- In 1973 under minimum need program the Kartar Singh Committee recommended the change of unipurpose workers to multipurpose workers (male and female). The ANM training period was reduced to one and half years from two years. Such worker is allocated to serve a population of 10,000 to 12,000. Therefore during this plan multipurpose worker training program was launched with the objective to retrain the existing cadre of vertical program workers and the various vertical programm were fully integrated into the primary health care package for rural population areas (Kartar Singh Committee, 1974).
- To increase the health manpower in rural areas, in 1977, created a new cadre of village based auxiliaries named as Community Health worker as a part time worker from the village trained for 3 months in preventive, promotive and curative skills both in allopathic and indigenous system of medicine supervised by multipurpose health workers. This was based on the recommendations given by Shrivastava Committee (Shrivastava, 1975).
- During this plan period, the national population policy was declared and more budget was allocated for family planning.

Rolling Plan (1978–1980)

In order to avoid the rigidity and fixing of targets of the five year plans and facilitate flexibility and economic status the rolling plan was initiated. It has three main plans proposed as:

1. The first kind of this proposed for the existing year' annual budget.
2. Second kind of this is a plan for a fixed number 3, 4 or 5 years. The period of the plan changes as per the requirement and the economic statue of the country.
3. The Third Plan is a for long, terms, i.e. for 10, 15 or 20 years. And there is no fixation of dates for its starts and ending. The main drawback of this plan was the targets are revised each year, it becomes very difficult to achieve them.

Sixth Five Year Plan (1980–1985)

During the Sixth Five Year Plan, there was an increase in cost of living because of elimination of price control. Food prices were increased because of closing of ration shops.

Sixth Five Year Plans: Impact on Health

To control over population, family planning activities were maximized in this period. Some of the developed states adopted family planning than the less developed regions that remained with high birth rate. National health policy came into being in 1983. Rural health care activities were prioritized and strengthened the health workers training program. Comparing other five year plans, the sixth plan brought a great outcome to the Indian economy by bringing the target growth rate from 5.2% to actual growth rate of 5.4%.

Seventh Five Year Plan (1985–1990)

The Seventh Five Year Plan focused on further economic growth of the country, by enhancing production level of industries through the support of technology production of food grains, and generating employment. The Seventh Plan had emphasized toward socialism and energy production. Social justice, removal of oppression of the weak, using modern technology, agricultural development, anti-poverty programmes, full supply of food, clothing, and shelter, increasing productivity of small- and large-scale farmers, and making India an independent economy were stressed in seventh five year plans' agenda.

The Seventh Plan was focused on achieving the prerequisites of self-sustaining growth by the year 2000. The plan envisaged the labor force to grow by 39 million people and employment to grow by 4% per annum. Voluntary agencies and general population contributed to the growth of sustainable economic growth. The target growth rate increased from 5.0% to the actual growth rate 6.01%.

Seventh Five Year Plans: Impact on Health

The main activities emphasized in seventh five year plans were:

- Development of community oriented health.
- Prioritized health services to the rural areas.
- Preparation and training of frontline health workers selected from the community and supervised by Multipurpose worker (MPW) and medical officers of PHC. The training of a large cadre of first level health workers selected from the community and supervised by MPWs and medical officers of the PHCs.
- More stress was given to integrate water supply, sanitation hygiene, nutrition and education for family planning and MCH.

Annual Plans (1990–1992)

Due to the political upheaval in the country the eighth plan could not start in 1990 and function till 1992 and were taken as Annual Plans. The Eighth Plan was finally launched in 1992 after the initiation of organizational adjustment policies.

Eighth Five Year Plan (1992–1997)

During the beginning of eighth plan, India confronted a great crisis in depletion of foreign exchange reserves, to correct the deficit of foreign reserves the country concentrated on developing, industries and India became the member of the World Trade Organization in 1995.

The eighth plan had the aims of, controlling population growth, poverty reduction, employment generation, strengthening the infrastructure, institutional building, tourism management, and human resource development. Peoples participation in administration was encouraged and Panchayati Rajs, Nagar Palikas and NGOs were involved. Energy was given priority and allocated 26.6% from the total budget.

Eighth Five Year Plan: Impact on Health

The plan accepted a new slogan instead of health for all by 2000 AD. It emphasized health for the under privileged. Private hospitals and private clinics for health care and privatization were encouraged. It insisted to maintain minimum standards of health care.

An average annual growth rate of 6.78% against the target 5.6% was achieved.

Ninth Five Year Plan (1997–2002)

The Ninth Five Year Plan focused on economic and social development. It supported social sector in the country to eliminate poverty. The Ninth Five Year Plan also encouraged joint partnership of the public and the private sectors in ensuring economic development of the country. In addition, the Ninth Five Year Plan witnessed the contributions towards development from the general public as well as governmental agencies in both the rural and urban areas of the country. During this plan Special Action Plans (SAPs) were evolved to achieve targets within the stipulated time with adequate resources. The SAPs supported the areas of social infrastructure, agriculture, information technology and Water policy. 8,59,200 crores were allocated during this plan for public sector. However the expenditure was more (49%) than the plan outlay (33%) of budget. In the total outlay, the center had a share of 57% while it was 43% for the states and the union territories.

The main objective of the Ninth Five Year Plan:

- To control over population.
- To create more employment by giving priority to agriculture and rural development.
- To make necessary needful to reduce poverty.
- To ensure availability of food and water for the poor.
- To ensure availability of primary health care facilities and other basic necessities for all rural population.
- To strengthen referral services.
- To promote primary education to all children in the country.
- To empower the socially backwards like Scheduled castes, Scheduled tribes and others.
- To promote self-reliance in terms of agriculture.
- To stabilize price and increase the growth rate and economy.

The following strategies adopted to achieve the above objectives

- Structural transformations and developments to enhance Indian economy.
- New innovative measures to meet the challenges in the economy of the country.
- Utilization of available resources effectively.
- Public private support to enhance employment.
- Promotion of exports.
- Strengthening electricity, telecommunication, railways services.
- Measures to enhance empowerment of socially disadvantaged population.
- Participation of Panchayati Raj institutions/bodies and Nagar Palikas in the development process.
- The Ninth Five-Year Plan achieved a GDP growth rate of 5.4% against a target of 6.5%. The agriculture industry grew at a rate of 2.1% against the target of 4.2%. The industrial growth in the country was 4.5% which was higher than that of the target of 3%. The service industry had a growth rate of 7.8%. An average annual growth rate of 6.7% was reached.

The target growth was 7.1% and the actual growth was 6.8%.

Tenth Five Year Plan (2002–2007)

The tenth five year plan aimed to achieve 8% GDP growth per annum. It envisaged to reduce poverty of the people by 5% by the year 2007. It had an objective to provide high quality of employment and reduce gender differences in wages and literacy. During this period 20 point program was launched.

The growth rate achieved was 7.7% as against the target growth rate of 8.1%. The total allocation of budget for this plan period was ₹ 43,825 crores in which ₹ 921,291 crores (57.9%) was distributed to central government program and the remaining ₹ 691,009 crores (42.1%) were distributed to states and union territories.

The Main Impact on Health in Tenth Five Year Plan

Draft of National Health policy 2001 was established during 10th five year plan.

Eleventh Five Year Plan (2007–2012)

The important characteristics of this plans were to enhance growth rate, reduce poverty, reduce gender-based inequality, enhance environmental sustainability, and empower the community through education, and training. The plan also aimed to increase growth rate in agriculture by 4%, industry by 10% and services by 9%. The total budget allocation for this plan period was increased from 0.9% to 3%.

Eleventh Five Year Plans: Impact on Health

- Reduce Total Fertility Rate to 2.1
- Standardize private sector health services and reform Medical Council of India (MCI) and other health councils
- Ensure women friendly, free, affordable, accessible and comprehensive care to marginalized population
- Ensure free ambulance referral or other transportation locally with proper reimbursement
- Full wages for all frontline health workers
- Initiation of policies on mental health, especially for women and adolescents
- Address occupational health hazards and needs of women working in mines, quarries, construction site, plantation, etc.
- Assure disease control and sanitation during disaster situation.

Twelfth Five Year Plan (2012–2017)

The Twelfth Five-Year Plan of the country had envisaged for the growth rate of 8.2% as against 8%. The plan is aiming at to reduce poverty rate by 10% by 2017 and by 9% annually. The plan also aims to increase to agricultural growth by 4%, provision of employment opportunity by creating 50 million work, and removal of gender and social disparity gap in education. The plan emphasizes to achieve universal road connectivity and electricity to all villages in India. Further the plan highlighted to provide access to banking services for 90% of households and welfare benefits to them by Aadhaar process.

Twelfth five Year Plan: Impact on Health

- Achieve the reduction of Maternal Mortality from 212 to 100, reduction of Infant Mortality from 44 to 25 and total fertility rate to 2.1
- Prevention and reduction of underweight children below 3 years from 40% to 23% and by average underweight to bring down to 29% by 2015 and 27% by 2017
- Raising child sex ratio 0–6 years from 914 to 950
- Reduction of anemia by simple and affordable intervention among women 15–49 years of age from 58.7% (2007) to 28% by the end of the 12th plan
- Operationalization of universal health plan through effective health insurance system
- Establish Health Information System (HIS)
- Develop health workforce for all health care facilities and CHC
- Provision of essential health care package to all patients whether they come for inpatient or outpatient care
- Regulation of food, drugs and medical practice
- Strengthening quality care by establishing AIIMS like institution in the country
- Promote health system research and implement research findings.

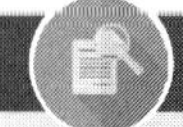

SUMMARY

✓ Nurses should know about the constitution of India which highlights Fundamental Rights of Indian citizen, that guarantees civil rights and focuses all Indians can lead their lives in peace and harmony as Indian Citizens. These include individual rights common to all such as all are equal before law, and everybody has freedom of speech and expression and to accept their own religion. Violation of these rights result in punishments as prescribed in the Indian law or other special laws, subject to discretion of the court. The Fundamental Rights are defined as basic rights that every Indian citizen has the right to enjoy for a proper and harmonious development of personality. These rights universally apply to all citizens, irrespective of caste, place of birth, religion, or sex. While caring patients nurses should keep the above in mind.

✓ The planning of the nursing component of health services forms part of health planning and this will enable the nurse administrator to participate effectively as a member of interdisciplinary team. Knowledge of health administration at national, state and peripheral level including public health arena and to understand the hierarchy, organization, staffing structure and functions at each level will enable the administrator in planning nursing services.

- ✓ The planning process highlighting five year plans, its allocation of budget and the progress made in each sector.
- ✓ This chapter emphasized the current five year plan and its goals for health care.

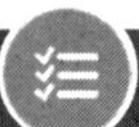

REVIEW QUESTIONS

1. Define constitution. Describe the fundamental rights as provided by Constitution to Indian citizen.
2. Describe the health administration at national level with hierarchy and functions.
3. Explain state health administration and its function.
4. Describe the rural district health administration and functions.
5. What are five year plans? Discuss the role of five year plans in improving health of Indian population.
6. Write short notes on the following:
   a. Constitutional amendments
   b. Union and concurrent list
   c. Community development block
   d. Primary health centre
   e. Twelfth five year plans
   f. Central Council of Health
   g. Municipal board and corporation.

SELECTED READINGS

1. 12th Five Year Plan http://12thplan.gov.in/ Draft 12th Five Year Plan Document; 09-12-2011. Steering Committees/Working Groups for 12th Five Year Plan (2012-17); 23-10-2011.
2. Anita Joshua, which bill is 100th amendment to constitution, The Hindu, National update, May 7, 2015.
3. Banerjee, D, 1973: Population Planning in India – National and Foreign Priorities, CSMCH, JNU, New Delhi
4. Batliwala, Srilatha, 1978: The Historical Development of Health Services in India, FRCH, Bombay
5. Chadha Committee, 1963: Special Committee for NMEP Maintenance Phase, MoHFW, GOI, New Delhi
6. CONSTITUTION OF INDIA (Updated up to (Ninety-Eighth Amendment) Act, 2012)
7. (Constitution of India Nov.1949)
8. Expert Committee on Public Health Systems, 1982, MoHFW, GOI, New Delhi
9. FYP I – IX, various years: Five Year Plans – First to Ninth, Planning Commission, GOI, new Delhi
10. Healthcare Administration- Evolution and Challenges | Via Hrx
11. http://bhpr.hrsa.gov/healthworkforce/supplydemand/nursing/workforceprojections/nursingprojections.pdf
12. http://india.gov.in/my-government/constitution-india
13. http://lawmin.nic.in/olwing/coi/coi-english/coi-indexenglish.htm
14. http://socialjustice.nic.in/pdf/constprovmsje
15. http://viahrx.com/healthcare-administration-evolution-and-challenges 17 May 2014.
16. http://www.aicte-India.org/downloads/engendering_XI_five_year_plan. pdf
17. http://www.aicte-India.org/downloads/engendering_XI_five_year_plan. pdf
18. http://www.cehat.org/go/uploads/Publications/a168.pdf Health planning in India
19. http://www.indiacode.nic.in/acts-in-pdf/2015/CONST100.pdf 29 May 2015
20. http://www.slideshare.net/mohmmedirfanmomin/health-system-in-india
21. https://en.wikipedia.org/wiki/Constitution_of_India
22. Kartar Singh Committee, 1973: Committee on Multipurpose Worker under Health and Family Planning, MoHFW, New Delhi

23. MoHFW, 1983: National Health Policy, Govt. of India, Ministry of Health and Family Welfare, New Delhi
24. MoHFW, 2001: Draft National Health Policy, Ministry of Health and Family Welfare, New Delhi
25. Mukherjee Committee, 1966: Committee to Review Staffing Pattern and Financial Provision under Family Planning Programme, MoHFW, New Delhi
26. One Hundredth Amendment - India Code
27. Population Census India 2011
28. Ravi Duggal, Health Planning in India, Expert Committee on Public Health System, 1993, MoHFW, GoI, New Delhi
29. Shrivastava Committee, 1975: Report of the Group on Medical Education and Support Manpower, MoHFW, New Delhi
30. The Future of the Nursing Workforce: National- and State-Level.

2

India's Health Care Policies

LEARNING OBJECTIVES

This chapter imparts learning about:

- Various Health Committees and their Impact on Nursing
- National Health Policies and their Implications on Nursing
- Introduction to National Population Policy and its Influence on Family Welfare
- Description of National Policy on AYUSH and Plans

VARIOUS COMMITTEE REPORTS ON HEALTH AND THEIR IMPACT ON NURSING

Introduction

Health of the people is very important for productivity and Nation's economy. Government of India constituted various health committees time to time to examine the health status of the people and invited recommendations to address the health needs and problem of the people of the country before and after the independence.

Health Survey and Development Committee, 1943–1946

This committee was constituted by the Pre-independent Government of India under Sir Joseph William Bhore, Indian Civilian Servant in the year 1943 popularly known as Bhore Committee. The committee submitted its report in 1946.

The committee established some of the objectives of the survey focused on:

- To asses and review the current health status of India
- To suggest for future development
- To review the activities falling within the scope of health administration
- To consider short-term goals which were expected to be achieved within 4–5 years
- To develop long-term goals to be achieved require longer period.

The committee submitted its report in 1946 comprising 4 volume.

The committee on survey observed that the Crude Death Rate was 22.4/1000, Infant Mortality Rate was 162/1000 live births, Maternal Mortality Rate was 20/1000 live births, life expectancy at birth was 27 years, incidence of communicable and infectious diseases were very high, and cholera and chickenpox were epidemic. The committee also observed many preventable health problems.

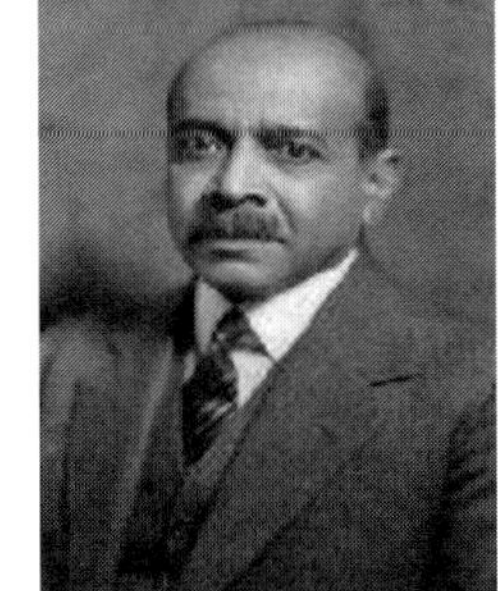

Fig. 2.1: Sir Joseph William Bhore

The Following Recommendations were made by Bhore Committee

Short-term Plan:

- Integration of preventive and curative services at all levels of administration need to be launched within 5–10 years.
- The committee suggested that for every 40,000 rural population, a Primary Health Center (PHC) to be established to meet the health care needs of the people. In addition to this, for supervisory, coordination and referral services a secondary health center to be established as referral institution.
- The primary health center to be manned by 2 medical officers, 4 public health nurses, one nurse, 4 midwives, 4 trained dais and 15 class IV employees.
- With the above recommendations, in All India Institute of Hygiene and Public health a certificate course on public health nursing started.
- The committee recommended the following long-term plan. It is also called three millions plan.
- The main recommendation in long-term plan was organization of three tier health care system in India.
- In first tier system, it was recommended that for every 10,000–29,000 rural population establishing: Primary health units with 75 bedded hospital manned by 6 medical officers, 6 public health nurses, 2 sanitary inspectors, 2 health zassistants and other supportive staff.
- Second tier system the focus was given to establish 650 bedded Regional Health Unit (RHU). This regional unit will serve for 30–40 PHCs as a referral center.
- Third tier system was recommended to cater the needs of 3 million population with a District Hospital with a bed strength of 2,500.
- To increase the manpower, a three months training program for social physician in social and preventive medicine was recommended.
- Integration of preventive and curative services was stressed in all health care facilities.
- In order to develop active participation of the community in local health care program the committee recommended to establish a village health committee comprising 5 – 7 individuals from the local community.
- Intersectoral coordination.
- Incorporation of public health nursing at graduate level.

Recommendations for Nursing

- With regards to nursing the committee recommended a stipend of rupees 60 per month for nursing students.
- For medical students an annual stipend of rupees 1,000 is recommended provided with the medical students consent to do public services after their completion of training.
- The committee further recommended to increase the number of trained nurses 7,40,000 by the year 1971. As per survey 7,000 trained nurses were existing and as per short-term objective it was estimated to have 80,000 nurses in the country.
- Preliminary training school to be established for nurses.
- Senior grade and junior nursing cadre stressed.
- As a long-term objective, the committee recommended to develop nursing colleges for professional education.
- To provide nursing services in male wards and OPD training of male nurses and employment was recommended.
- Need to train public health nurses was emphasized.
- Nurses who were already trained in nursing and midwifery were eligible for such course. The public health nursing training program should be based on preventive care in nature.
- The committee recommended one midwife for 100 births. To make up this ratio 1:100 birth additional 1,00,000 midwives should be trained as against 5,000 midwives existed.
- The training centers to be developed with good infrastructure to train midwives with proper curriculum.
- Until the required midwives are available in the country, Dais training program recommended to continue.

Health Survey and Planning Committee, 1959–1961

The Government of India constituted Health Survey and Planning Committee in 1959 under the chairmanship of Dr A Lakshmanswamy Mudaliar, the then Vice Chancellor, Madras University with the following objectives:

- To evaluate the medical relief and public health activities done after the recommendation reports made by the Bhore committee.
- To analyze and assess the projects of the first and second five year plans.
- To recommend for the country's future development health plans.

The following are some of the observations made by the committee presented in their report in 1961

- The country is not facilitated with basic health care amenities.

- Hospital and beds are available more in urban areas than in rural areas.
- The primary health centers provided inadequate quality of health services because of its poor functioning, lack of resources, understaffing, and inadequate referral procedure.

Mudaliar Committee Recommended the following

- To compile the progress made in the country by two five year plans.
- District hospitals need to be strengthened by providing specialized services so as to cater as focal point of regional.
- There should be regional organization in each state to coordinate between the regional head quarters and the districts. In order to supervise 2–3 district medical health officers, a Regional Deputy or Assistant director to be employed.
- 40,000 is population allocated for each primary health center.
- The committee recommended to reinforce the recommendations made by Bhore committee such as integration of medical and health services to strengthen the quality health care provided by PHCs.
- The committee stressed to establish an All India Health Service on the pattern like Indian administrative service.

The following are the recommendations made by this committee for nursing and hospitals

- The committee recommended the ratio of bed to population, i.e. 1:1000 population and 600–800 beds for district hospital or Taluka hospital for providing and improving quality health care to community.
- To reinforce Bhore committee recommendation allocation of 10 beds suggested in PHCs and integration of medical and health services should be realized.
- The committee strongly recommended to post Lady Health Visitors (LHVs) and midwives to take care of the health of the children, their personal hygiene, and nutrition. They are also be made responsible for health education.
- The committee envisaged three grades of nurses:
  - Basic nurses with 4 years training eligible after matriculation or equivalent.
  - Auxiliary nurse midwife with 2 years training.
  - Professional nurse with a degree with 4 years training with higher secondary or preuniversity examination as eligibility.
- Eligibility criteria for age is 17 years for admission. The states where students are not available or difficult to get, 16 years of age could be eligible for degree course, instruction medium is english and for diploma program english medium is preferred.

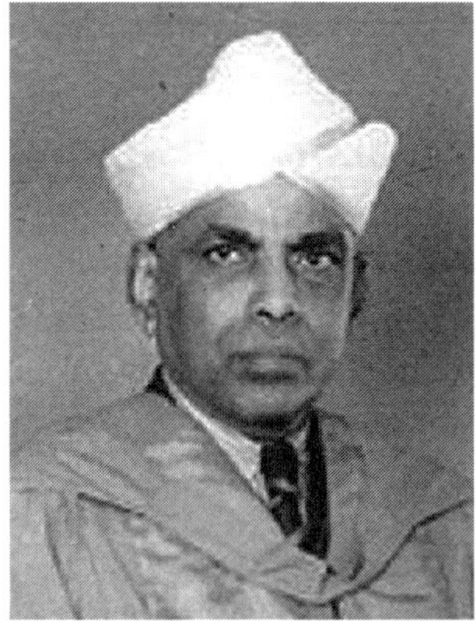

Fig. 2.2: Dr A Lakshmanswamy Mudaliar

- Regarding the training program for nurses, the committee recommended a nursing school attached to a district hospital with minimum 75–100 beds should be available, student nurses should not be utilized for service purposes.
- District hospitals with a bed strength of 75–100 should be utilized to train more nurses.
- Student nurses should be provided with free accommodation, free supply of uniforms, laundry arrangements, free books, free medical services and medical checkups.
- The committee further recommended for provision of separate budget for each school of nursing. In order to look after and advise the admission and welfare of the student nurses, there should be a nursing advisory committee in each school.
- The ratio of auxiliary nurse midwife to population should be 1:5000 by the end of 15 years.
- In order to replace Dais, sufficient number of midwives needs to trained.
- Emphasis was given to train male nurses for special service units.
- The committee also recommended for higher education and specialization in nursing such as the general sick nurse, public health nurse, pediatric health nurse, mental diseases nurse, theater sister, nursing administrator, etc.

Chadha Committee Reports, 1963

In 1963, a committee was constituted under Dr MS Chadha, Director General of Health Services by government of India to assess the preparation made for launching the maintenance phase of malaria eradication program. The main aims of the committee were:

- To study the requirements in relation to planning and setting priorities for maintenance phase of

Malaria Eradication Program (MEP) by primary health centers.
- To calculate and suggest staffing pattern required for the malaria eradication programme including for other health activities.
- To suggest the ways and means to utilize the technical and supervisory staff of the National Malaria Eradication Program (NMEP) after the MEP is achieved.

The following Recommendations made by Chadha Committee

- Basic health workers posted for 10,000 population at Block and District level to be assigned for maintenance phase work of Malaria Eradication Program.
- In order to implement malaria activities, home visiting once a month to be done by basic health workers.
- For family planning and vital statistics Basic Health Worker (BHW) to function as Multipurpose Health Worker (MPHW) 3–4 BHW to be supervised by Family Planning Health Assistant (FPHA).

Dr Mukherjee Committee Reports, 1965

In 1965, Shri Mukherjee, the then Secretary of Health to the Government of India, was appointed as a chairman to evaluate the plan of operations for the family planning programme in the country on the basis of the Central Family Planning Council meet held at Madras. In 1965, the Indian Council of Medical Research (ICMR) Director declared that that Lippes Loop was safe family planning method and IntraUterine Contraceptive Device (IUCD) was introduced into the family planning programme. The committee recommended to bring down the birth rate from 41 per 1000 to 25 per 1000 within a period of 10 years. The committee also reviewed on additions and changes are necessary, for staffing program and funding, etc. due to new strategy of IUCD.

The following Recommendations made by Mukherjee Committee, 1965

- All program should be target oriented.
- Need to strengthen education and publicity works and involve other organizations of health for better outcome.
- In state health directorate of the government, there should be a strong executive wing to deal with family planning.
- The committee accepted the existing Urban Family Welfare Planning center.
- BHW to be utilized as MPHW for all general care services. FPHA is responsible only for family planning work but not necessary to supervise BHW as suggested by previous committee.
- The committee also recommended to delink malaria activities with family planning program.

Dr Mukherjee Committee Reports, 1966

In June 1966, at Bangalore the 13th Meeting of the Central Council of Health was held. It was observed that the states were unable to take up the activities of maintenance phase of malaria program along with small pox, leprosy, FP, and trachoma program. Therefore a committee was established in 1966 by the government of India under the chairmanship of Shri B Mukerji, the then Union Health Secretary with the objectives of reviewing the staffing pattern the primary health centers and to recommend the minimum staff required of various cadres within the district to provide an integrated health services like vigilance services in the maintenance phase of National Malaria Eradication Programme, smallpox eradication, tuberculosis, leprosy and trachoma control, program etc. The other aims specified by this committee were recommend for:

- The pattern of central assistance for the states
- Types of basic health services to be provided at block level
- Ways and means to strengthen at higher level health facility
- More BHW to cater block level activities because lack of adequate BHW may not be able to complete the tasks.

The Recommendations made by Mukherjee Committee, 1966

- Enhance integration of medical and public health and provide care with Integrated approach in all health care facilities at all levels.
- Appointing separate staff for the maintenance phase activities along with the existing large number of basic health workers at the periphery and emphasis was given to provide domiciliary services.
- The committee further recommended that for every 10,000 population, one basic health worker to be posted.
- At the district level more integration of services being recommended and family planning program to be given more attention.
- The committee suggested that state government should plan strategies to strengthen health services at zonal, state and district level.

Recommendation for Nursing

- Sanctioning more posts of lady health visitors
- For every two subcenters one Family Planning Female Workers (FPFW) is recommended

- In order to motivate couples for acceptance IUD, part time workers were recommended for motivating population for acceptance of IUD.
- For family planning motivation activities, education leaders to be appointed for motivational campaigns at block and district levels and be paid honorarium of ₹ 600 per annum.
- Honorarium was also recommended to government doctors and to part-time private medical practitioners as ₹ 100 to motivate couple for family planning.

Jungalwalla Committee on Integration of Health Services, 1967

In 1967, Dr N Jungalwalla, the then Additional director General of Health Services Committee on Integration of Health Services was appointed by the government of India with the aims to examine the problems of health services, service conditions and private practice.

The committee clarified the nature of integrated health services that is a service with a unified approach for all problems to avoid the services in fragmentation.

The committee observed that in some states integration of medical care and public health was integrated, some places it was found as separate services and some places it was proposed to integrate in state and periphery.

Jungalwalla Committees Recommendations (1967)

- Integration of health services from state to the periphery.
- Integration of preventive and curative services at all levels.
- Integration of medical services and public health personnel on rotation.
- The committee recommended integration of functions and methods, organization of health services and the personnel providing these services and their administration.
- Emphasized on unified cadre of personnel for better integration.
- Recognition for seniority and recognition of additional qualification for salary decisions.
- Provision of equal pay for equal work special pay for specialized work.
- Private practice to be discontinued.
- All personnel to be provided with good service conditions.
- States are responsible to develop their own health strategies.

Kartar Singh Committee on Multipurpose Workers Under Health and Family Planning 1972

The Government of India appointed Kartar Singh the then Additional Secretary, MOHFP in 1972 and the committee submitted its report in 1973 when there was a growing demand for increase of staff under each program and to reduce population/area covered by each health worker.

- The committee emphasized for integrated health services at the peripherals and supervisory levels.
- Focused on the feasibility of Multipurpose Health Workers (MPW) and their training needs.
- Effective integration by using mobile services.
- Multipurpose workers will be the right personnel for complete coverage of population.
- Female Health Workers (FHWs) replaced the current Auxiliary Nurse Midwives (ANMs) It was a redesignation of ANM.
- The unifunctionary workers like BHW, Malaria surveillance workers, vaccinators, FPHAs replaced by MHWs.
- Existing Lady Health Visitors (LHV) designated as Female Health (FH) supervisor and placed in malaria maintenance phase areas and small pox controlled areas.
- The committee stressed the need for job description of health workers and health supervisors.

The following Recommendations made by Kartar Singh Committee 1973

The Focus of Recommendations

- *Center to periphery:* More attention is paid to rural health infrastructure than establishing more medical colleges.
- *Specialization to generalization:* More attention is paid to develop a generalist who can take care of all problems in the family than that of specialist who take care one aspect or problem.
- *Unifunctionaries to multifunctionary:* BHW, Malaria surveillance workers, vaccinators, trachoma workers FPHAs replaced by MHWs.
- The two years ANM training program is reduced to one and half year program.
- For every 50,000 population there should be one PHC for complete coverage. Each primary health centre to be divided into 16 subcenters each comprising a population of 3000 to 3500 depending upon geographical nature and means of communications.

- Each subcenter to be manned by one male and one female health worker. There should be one male health supervisor to supervise the work of 3 to 4 male health workers; and a female health supervisor to supervise the work of 4 female health workers. Existing lady health visitors to be designated as female health supervisors. These personnel are to be supervised by the Medical Officer in-charge posted at the PHC.
- The committee recommended to implement all the health care activities proposed by fifth five year plan.

Shrivastava Committee, a Group of Medical Education and Support Manpower, 1975

There was a drastic imbalance observed by the Government of India in Medical education system between rural and urban aspects of care. It concentrated more on urban orientation like curative care, highly sophisticated diagnostic and treatment modalities where as training in the fields of nutrition, family welfare planning, and maternal and child care were lacking which are basic to rural health. The committee recommended more emphasis to be given in undergraduate medical education with emphasis on community rather than on hospital care and the importance of integrating teaching of various aspects of family and community health.

Keeping the above factors, the MOHFP, Government of India appointed Shrivastava committee–A Group on Medical Education and Support Manpower in 1974 and submitted report in 1975.

The purpose of the committee were

- To design a suitable curriculum for training a cadre of Health Assistants.
- To suggest steps to improve current medical education program according national health care requirements.

The following Recommendations made by Shrivastava Committee in 1975

- Establishing the basic health services (including nutrition, health education and family planning) within the community and training the personnel needed for the same.
- To provide complete health care to the population like professionals creation of new cadre of Village Health Guide (VHG) or community health volunteers from the community like teachers, postmasters, gram sevaks. Placing the health in the hands of the community by creating Primary health care trained workers.
- Creation of posts of MPW and Health Assistants (HA) in between the VHG and Medical Officer (MO) in-charge of PHC.
- Strengthening of upward and downward referral services PHC to tertiary health facilities and vice versa.
- Reorganization of medical education system to meet the national health care needs.
- Establishment of the Medical and Health Education Commission.
- Organization of the basic health services (including nutrition, health education and family planning) within the community itself and training the personnel needed for the purposes.
- Creation of Village Health Guide (VHG) or community health volunteers from the community itself like teachers, postmasters, gram sevaks who can provide comprehensive health services as paraprofessionals.
- Primary health care be provided within the community itself through specially trained workers so that the health of the people is placed in the hands of people themselves.
- Organization of an economic and efficient programme of health services to bridge the community with the first level referral Center, viz. the PHC.
- Creation of MPW and Health Assistants (HA) in between the VHG and Medical Officer (MO) in-charge of PHC.
- The creation of a National Referral Services Complex by the development of proper linkages between the PHC and higher level referral and service centers.
- To create the necessary administrative and financial machinery for the reorganization of the entire programme of medical and health education from the point of view of the objectives and needs of the proposed programme of national health services.
- The committee further recommended an establishment of 'The Medical and Health Education Commission' in the country.

Rural Health Scheme, 1977–1978

During 1977—1978, A 'Rural Health Scheme' was established by the government of India based on Dr Shrivastava committee's recommendation. In this scheme, the major activities are focused on report of the group of Medical education and support Manpower (Srivastava committee), Ministry of health and Family welfare, Government of India, New Delhi, 1975.

Reorientation of Medical Education (ROME) in which the training of undergraduate medical students and interns will be at primary health centers. Thus, this scheme has a vision to involve medical colleges in rural health care services.

Report of the Working Group on Health for all by 2000

In 1980, Kripa Narain, the secretary, MOHFW and President, AIIMS was appointed by planning commission following the acceptance of commitment of Health For All (HFA) by 2000 to assess the progress made as per the previous committee. The committee submitted its report in 1981. The committee was aiming at:

- To assess the existing health status, implementation of program and methods of evaluation to justify them.
- In order to establish a strong basis to implement HFA 2000, formulating plan outlines for 1980–1986 for health sector.
- To recommend specific program for the under privileged like rural, tribal and weaker sections.
- To reassess components of health on minimum needs programme.

The working group made the following recommendations:

- Minimum Needs Programme needs to be reviewed.
- Medical experts with specialization in curative care and public health to be available in PHCs of each district.
- An epidemiological section to be facilitated for 5 lakhs population in subdivisional health center.
- The block community health center having 1,00,000 population specialists services to be made available.
- Establishment of primary health center to cater 30,000 population in rural and 15,000 in hilly area. These PHCs need to provide preventive, promotive and curative services.
- Health subcenters to be set for every 5000 population and for 2500 population in hilly areas. It should be staffed by one MPW(F), MPW(M) and one part time attendant.
- Each village: One health volunteer to be posted.

OTHER IMPORTANT COMMITTEES

Sokhey Committee (1947)

- The committee recommended to develop standards for nutrition and diet to the population irrespective of their class in the society.
- The committee further suggested strategies for guarding against epidemic diseases and identification of causes of maternal and infant morbidity and mortality.
- In order to reduce mortality the committee suggested establishing health units, consisting adequate manpower like physician, nurses, surgeons, hospitals and dispensaries, sanatoria and nursing homes; health insurance; medical training and research; compilation of vital statistics, including those of birth and death rates.
- The committee recommended cultivation of the medicinal plants and enhance production of medicines to preventive or curative support, and scientific and surgical equipment and accessories of the National Health Services.

Chopra Committee (1948)

This committee recommended integration of medicine and multidisciplinary approach of research to enhance indigenous and modern medicine.

Balwant Rai Mehta Committee (1952)

The committee was appointed to evaluate outcome of Community Development Programme initiated in 1952. Unfortunately, the program was found to be an utter failure because of lack of initiation from local community.

Renuka Roy Committee (1960)

This committee concentrated on school health program and suggested enhancing preventive care through schools, facilitating mid day meals, and integration of health education as part of curricular activities.

Jain Committee (1966)

This committee was assigned to evaluate the functioning of different hospitals and central health services.

Krishnan Committee (1982)

The committee was chaired by Shri Krishnan to review the health services available in urban areas and cities.

Dr Shanthi Lal J Mehta Committee (1983)

The committee was established to review medical education.

H Bajaj Committee (1987)

The committee was established to assess the health manpower planning, and procedures relating to admissions to undergraduate and postgraduate courses:

- The committee reviewed the duration of the undergraduate course and internship and postgraduate courses and their thesis.
- The committee further assessed the residency program and suggested strategies to improve the undergraduate and postgraduate education in the country.

Report of the National Commission on Macroeconomics and Health (2005)

This committee was constituted under chairmanship of P Chidambaram, the Finance Minister and Dr Anbumani Ramadoss, the Health Minister.

The Committee Recommended the following:

- Reduction of household expenditure on health care by developing alternative strategies in health financing.
- To make the health care delivery system more accountable, need for restructuring current primary health care system.
- Reduction of high-risk conditions and bring down the disease prevalence risk.
- Develop and formulate institutional frameworks for enhancing quality for effective monitoring, develop more skilled professionals and enhance technology.

COMMITTEE CONSTITUTED BY GOVERNMENT OF INDIA WITH REGARD TO NURSING AND NURSING PROFESSION

Shetty Committee, 1954

The Government of India constituted a committee under the chairmanship of Mr Shetty and Ms Adranvala as the member secretary to review the conditions of the nursing profession on May 19th, 1954.

Recommendations of Shetty Committee

- The committee recommended that a State Nursing Superintendent (SNS) to be appointed in each state.
- The committee focused on amalgamation of public health in nursing education and combining the nursing services with the public health program.
- The ratio of midwife to birth was suggested as 1:100 birth in rural area and 1:150 birth in hospitals and to be for every 10,000 population one public health nurse or health visitor to be appointed.
- In existing training centers more staff to be recruited for training and supervision.
- Additional posts of nurses and public health nurses in hospitals and in community to be created.
- Conditions of nurses training centers to be improved.
- Married women, unless widowed and separated from husbands are not eligible for nursing training.
- Indian Nursing Council (INC) regulation should be strictly followed for admission criteria for nursing.
- Medium of instruction should be decided by each state.
- Establish a counseling cell in all nursing school and counseling to be done by an experienced nurse.
- During training, student should live in hostel.
- Nursing personnel should be selected by qualified nurses, and nurses should be provided with residential quarters.
- In order to bring quality patient care, all the infrastructure facilities, equipment and supplies and other improvement in working conditions for nurses to be facilitated. Adequate staff to be appointed. During illness, nurses should be given adequate treatment and periodical medical checkup for nurses recommended. In order to have job security provision of pension or provident fund to be provided for nurses.
- The committee further recommended to provide for in-service education program or refresher courses for all categories of nurses to update their knowledge.
- Those nurses have family responsibilities to be provided with part-time jobs. The committee recommended to have exchange program for nurses between states.
- As per the job opportunities and proportion men nurses must be recruited.
- The committee suggested to reduce the period of training of ANM from 2 years to 1.5 years.
- In order to strengthen the training for health and family planning the committee recommended to set up a training department at the Ministry of health and family welfare.

Bajaj Committee Report, 1986–87

In 1986, a committee on Health Manpower, Planning, Production and Management was established by the Ministry of health and family welfare, Government of India, Professor J S Bajaj, Professor of Medicine, AIIMS, and New Delhi was the chairman of that committee.

The Committee made the following Recommendations

- Establishing national policy on education in health services.

- Developing a curriculum for school teachers.
- Utilizing the services of Indian system of Medicine health care.
- Emphasized the need for continuing education programme for the health personnel.
- Hospital nursing services need man power planning.

Manpower Requirement as Recommended by Bajaj Committee (2001)

Hospital Nursing Services

The following are the norms recommended by the above committee:

- Nursing superintendent — 1:200 beds
- Deputy nursing superintendent — 1:300 beds
- Departmental nursing supervisors — 7:1000 + 1 Addl:1000 beds
- Head nurses — 8:2000 beds
- Staff nurse for wards — 1:3 (1:9 for each shift)
- OPD, blood bank, X-ray, diabetic clinics — 1:100
- For ICU (8 beds ICU) — 1:8 (1:3 for each shift)
- For specialized departments and clinics, OT, Labor room — 8:200

Community Health Nursing Services by 2000 Infrastructure Requirement

- Community health centers — 7436
- Primary health services — 26439
- Population recommended for plain area — 30000
- Population for difficult area subcenters — 20000
- Subcenters required — 163941
- Population for plain area for subcenter — 5000
- Population for difficult area — 3000
- For Primary health Centers midwives ANM required — 26439
- Community Health Centers midwives ANM required — 52052

The Committee Presented Total Manpower Requirement in Nursing Services

- Nurse midwives — 664623
- Subcenters ANM/FH worker — 323882
- Health supervisor — 107960
- Community Health centers Nurse Midwives — 26439
- Primary Health Center PH Nurse — 26439
- Public Health Nurse Supervisor — 7436
- District Public health nursing officer — 900

High Power Committee on Nursing and Nursing Profession Report on Nursing, 1989

A high power committee on Nursing and Nursing profession was constituted by the Government of India in July, under the chairmanship of Smt Sarojini Varadapan and Smt Rajkumari Sood, the nursing advisor to Government of India as the member secretary.

High Power Committee Recommended the Following Aspects of Nurses and Nursing Profession

- This committee focused on Working conditions of nursing personnel including employment and, job description working hours, working facilities, salary and allowances.
- The committee also recommended for special allowances for nurses such as; uniform allowance, washing, mess allowance, etc.
- With regards to promotional opportunities, should be based on merit cum seniority. Open selection should be made for promoting the senior most administrative and teaching posts.
- In terms of career development, it is recommended only after competition of 5 years of regular service opportunity to be given. Nurses should be allotted accommodation near to the work place. During calamities and odd hours of duty, transport facilities to be given to nursing personnel.
- Those nurses showing exemplary services to be facilitated with incentives by awards, special increment, or promotion who are working in hospital or community of each state or district to be worked out.
- All nursing personnel like central government to be given free treatment if they are exposed to occupational hazards. Hospital should provide welfare services to all nursing personnel.
- The committee suggested two levels of nursing personnel:
  - *Professional nurse:* A degree level nurse admitted with 12 years of schooling with science group, had undergone training for 4 years.
  - *Diploma nurse:* 10 years of schooling with 3 years training should be trained in schools of nursing attached to medical college hospitals.

- There should be a separate budget for each nursing school. The principal of the school should be the drawing and the disbursing officer.
- ANM nursing schools to be attached to district hospitals.
- The committee recommended to continue with the post certificate BSc Nursing degree program. The current postgraduate nursing programme needs to be strengthened and number of postgraduate institution in nursing needs to be increased including Doctoral program.
- For all levels of nursing education financial assistance should be provided from central government.
- Selection of nursing should be based on merit and aptitude.
- The committee further recommended to strengthen nursing schools by facilitating adequate infrastructure and adequate budget for libraries and teaching equipment as recommended by Indian Nursing Council Norms. Students should be given proper accommodations in the hostel.
- The learning for students should be under the supervision of tutors/clinical instructors and to take place in wards.
- Community nursing experience should be provided as per INC requirements. Necessary transport to be given for students for community health nursing experience.
- With regards to faculty in school of nursing, INC norms to be followed.
- In terms of specialty courses at postgraduate education the committee recommended special centers of excellence, e.g AIIMS, National Institute of Health and Family welfare, RAK College of Nursing and several other institutions may develop courses on nursing administration for senior nursing personnel.
- For higher education in nursing training in abroad to be facilitated.
- ***Continuing education:*** Each state to develop definite policies to depute 5–10% of staff for higher studies. Provision for training reserve is made in each institution.
- Deputation for higher study is to be made compulsory after 5 years.

These committees are appointed from time to time by Government of India to look into the issues of the health care administration. Recommendations made by these committees were very helpful to make an excellent change in nursing profession in specific and our health care delivery system in general.

NATIONAL HEALTH POLICIES

In 1978, the Joint WHO UNICEF international conference held at Alma-Ata (USSR). Based on Alma-Ata Declaration, WHO and UNICEF called all the governments of the world countries to establish national health policies according to their own resources to maintain and sustain primary health care as a part of national health system. India became one of the countries to accept Alma-Ata Declaration.

National Health Policy of 1983

The Government of India formulated its first National Health Policy (NHP) in 1983 as a commitment to the Alma-Ata Declaration to achieve 'Health for All by 2000'. It accepted that health was fundamental central to development of any country and had a focus on access to health services, and ensuring cooperation of the community. The policy recognizes that promotion of nutrition, prevention of food adulteration and maintenance of the quality of drugs, water supply and sanitation, environmental protection; immunization programme, maternal and child health services, school health programme, and occupational health services as prime attention for inputs required for enhancing health care. The policy also emphasizes for reorientation of the existing health personnel and inclusion of various Indian systems of medicine and health care at all the levels, in the over-all health care delivery system, focusing to the preventive, promotive and public health objectives.

The Salient Features of the 1983 Health Policy

- It was critical of the curative-oriented western model of health care.
- It emphasized a preventive, promotive and rehabilitative primary health care approach.
- It recommended a decentralized system of health care, the key features of which were low cost, use of volunteers and paramedics, and community participation.
- It recommended for an expansion of the private curative sector.
- The policy recommended the setting up of establishment of a nationwide network of epidemiological stations that would facilitate the integration of various health activities. NHP 1983 emphasized for providing primary health care with special focus on prevention, promotion and rehabilitation.

NHP 1983 Suggested Planned Time Bound Attention to the following

- Nutrition, prevention of food adulteration
- Maintenance of quality of drugs

- Water supply and sanitation
- Environmental protection
- Immunization programme
- Maternal and child health services
- School health programme
- Occupational health services
- For better programme planning NHP 1983 recommended an effective Health Information System (HIS) to be launched.

National Health Policy, 2002

Policy means a guidelines, which provides the scientific outline and rationality of decision-making for the achievement of desired goals.

It is the statement that guides the functioning of an organization. Public health policy helps to enhance the health conditions of people who lives under the health care unit. It focuses on ensuring safe, adequate and sustainable livelihood lifestyle and healthy environments, including housing education, nutrition, childcare, reproductive health, transportation, information and communication, community and personal social and health services. The adequacy of the health of the population reflects on the country's health policy.

Objectives of National Health Policy, 2002

- To achieve good health amongst all the population of the country at an acceptable standard.
- To strengthen decentralizing public health system by setting up new infrastructure that is accessible in deficient areas and by enhancing the infrastructure in existing institutions.
- To ensure accessibility of health services to all population.
- To enhance the contribution of the private sector in providing health service for the population group which are affordable to general population.
- To increase health system support from central government.
- For effective health services strengthen the state level health care delivery system.
- To effective use of allopathic medicine with rationale for using them.
- To increase the access of traditional medicine which are tested for their safety.

The Policy Formulated the Following Goals to be Achieved 2000–2015

- Enactment and regulation for minimum standard for clinical field in medical institution by 2005.
- Eradication of polio, yaws, leprosy, kala azar and lymphatic filariasis.
- Increase allocation of budget for health sector from 5.5% to 7%.
- The committee strongly recommended for setting up an integrated system of surveillance, and focused National Health Accounts and Health Statistics
- For medical research 1% of the total budget needs to be allocated.
- By the year 2007 decentralization of implementation of public health program needs to be completed.
- By 2010 the committee stressed to achieve of zero level growth of HIV/AIDS.
- Mortality due to tuberculosis, malaria, other vector and water borne diseases to be reduced by 50% by 2011.
- Prevalence of blindness to be reduced to 0.5% by 2011.
- IMR to 30/1000 live births and MMR to 100/Lakh live births to be brought down.
- From < 20% to > 75% increase utilization of public health facilities.
- Increase health expenditure by government from the existing 0.9% to 2.0% of GDP health expenditure.
- 25% of share of central grants to total health spending to be increased.
- ***Financial resources:*** 55% total public health investment for the primary health sector, 35% for secondary sector and 10% for tertiary sector has been allocated as per NHP 2002.
- ***Delivery of national public health programs:*** NHP 2002 focuses for a scientific designing of public health projects to reach for the population from center to periphery level by its vision of strengthening public health administration.
- ***The state of public health Infrastructure:*** With the belief that NHP 2002 emphasized a decentralized public health system that will ensure a more effective supervision of the public health personnel through community monitoring, than has been achieved through the regular administrative line of control.
- ***Extending public health services:*** NHP 2002 advocated to include Indian systems of Medicine and Homeopathy Practitioners as registered Practitioners along with the expansion of medical practitioners to provide health care.
- ***Role of local self-government institutions:*** NHP 2002 lays great emphasis upon the implementation of public health programs through local self-government institutions.
- ***Norms of health care professional:*** Minimal statutory norms with constant monitoring for the appointing

doctors and nurses in medical institutions need to be introduced urgently under the provision of the Indian Medical council Act and Indian Nursing Council Act, respectively.

- *Education of health care professional:* The committee strongly recommended medical research and geriatric concern. This policy also stresses creation of additional PG seats in deficient specialties. It suggests for a need based, skill oriented syllabus with a more significant component of practical training to be implemented.
- *For discharging public health responsibilities in the count:* NHP 2002 recommends specialization in the disciplines of Public Health and Family Medicine where medical doctors, public health engineers, microbiologists and other natural science specialists can take up the course and work as a public health team.
- The policy strongly advocated a need for specialists in 'public health' and 'family medicine'.
- *Nursing personnel:* NHP 2002 recognizes acute shortage of nurses trained in the areas of super specialty disciplines. It recommends enhancing nursing personnel in public health delivery centers and establishment of training courses for super specialties.
- *Use of generic drugs and vaccines:* This policy emphasizes on the need for basic treatment regimens, in both the government and private sector, and a limited number of essential drugs of a generic nature.
- *Urban health:* Primary center as first tier health facility that cover 1 lakh population should have OPD facilities and provision of essential drugs. It has the responsibility to carry out national health programmers.
- General hospital serves as second tier health facility is to function as a referral centre to primary centre. A fully equipped infrastructure for trauma care network to be facilitated in this care facility to reduce accident mortality is also recommended.
- *Mental health:* The policy recommended to decentralize mental health service for diagnosis and treatment by general duty medical staff. It also recommended ensuring the human rights of mentally sick patients.
- *Information education and communication:* According to NHP 2002, the school children must be made aware of health promotion concepts through folk tradition street play like media and communication. It will help in bringing health seeking behavior, which is the most cost effective intervention where the school children extends health awareness to family and community.
- *Health research:*
  - The policy recommends an increase in government funds and health resources to 1% of total health for medical research by 2005 and up to 2% by 2010.
  - New therapeutic drugs and vaccines for tropical disease needs to be prioritized.
- *Role of private sector:* The policy appreciates the participation of the private sector in health activities conducted at primary, secondary and tertiary level. The committee recommended a regulatory mechanism and accreditation standard of private sector for the conduct of clinical practice. The policy further stresses a social health insurance scheme for the needy population. It emphasizes need for standard protocols in practice by health professionals. The policy recommended tele-medicine in tertiary health care services.
- *Role of civil society:* The policy recommended participating in all disease control program by NGO.
- *National disease surveillance network:* This policy recommended the functioning of an integrated disease control strategy by public health surveillance network along with information from private health care institutions and practitioners by 2005.
- *Health statistics:* As an immediate task, NHP 2002 recommended to develop full baseline data of tuberculosis, malaria and blindness by 2005, and in the long-term develop data of cardiovascular diseases, cancer, diabetes, accidents, hepatitis.
- *Women's health:* The policy strongly recommended for developing measures for women empowerment.
- *Medical ethics:* The policy recommended modification of code of ethics by medical council of India. The policy further recommended the need to monitor on gene manipulation and stem cell research.
- *Enforcement of quality standards for food and drugs:* NHP 2002 recommended to strengthen food and drug administration with reference to laboratory facilities and technical expertise.
- *Regulation of standards in paramedical disciplines:* The policy recommended monitoring training institutions that have established recently in larger number. Since there is no strong regulatory control over these institutions the policy strongly suggested to develop Statutory Professional Council for paramedical discipline.
- *Environmental and occupational health:* NHP 2002 has recommended for an independent state policy

and programme for environment conditions like unsafe drinking water, unhygienic sanitation and air pollution. The policy further focused on child labor and substandard working environment causing hazards and illness to be taken care of.

- *Medical facilities to users from overseas (Health Tourism):* The NHP 2002 Strongly encourages medical tourism

Achievements 2003

- The Government had successfully enacted legislation for regulating minimum standard in clinical practice for Medical institution 2005.
- Yaws has been declared eliminated however confirmation of complete eradication of poliomyelitis is not ensured
- Leprosy has been declared eliminated from the country as per WHO criteria.
- Inspire of setting up of Integrated Disease Surveillance Project, establishing of National Health Accounts and Health Statistics is still moving in a low pace.
- No changes had been observed in increasing budget from 5.5% to 7% spending on state health sector:
- The total health budget has not been increased in spite of 1% of the total health budget for Medical Research has been targeted.
- National Rural Health Mission has been launched in 2007 as a result of implementation of decentralization of public health program.
- One of the important achievement is achievement of zero level growth of HIV/AIDS.

The following goals were not achieved by 2005

- Eradication of poliomyelitis
- Establishing an integrated system of surveillance, and National Health Accounts and Health Statistics.
- Increase of budget allocation from 5.5% to 7%.
- Allocation of 1% of the total health budget for Medical Research.
- Decentralization of implementation of public health programs.

Draft on National Health Policy, 2015

In December 2014, the central government made the draft on National Health Policy 2015. As a first step in accomplishing universal health coverage focusing health as a fundamental right. The current government spending on health care is a dismal 1.04 per cent of gross domestic product (GDP), one of the lowest in the world; this is to ₹ 957 per capita in absolute terms. The draft policy is aiming at allocating an increase in government spending to 2.5 per cent of GDP (₹ 3,800 per capita) in the coming five years around 63 million people are suffering from poverty every year because of the failure of public health care system that is unable to provide affordable and accessible health services to the people.

Draft on National Health Policy 2015 envisages different approach based on the philosophy that health will be recognized as a fundamental right and objective of this draft will be universal health coverage. Being health is a state subject, adoption and implementation should be by States.

NATIONAL POPULATION POLICY

In 1952, India was the first country in the world to launch a national programme, emphasizing family planning is vital for reducing birth rates for stabilization of population which in turn will influence the national economy. Though a drastic decline in death rate was observed after 1952. The birth rate was static. In 1976, during emergency, the Government of India launched National Population Policy with the aims of:

- Proposing legislation by the government to raise the age of marriage to 18 for girls and 21 for boys;
- Special measures to raise the level of female education in the states by the government
- Provision of monetary compensation from May 1, 1976, as ₹150 for sterilization (by men or women) if performed with 2 children, ₹ 100 if performed with three living children and ₹ 70 if performed with four or more children.

Achievement of National Population Policy

After a period of five decades, after launching the national family welfare programme, India has achieved the following:

- Crude birth rate reduced from 40.8 (1951) to 26.4 (1998) according Statistical registration service; (SRS)
- Infant mortality rate reduced (IMR) from 146 per 1000 live births (1951) to 72 per 1000 live births in 1998,as per SRS
- Couple protection rate increased 4 times (CPR) from 10.4 percent (1971) to 44 percent (1999)
- Crude death rate reduced (CDR) from 25 (1951) to 9.0 (1998), as per SRS
- From 37 years to 62 years; life expectancy increased
- There was an universal awareness observed and achieved to the maximum for the need and methods of family planning

- Reduction of total fertility rate was observed from 6.0 (1951) to 3.3 (1997,as per SRS).

The National Population Policy, 2000 (NPP 2000) emphasized the commitment of Government towards motivating couples for voluntary consent and informed choice while accepting reproductive health care services and target free approach in conduct of family planning services.

The NPP 2000 also prepared a policy framework for forwarding goals and prioritizing strategies of reproductive and child health needs, achieve Total Fertility rate (TFR) by 2010, child survival, maternal health, contraception, increasing outreach and coverage of a comprehensive reproductive and child health services by government and public private partnership.

Goals to be achieved in each case by 2010 are formulated as follows:

- Achieve the unmet needs for basic reproductive and child health services, supplies and infrastructure for family planning.
- Compulsory and free school educations up to age of 14 and reduce drop outs below 20% at primary and secondary schools boys and girls.
- One of the goals to be achieved was reduction of infant mortality rate to below 30 per 1000 live births.
- Reduction of maternal mortality ratio to below 100 per 100,000 live births was important goal of NPP.
- Achievement of universal immunization of children against all vaccine preventable diseases was one of the targets.
- Age for marriage for girls to be delayed not earlier than 18 preferably 20 years of age.
- Institutional deliveries to be achieved by 80% and deliveries by trained personnel 100%.
- Achievement of universal access to information/ counseling, and services for Family planning, fertility regulation and contraception of choices are important goals of NPP.
- To have proper statistics 100 per cent registration of births, deaths, marriage and pregnancy is targeted.
- Reduction of spread of AIDS, reproductive tract infection and sexually transmitted diseases.
- Prevent and control communicable diseases.
- Promote Indian Systems of Medicine (ISM).
- Promote the small family norm to achieve target rate of TFR.
- Promote the small family norm to achieve target rate of TFR.

Table 2.1: National population, family welfare vital statistics 2011

S.No.	Indicators	2009	2011
1.	Population		21.21 Billion
	Male (51.54%)		623..72 Million
	Female (48.46%)		586.47 Million
2.	Growth rate	21.5%	17.64%
3.	Sex ratio (female per 100 male)		940
4.	Overall literacy rate		74.04%
	Male		82.14%
	Female		65.64%
5.	Birth rate per 1000 population	22.5	
6.	Death rate per 1000 population	7.3	
7.	Total fertility rate	2.6	
8.	Maternal mortality rate/10000 population	212	
9.	Infant mortality rate/1000 birth	50	
10.	Child mortality 0–5 years/1000	14.1	
11.	Couple protection rate in %		40.4
12.	Life expectancy Male Female	 63 66.7	
13.	Neonatal mortality Rural Urban	 38/1000 21/1000	
14.	Post neo mortality	16/1000	
15.	Perinatal, mortality	35/1000	
16.	Still birth	8/1000	
17.	Institutional deliveries		78.1

The vast population of India is her greatest asset if they are provided with the means to lead healthy and economically productive lives. Population stabilization is a multispectral approach requiring constant and effective coordination at all levels of the government and society. Today we need, increasing availability of affordable reproductive and child health services, family welfare service delivery at village levels, may enhance early achievement of the sociodemographic goals.

NATIONAL HEALTH POLICY ON AYUSH AND PLANS

AYUSH stands for Ayurveda, Unani medicine, Siddha, and Homeopathy. From ancient times AYUSH was practiced in India. Now it is universally accepted. The basic philosophy of AYUSH system lies in preventive and promotive health care, diseases and health condition relating to women and children, noncommunicable diseases, stress management, palliative care, rehabilitation, etc.

AYUSH has very little side effect. In March 1995 the department of Indian system of medicine and homeopathy was renamed as AYUSH by the Government of India.

The main aims of AYUSH are:

- Enhance and upgradation of AYUSH educational standards
- Quality control and standardization of drugs
- Improving the availability of medicinal plant material
- Research and development in AYUSH
- Awareness development of efficacy of systems.

Objectives of national policy on AYUSH 2002 including promotion of good health and expand the outreach of health care ensuring affordable AYUSH services to population; provision of availability of drugs and integration of AYUSH in health care delivery system and national programmes. Plans for AYUSH and infrastructure comprising of Medical colleges, for training, placement of registered medical practitioners in hospitals and dispensaries, and developing drug manufacturing unit is available in the country. The facilities available in the country are:

- Institutionally trained practitioners: 488714
- Non Institutionally qualified practitioners: 200088
- Number of colleges: 437
- Admission capacity per annum in UG colleges: 23280
- Number of drug manufacturing units: 9832
- Number of hospitals: 3841
- Number of beds in hospitals: 65753

National institute setup by the central government for AYUSH

- National Institute of Ayurveda, Jaipur, Rajasthan
- National Institute of Unani Medicine, Bangalore, Karnataka
- National Institute of Homoeopathy, Kolkata, West Bengal
- National Institute of Naturopathy, Pune, Maharashtra
- Morarji Desai National Institute of Yoga, New Delhi
- National Institute of Siddha, Chennai, Tamil Nadu
- National Ayurveda Hospital, New Delhi.

Statutory Regulatory Bodies of AYUSH are a) Central Council of Indian Medicine (CCIM), b) Central Council of Homeopathy (CCH) to formulate standards of education, and to ensure adherence to laid down standards. The council also recommends to the Central Government for recognition and withdrawal of medical qualifications awarded by Universities if standards are violated.

The Following are the Priority Program of AYUSH

- Standardization of Education and Continuing Medical Education (CME)
- Medicinal plant sector
- Research and Development
- Information, Education and Communication (IEC) and international collaboration
- Standardization and Quality Control of Ayurveda, Siddha, Unani and Homeopathy drugs
- Mainstreaming of AYUSH in National Health Care Delivery System.

Schemes for strengthening AYUSH

- Strengthening of existing Under Graduate Colleges.
- Assistance to Postgraduate Medical Education
- Reorientation Training Programme of AYUSH Personnel
- Short-term Continuing Medical Education (CME) Programme for General AYUSH Practitioners
- Scheme for Renovation and Strengthening of AYUSH Teaching Hospital
- Scheme for Establishing of Computer Laboratories with internet facilities in selected AYUSH Colleges
- Upgradation of AYUSH colleges to the status of State Model Institute of Ayurveda, Siddha, Unani and Homeopathy.

SUMMARY POINTS

✓ In the development of nursing as a profession and practice discipline, the recommendations of various health and nursing committees contributions are immense. Bhore committee, Mudaliar committee and Shetty committee constituted by Government of India with regards to nursing and nursing profession, Bajaj committee on health manpower planning and High power committee on nursing and socioeconomic conditions are still utilized by our planners and council of nursing as guideline for developing nursing program in the country.

- ✓ With regards to national health policies (1983, 2002 and the draft plan for 2015 emphasizes maternal and child nursing and public health nursing at the grass root level.
- ✓ Population policies reminds the achievement of national family welfare program and the scope of a nurse in achieving the goal of family welfare.
- ✓ National policy on AYUSH provides nurses expanded role and in many states Ayurveda nursing program in graduate level are planned.

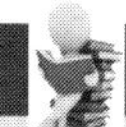

REVIEW QUESTIONS

1. Discuss the various health committees and their contributions to development of nursing in India.
2. Describe High power committee recommendations for nursing.
3. Define policies Explain National health policy 2002.
4. Explain the achievement of national population policy 2000.
5. Discuss National policy on Ayush and its plan.
6. Write short notes on:
   a. Mudaliar committee report on Public health
   b. Importance of Minimum need program by Kartar Singh committee
   c. Shrivastava committee reports
   d. List policy statement of AYUSH and action taken
   e. Committee on hospital bed standard or ratio of nurse: patients
   f. Multipurpose health worker.

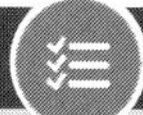

SELECTED READINGS

1. AYUSH Mission, Department of AYUSH, Ministry of health and Family planning Govt of India, 2014
2. Bhore committee,1946 | National Health Portal Of India, http://www.nhp.gov.in/bhore-committee-1946 pg Last access Apr 3, 2015
3. Editorial, A step in the right direction. The Hindu, Jan 3, 2015
4. Features of the Population Policy of the Govt, of India http://www.yourarticlelibrary.com/population/features-of-the-population-policy-of-the-govt-of-india/5605/
5. High Power Committee on Nursing and Nursing Profession http://www.communityhealth.in/~commun26/wiki/index Last access Nov 22, 2012.
6. Highlights on National Population Policy, 2000 | India http://www.yourarticlelibrary.com/law/highlights-on-national-population-policy-2000-india/31384/
7. Highlights on National Population Policy, 2000 | India http://www.yourarticlelibrary.com/law/highlights-on-national-population-policy-2000-india/31384/
8. National Health Policy (1983) - communityhealth.in. http://www.communityhealth.in/~commun26/wiki/index.php, National_Health_Policy_(1983) last access Jan 15, 2013 .
9. National Population Policy 2000 - National Commission On Population http://populationcommission.nic.in/Publication/2011
10. Priya daharshini National Health Committee Reports http://www.slideshare.net/cpdarshini/national-health-committee-reports last access Aug 27, 2011
11. Ravi Duggal. Health planning in India http://www.cehat.org/go/uploads/Publications/a168.pdf last..access on 3 Feb 2014.

12. Report of the High Power Committee - of Planning Commission http://planningcommission.nic.in/reports/publications/pub95_hghpwr.pdf Government of India:1995
13. Sabitha Jain, Health committees http://www.slideshare.net/sabithajain/health-committees last access Oct 6, 2013
14. Sheila Seda. Making India a healthier nation, The nursing Journal of India, Vol CIII:No.2 last access ; April, 2012
15. State Institute of Health and family welfare, Jaipur. Public health care in India-An overview. http://www.authorstream.com/Presentation/abdoctor-1176195-public-health-care-in-india/Sep 6, 2011
16. Statistical division, Government of India, Ministry of health and family welfare 2011

UNIT II
INTRODUCTION TO NURSING SERVICE ADMINISTRATION

3. Nursing Administration and Management

4. Role of a Nurse Administrator and Manager in a Hospital

3

Nursing Administration and Management

LEARNING OBJECTIVES

This chapter imparts learning about:

- Introduction to Nursing
- Definitions, Concepts of Administration and Management
- Description of Various Theories of Management
- Explanation of Significance, Elements and Principles of Administration
- Description of Functions of Administration
- Discussion on Principles and Functions of Management
- Research Highlights

INTRODUCTION TO NURSING SERVICE ADMINISTRATION

Nursing is a practice discipline. The nurse works in an environment that is constantly changing to provide quality patient care. The philosophy of nursing is caring, comforting and nurturing that is based on the health needs, nursing problems, nursing diagnosis and plan for nursing intervention and evaluation of the care given. As medical advancement and specialization are becoming complex the dimension of nursing service, education and administration also becoming more challenging. Nurses are the vital part of health care delivery system. They provide comprehensive health services that include preventive, promotive, curative, restorative and rehabilitative care.

Nursing is confronted with independent, interdependent and collaborative care activities for patients of all age group of individuals, male and female, sick or well, individuals and families in all health care settings. Nursing includes provision of quality care, teaching the individuals and families, advocacy, counseling and guidance, providing safe environment, participating and implementing policies and conducting clinical research. Administration is an art and science. The effective leadership of an administrator is the key to the success and progress of any organization.

THE DIFFERENCE BETWEEN MANAGEMENT AND ADMINISTRATION

People view administration and management differently. The American Authorities view administration is the top level function and the management is low level function. Whereas European Authorities view management as a comprehensive term and administration is a part of management. Currently, we use administration and management interchangeably.

Nursing management is a process of planning, organizing, leading and controlling the efforts of the members of the organization and thus it is the effective utilization of available resources to achieve the preset goals of the organization that is to bring better quality patient care outcomes. Management and administration are two different concepts and levels of organization. The administrator is on the top level of the organization, who makes administrative decisions. They are involved in policy making, and establishing aims and goals for the organization such as the hospital or college of nursing. Manager is posted in the middle level of the organization who mainly engaged in implementation of the policies of the organization developed by the administrator.

Management is the art of getting the work done through the members of the health team by directing and controlling their efforts to achieve the organizational goals. Administration consists of individual who owns the establishment and receive the benefits/profits from the establishment whereas the management consists of group of personnel who is an expert and functions to achieve the goals and objectives of the organization.

Administration plans and organizes whereas management motivates and control the organization.

Difference Between Nurse Administrator and Nurse Manager

The nurse administrator and the nurse manager's positions are not the same. There is a difference in their functions, responsibilities, salary benefits and positions. In the hierarchy, a nurse administrator is responsible for the entire hospital nursing service department like all the wards, operation theater, outpatient departments, etc. (e.g. a Principal is responsible for all the departments of the college of nursing like medical-surgical department, pediatric department, etc.), while a nurse manager is only responsible for her or his nursing unit or units under her care within the hospital or college of nursing. A nurse administrator often reports to the chief executive officer in the organization like medical superintendent or chief medical officer, while nurse unit managers usually report directly to the nursing superintendent or nurse administrator.

MANAGEMENT THEORIES

Management theories are implemented to help increase in organizational productivity and service quality. Not many managers use a singular theory or concept when implementing strategies in the workplace: They commonly use a combination of a number of theories, depending on the workplace, purpose and workforce. Contingency theory, chaos theory and systems theory are popular management theories. Theory X and Y, which addresses management strategies for workforce motivation, is also implemented to help increase employees productivity.

Management theories are developed based on three approaches.

The Classical Approach

The classical approach to management theory evolved in the nineteenth century and was applied in administration till twentieth century. The administrators during this period confronted with various issues and challenges in administration. In order to overcome those issues administrators identified efficient method, that included a scientific approach which was justified to some extent.

The classical approach includes the following three theories:

Scientific Management by Frederick W Taylor 1856–1915

Scientific management theory is also expressed as Taylorism. It was a scientific approach that was used to enhance labor productivity. One of Taylor's philosophies was man who was given importance in the past history and in future history system will take the importance'.

The General Concept of Scientific Management

The main concept in this theory was to develop and train employees for performing the given task by a standard method. To do this the managers identified and established meticulous protocols/procedures that were based on each organizational task. The employees were given a good work environment. According to the capacity of the employees selected tasks were assigned to each one of them. Those employees demonstrated good mental and physical health were assigned specific tasks. When the outcome was good, increased wage and incentive were given to the employees. Because of improved benefits, the employees were satisfied and motivated to bring better outcome.

Disadvantages of Scientific Management

The major drawback of this theory was dehumanization as it was focused more on outcome than the individual social needs. Employees worked like machines and were more coerced to bring more output. There was no chance for the employees to demonstrate their talents and bring innovation.

Administrative Principle by Henry Fayol 1841–1925

Fayol's theory of administrative principle emphasized the importance of both the employer and the employees in an organization. This theory worked with four basic principles. They are:

1. *Unity of command:* Each employee takes instruction from only one superior.
2. *Division of work:* The employees were given task based on their expertize competency.
3. *Unities of direction:* The related activities of an organization were combined under one supervisor/ manager.
4. *Scalar chain:* The hierarchical structure of an organization starting from administrator to the employee working at the bottom level, for example nurse administrator to staff nurse.

Administrative Principles

According to Fayol's theory there were five basic functions or elements of management:

1. Planning
2. Organizing
3. Controlling
4. Coordinating
5. Commanding (leading/directing).

Mary Parker Follett (1868–1933) contributed further to the administrative principles emphasized on the common interests of the employees in preventing organizational conflict and developing trust, confidence and respect to the employer as well as the employee.

Chester I Bernard (1886–1961) established the concept of informal organization where the employer and employee worked informally and demonstrated a working bond.

Bureaucratic Organizations by Max Weber 1864–1920

Weber's theory emphasized on the hierarchical positions that is structured where there is line of authority. Employees are selected by competency and skills for employment and the promotion is based on achievement of the employee.

Good bureaucracy has no chance for corruption, favoritism and misuse of power and authority. Sometimes bureaucracy would be taken for civil service (governmental organizations) but actually is being used in larger organizations. Bureaucracy is rigid system.

HUMAN RESOURCE APPROACH TO MANAGEMENT

The human resource approach to administration emphasized that in order to bring the full potentials and skills of an employee the administrator should assign the task in such a way that the employee does his job independently and achieve his goals to the maximum. This approach comprises the following three theories:

Hawthorne Studies by Elton Mayo

Elton Mayo conducted studies at the Hawthorne Works of the Western Electrical Company at Chicago with the aims of organizational outcome for five years. Six women were selected as sample size for the study and these women were given different work conditions such as improvement in payment mode of salary, break for rest during work in different timing with satisfying duration, food supply and refreshments in between work and the study observed that the productivity and employee morale of the group.

Elton Mayo and his team understood that, the women perceived importance in the organization, there was an improvement in the interpersonal relationship among women which in turn encouraged them to work in their own work pattern and style of work, the working environment became more positive and pleasant.

With the result of the changed intervention in the organization, Mayo determined that job satisfaction must depend upon the flexible/informal social relationships between employees and the social relationships between employees and employers.

The studies by Elton Mayo concluded that when individuals work in group they develop a work pattern in their social world because work is a group activity. The employees' need safe and secured work environment, approval for the good work done by them, and a sense of belongingness to the organization are more important for good organizational outcome. The study also concluded that any conflict in the organization affect the employees' work. There is an impact of inside and outside social demands on employees' attitude. The employees' attitude and performance is affected by the social control created by the informal group in the organization. A planned and developed collaboration of work can resists the negative effect and bring cohesion within the organization. Adaptation of the individual from home environment to work place with advanced technology affect the disruption of the social organization.

Maslow's Theory of Human's Needs

Maslow's hierarchy of needs is psychological theory that explains each individual is motivated by his needs. One of the challenging responsibilities of an administrator is motivating the employees effectively. Motivation refers to the psychological processes that stimulate excitement of voluntary actions aimed to achieve the goal. Since motivation is highly individualized, managers use a wide range of activities to enhance employees motivated and happy. Therefore, it is essential for managers to understand the psychological processes involved in motivation so that they can effectively direct employees to achieve organizational goals.

McGregor's Theory (X–Y Theory)

In 1960 Douglas McGregor, an American psychologist authored a book '*The Human Side of Enterprise*' described the characteristics of people in the work place. Based on the belief of theory X and theory Y, people who are basically lazy and avoid work responsibilities are categorized in X theory and people who are innovative and enjoyed their work are categorized in Y theory.

The difference between X and Y theory managers:

X Theory

- Manager is a strong authoritarian leader shows poor outcome in administration
- Exercises coercive power
- Stereotype, not interested in advanced techniques in organization
- Forces the employees to get good results
- Not committed to work
- No sharing with employees, arrogates with employees
- The manager uses punishment and disciplinary action when the work is not done
- Concentrates on monetary gain
- One way communicator
- Conflict is intolerant
- Performance appraisals occur on a regular basis.

Y Manager

- Demonstrates rewarding leadership
- Work with employees to bring better outcome uses participative power
- Innovative, and creative, uses the best techniques in administration
- Motivates and support the employees to get good results
- More committed in work
- Accepts and shares the responsibility
- Encourages and allows the employees to develop and grow
- Demonstrates participatory decision making and accepts constructive suggestions from employees
- Conflicts often resolved through negotiation
- Performance appraisals and promotions done regularly
- Various studies have demonstrated that the organizational success depends upon the administrators leadership styles.

MODERN APPROACH TO MANAGEMENT

Modern approach includes the following three theories and their contributors:

Open Systems Theory

This system explains a group of units with a common goal in a system interacts with other system accepts their inputs, makes changes and transforms them into outputs with mutual effects.

Contingency Theory

The contingency approach is based on management effectiveness and contingent or dependent upon the managerial behavior and organizational environment or specific situation. The manager changes his leadership behavior according to changing environment.

Japanese Management Style Theory Z

Japanese management system was concerned about the competitiveness of American companies led clues to evaluate Japanese management practices to achieve success in their industries. It was in this situation William Ouchi developed 'Z' theory and introduced into Japanese industries. Theory Z is an extension of motivation and assumes that bigger establishments are human systems and their effectiveness depends on the quality of humanism used. A z theory) has the following distinguished feature:

- Mutual trust between the employer and employees
- Strong bonding between the management and workers
- Employee employer participation
- Integrated organized work pattern
- Coordination with various departments in organization
- Informal control over employees
- Development of human resource system.

SIGNIFICANCE, ELEMENTS AND PRINCIPLES OF ADMINISTRATION

Administration is an enabling process it covers the whole art of carrying to effect any policy plan, or undertaking whether conceived by government, public or private agency. It may how ever go further than the simple executive function of applying rule to given cases it include leadership, policy making and planning (Goddard, 1979).

According to Simon, 'Administration can be defined as the activities of groups cooperating to accomplish common goals' (Simon, Smithburg, Thompson, 1950).

In another definition, administration is defined as 'an activity or process mainly concerned with the means for carrying out prescribed ends.' (Pfiffner and Presthus, 1967).

According to Waldo 'administration is a type of cooperative human effort that has a high degree of rationality.' (Waldo, 1955).

From the above concepts of administration, it is clear that in an establishment administration is highly significant. In order to achieve the goals of establishment administration is a means by planning, policy making and decision making activity with the help of group of people.

Elements of Administration

Henri Fayol classifies the key functions of management into five main elements:

1. *Planning:* Forecasting to the operation of an organization. Good planning involves experiences, unity, continuity, flexibility, precision and leadership in administrator.
2. *Organizing:* Material organization, human organization and finance organization requires leadership, and good organizational structure.
3. *Commanding:* Rests on certain personal qualities and knowledge of general management in an administrator
4. *Coordinating:* Coordinating by integrating subordinates and keeping balance among material, social and functional parts in an establishment.
5. *Controlling:* It is very important to verify whether activities take place in conformity with the plan adopted, instructions issued and principles established.

Principles of Administration

The basic and important aspects of administration are called as the principles. These are the protocols or guidelines which guides the administrator in the administrative process to achieve the goals of nursing service administration

- *Hierarchy:* It is the organizational structure depicting position of each employee from the top level administration to the bottom of the administration. The nursing superintendent at the top level of hierarchy and the staff nurse may at the bottom level positioned in hospital nursing hierarchy.
- *Control:* The decision making and various controls are made by the head of the institution that has many departments.
- *Unity of command:* In this principle one employee is accountable to one supervisor.
- *Delegation of authority:* The head of the institution divides the authority to various departmental heads. This suggests increase number of employees are answerable to their work that in turn enhance in the smooth running of the organization.
- *Specialization:* Each worker is assigned his work according to his skill and expertise and according to his training and specialization for efficiency and effectiveness.
- *Objective:* Each employee is to be informed about the nature of job and the objective of the establishment to achieve the goal.

FUNCTIONS OF ADMINISTRATION

The administration process include planning, organizing, staffing, directing , coordinating reporting and budgeting.

Planning is the first phase of administration in forecasting the activities required to achieve the goal of establishment. The administrator determines in advance what is to be done for the present and for the development of the future. It is an intellectual activity that helps to eliminate uncertain failure in future. Good planning facilitates coordination, utilization resources to the maximum, and lays foundation for achieving organizational goals.

Organizing is the act of rearranging elements following one or more. Organizing can also be defined as to place different objects in logical arrangement for better searching. It is the synchronization of various parts to whole in order to achieve organizational goals. Organizations are groups of people organized for some purpose, such as business or political activities. Staffing is a term used in the sphere of employment. It has been applied to more than one aspect of the working environment.

Staffing is also known as human resource management. It include various activities such as recruitment, selection, orientation, training and retaining nurses in sufficient quality and quantity for the smooth running of the organization. A good staffing brings a positive impact on quality patient care outcome. Calculation of staffing according to the needs of the organization is an important function of the administrator. The administration needs to define their job description with mental and physical abilities required to perform the particular job. The nurse administrator plans for in-service education program for updating the knowledge of nurses employed in the establishment. Periodical ongoing performance appraisal is one of the important activities of staffing from an organization. A staff policy manual helps the nurses regarding their salary, benefits, promotion and retirement procedures, etc.

Directing means giving instructions, guiding, and counseling, motivating and leading the nursing staff in the organization to perform their job and to achieve organizational objectives. It is a fundamental function of the administrator Whether it is a ward/unit, whether it is a hospital direction is an activity that flows from the higher level to bottom level. It is a continuous activity initiated by the top level manager or supervisor.

Coordination: This activity is very important for the successful organization. The administrator maintains inter and intra departmental coordination of all activities pertaining to nursing service administration along with organizing, monitoring and controlling.

Reporting is a brief guide to enterprise reporting. It is intended to help people who have to rapidly come to grips with concepts in enterprise reporting.

Budgeting is the process of creating a plan to spend money. Creating this spending plan allows to determine in advance whether there is enough money to do the things needed to do. Budgeting is simply balancing expenses with income. If they do not balance and the administrator spends more than she/he make, and there will have a problem. Many people do not realize that they spend more than they earn and slowly sink deeper into debt every year.

PRINCIPLES AND FUNCTIONS OF MANAGEMENT

Principles of Management

Principles are guidelines and thought to action. Managerial principles are essential factors for decisions for action to be taken by the administrator.

The following are the important characteristics of management and are explained as principles of management:

- *Management is a process:* As a process management constitute of planning, executing and controlling the activities of an establishment. These are series of action coordinating the human and material resources to achieve organizational goal. The manager's decision is important in each activity of the process to enable the goal achievement.
- *Management as a Profession:* Like any other profession management also considered as a profession. A manager is a person who is qualified to manage an establishment because he/she had undergone training for a particular duration of time from a recognized management institution. He/she has professional knowledge, professional attitude and professional skills that is required to carry out management functions. A manager is well-versed with his tasks and responsibilities to achieve the organizational objectives.
- *The decision:* Within the framework of the area of service, all matters relating to administration, decision is taken by the manager effectively as he/she is the top level personnel in his/her department or unit. An effective manages encourages participatory decision making to resolve problem. Decision-making is soft skill in administration is also termed as social skill.
- *The objectives:* These are defined in the planning phase itself. They may be long-term or short-term objectives. The manager has a responsibility to concentrate all administrative tasks, activities and decision to achieve the objectives that are determined.
- ***Actions relate to the utilization of resources.*** For effective management resources are very important. Man, money, material and time resources are in scares in health care industry. Some managers use improvisation of resources to achieve the goals. Efficiency is observed when the manager utilizes the minimum resources to achieve for maximum outcome.
- *The economic achievements:* An establishment is measured by periodical assessment and evaluation based on the criteria laid down to achieve the objectives. The review must focus on activities that are taken based managerial decision.
- *To maintain the recurrent action and interaction:* The manager needs to interact with the employees as a continuous process.
- *The management process is future oriented*: Because whatever planning is done, that will focus the needs of today and forecast the needs for tomorrow.

Functions of Management

The five fundamental functions of the management:

1. *Planning:* Planning is a key activity of all managers. The manager in a unit or department plans all the activities to bring quality outcome for example the head nurse or unit incharge plans all the activities for patients care daily, weekly and monthly as well as yearly. It is planning the work with the direction and guidance of head nurse working together with all others in that ward because the others are responsible to carry out the plan. It is the duty of the head nurse/ unit managers to clarify the objectives and set goals for each department. The head nurse also develop policies and standard procedures, strategies and schedules to guide the staff nurses who do the work.

The plan is always flexible according to the changing needs of the establishment. The ultimate goal is to bring quality patient care.

2. *Organizing:* In order to carry out the plan, organization becomes necessary. In order to bring coordination, the tasks are delegated to the employees according to the level of preparation and position in organization. A manager must perceive organization as a social group composed of human beings. The employees are influenced by managerial actions and decisions. Therefore the manager has to be humane.
3. *Leading:* A manager is essentially a leader. Framework for nursing leadership requires a conceptualization of the various functions, roles, and responsibilities of the nurse manager and must also provide leadership if the team working with him/her. In an organization both the manager and employees are to work as a team to achieve the desired results. Good interpersonal relationship helps in team building that is an asset to management. A manager always respects the interests and motivation of the employees and foster the development of their knowledge, attitude and competence. That in turn enhances organizational success.
4. *Measuring and Controlling:* A manager has to evaluate the progress and achievement of the department by measuring the objectives periodically. Necessary corrective planning needs if the objectives are not achieved.
5. *Framework:* In all unit there must be a frame work for the employees. The framework must have systems and procedures, infrastructure for future expansions and the documentation or connectivity through network must help the employees to carry out the work without any problems. This helps the employees to organize their work, think in an orderly fashion and to provide a systematic work culture. Generally, the frame work is developed by the top level administrators for all the departments of an establishment.

BOX 3.1: Research highlight

A study on head nurse role was conducted using a self-logging technique for a two week period. A sample list of activities was provided. It was found that head nurse activities centered in three different areas: hospital-related management functions, the role of the charge nurse performing patient care management functions, and the role of the staff nurse providing direct patient care (Baker and Ganti 1980).

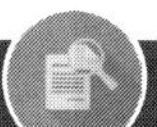

SUMMARY POINTS

- ✓ Nursing is a caring discipline. In order to provide quality patient care and to bring quality health care outcome, the nurse administrator has to plan, organize and execute systematically man, money and materials.
- ✓ As medical advancement and specialization are becoming complex complex the dimension of nursing service, education and administration also becoming more challenging. Nursing services as the part of the total health organization which aims to satisfy major objective of the nursing services and to provide provide prevention of disease and promotion of health.
- ✓ Though administration and management is used interchangeably, there exists a major difference. A nurse administrator is usually responsible for a group of departments, an entire hospital or several hospitals, while a nurse manager is more likely to have the responsibility for one or more nursing units within a hospital or other health care organization. A nurse administrator often reports to the chief executive officer in the organization or to a vice president directly below the CEO, while nurse managers generally report directly to the nursing administrator.
- ✓ The knowledge of principles and functions of administration and management are very important for a nurse administrator and nurse manager for the smooth running of the hospitals or ward units.
- ✓ Various theories in administration and management explain about human engineering process where the administrator or manager functions as a leader and the leadership styles based on the theory what she or he is adopting for the successful administration or management.

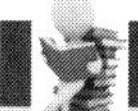

REVIEW QUESTIONS

1. Define administration and management.
2. Differentiate management and administration.

3. Discuss various management theories.
4. Describe various principles and functions of administration.
5. Explain functions of management.
6. Write short notes on:
    a. Classical theories of management
    b. Maslow's theory
    c. X and Y theory
    d. Functions of management
    e. Management principles
    f. POSDCORB.

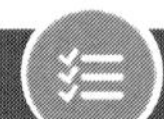

SELECTED READINGS

1. Barker. M, A R Ganti. An in-depth study of the head nurse role. Supervisory Nurse: 1980; 11:(11) 16-21
2. Basic management models and theories associated with motivation ... http://www.healthknowledge.org.uk/public-health-textbook/organisation-management/5c-management-change/basic-management-models Management and Change:
3. Goddard H A >, Principles of nursing service administration, WHO Monogram series Genewa: WHO 1979
4. Historical and Contemporary Theories of Management - http://managementhelp.org/management/theories.htm
5. http://www.differencebetween.info/difference-between-management-and-administration Difference between Management and Administration.
6. http://www.differencebetween.net/business/difference-between-management-and-administration/
7. Management Theories and Concepts at the Workplace | Chron.com http://smallbusiness.chron.com/management-theories-concepts-workplace-17693.html
8. Management theories, roles, motivations, and communication http://www.engr.sjsu.edu/epeterson/Avia179/docs/Chap3.pdf
9. Modern Theory of Management - Video and Lesson Transcript | Study http://study.com/academy/lesson/modern-theory-of-management.html Modern management theory has changed the way managers look at their jobs.
10. Principles of administration applied to nursing service ... https://www.facebook.com/.../Principles-of-administration- applied-to-nursing.
11. Agrawal V K, Vashistha R. POSDCORB- Managerial view, Indian Journal of Research, Vol 31:4 May2013
12. Newman W H, Summer C E, Warren E Kirby. The Process Of Management 1970 Edition The Practice Of Management By Peter F Drucker (Reprinted 1997)

4

Role of a Nurse Administrator and Manager in a Hospital

LEARNING OBJECTIVES

This chapter imparts learning about:

- Role of Nurse Administrator in a Hospital
- Role of a Nurse Manager
- Research Highlights

INTRODUCTION

The health care delivery system is more challenging today than ever before. It requires strong, committed and leading nursing professionals who can create effective and positive work environment and resources for quality health care delivery, while leading a committed efficient work force of nurses. This allows for best possible patient care in any health care facility, from a small private hospitals to large medical college hospitals and corporate governed hospitals.

ROLE OF NURSE ADMINISTRATOR IN HOSPITAL

Nursing administration is a broad concept term that consists a large nursing professionals who are intelligent, knowledgeable of leadership practices. As such, nursing administration, or leadership, may refer to a number of management supervisory and executive connotations. The term 'role' means 'part played by a person. The nurse administrator exercises varying role for the smooth running of the hospital.

Ensuring Patients' Welfare and Safety

The nurse administrators are concerned with facilitating the highest quality and safe care to the patients and their families from the nursing personnel. She ensures that her patients and families are facilitated with quality and safe care environment.

Supervising Employees

In terms of supervision, the nurse administrator supervises the staff nurses, head nurses and other nursing personnel including student nurses sometimes posted in the ward for clinical experiences.

Staffing Functions

In relation to staffing she actively engaged in recruitment and selection of new nursing personnel, prepares schedule for their duties, plans for in-service education program for staff development, carries out performance appraisal of nursing personnel, and conducts counseling and guidance for nurses as needed. It is also her responsibility to update the registration, credentials and certification of nursing personnel. Her role as mentor and role model helps nurses to carry out their job competently.

Communicator-Representing Employees

The nurse administrator is essentially an effective communicator. She ensures upward, downward and lateral communication among all health care professionals effectively to strengthen organizational effectiveness. She acts as a liaison officer between the nursing staff and senior managers of the organization. To maintain effective communication she demonstrates leadership qualities, and negotiation skills. She always stands for nurses and nursing decision by representing nurses.

Budgeting and Business Decision-making

The nurse administrator's one of the functions is budgeting. She makes budget proposals for nursing service department and nursing personnel. She carefully executes the budget obtained. She represents in budget planning committee. Since the budget controls the organization, the nurse administrator ensures that patient needs are met first and is also responsible for making sound business decisions in deciding and purchasing equipment and supplies and linen, etc. for patient care. The nurse administrator is responsible for helping in auditing of nursing service department.

Policy Making

In formulating and carrying out policies, the nurse administrator ensures that all nursing staff are well-acquainted with policies of nursing service department and organization and practice guidelines. She evaluates the outcome of policies and suggests for amendments if any.

Supervisory Role

The nurse administrator makes assignments for the nurses and she supervises the nursing personnel whether they are implemented and assesses nurses experience, types and number of patients assigned for care. She is committed to develop staffing pattern and scheduling for all nursing personnel in each ward. She confirms that nurses carry out their job effectively to achieve the hospitals goals as per the job description. Limitations of the nurses in implementation of the assignment are reviewed and necessary remedial measures are taken immediately by the nurse administrator.

Mentor and Coach

Nurse administrators play a mentoring and coacher's role, especially to novice nurses when they newly posted in hospital unit. They are frequently supervised closely, appreciate them for a job well done and offering suggestions and advice for improving the quality of care if they need improvement. The senior nurses are also guided, whenever they need it.

Leadership and Conflict Management Role

Effective nurse administrators establish vision, mission statement and formulate philosophy of the hospital. She as a leader develops values of nursing and the values of organization. The vision, mission, values and philosophy is communicated to all nurses. Through job description, she affirms the duties and responsibilities of each cadre of nurses. This way she prevents role conflict. She organizes nursing and patient care conferences to manage conflict regarding care conflicts and interpersonal conflicts. However, even in teams who normally work well together, conflicts occasionally arise. It is the nurse administrator's responsibility to defuse the conflict before it becomes detrimental to the team or hinders patient care. She may call in the conflicted parties for a meeting, encouraging them to discuss their dispute and creating a plan for resolving the conflict in a way that benefits the individual nurses, the team nurse manager and patients.

Public Relation Officer

A nurse administrator role as public relation officer is very important. When patients or their families have problems about the quality nursing care she clarifies the problems and makes possible solution for patients and family. The nurse administrator listens, shows concern, investigate, resolve and implement resolution during her meeting with the patient or family member.

Academic Role

The nurse administrator maintains integration of academic and clinical activities for students and ensures that students are given all facilities for their clinical learning. The nurse administrator plans, organizes and evaluates in-service education program for nurses and encourages and facilitate nurses to attend various educational programes like workshops, conferences, and seminars. She or he acts as member of Ethical Committee for the approval of research of nurses or students.

Research

The nurse administrator participates in research work or conducts research, inculcates interest among nurses to read research journal. As a professional, she promotes evidence-based practice in clinical setting (the detail functions of nurse administrators will be discussed in later chapters).

ROLE OF NURSE MANAGER IN HOSPITAL UNIT

Nurse managers function in a ward unit in a hospital, such as med-surg unit, operation theater or postoperative unit. These unit managers are responsible for nursing care of patients and unit administration. They supervise nursing personnel and solve problem concerned with unit management or nursing care. They are expert nurses with specialized nursing knowledge, strong in communication skills and the ability to administer the unit.

Administrative Role

Nurse managers are responsible for patients admitted in different units such as medical unit, surgical unit, post-operative unit, CCU, ICU casualty or emergency room. The unit managers plans therapeutic environment for patients in the unit. They schedule the duties for staff nurses and assign tasks for each shift. They supervise the nursing personnel in their work.

Administrative Role in Policy Implementation

Nurse managers are responsible to implement unit policies. They ensure that the patient care for 24 hours are provided by trained and registered nursing personnel. They plan and organize daily, weekly and monthly work. Maintaining equipment and supplies, by requisition, standardization, exchange, condemnation, are important tasks of nurse manager including inventory keeping and stock keeping. They collect work reports from nursing personnel under her regarding their day-to-day activities and maintain a record of them.

Nurse managers keep update with trends in nursing, accept and implement innovative ideas and research, and work together to achieve the goals of the hospital by providing quality and effective care. They are the leaders who guide, lead and support nurses to contribute towards the success of the organization.

Patient Safety and Quality Care

The nurse manager maintains therapeutic environment to patients under her care. The best practices evidence-informed are promoted while caring patients. Periodical evaluation of managing care and performance appraisal of nurses are focused in managing units.

Supervisory Role

The nurse manager is responsible for supervision of nursing practice. She supervises the quality of care, needs and problems of patients and utilization of resources for patient care adequately in her/his unit. Periodical nursing care conferences enable her to know her nurses need and she rectifies accordingly.

Communicators Role

The nurse managers communicate and achieve the organizational goals to first level nurses and remove those factors which are obstructed to their clinical nursing practice. They keep updated with current advancement in health care delivery, technology and regulatory requirements including nursing ethics.

Educator's Role

Most nurse managers play an important role in nurses' education and patient's education. She allows the nurses to participate in in-service education program by relieving them from duty for their personal development and professional growth. If the school of nursing is affiliated with the hospital and student nurses are posted in her unit, she plans for their clinical experiences by collaborating with the teachers of school of nursing and helps in assigning patients to learn procedures, health teaching and gives an evaluation report to the teacher regarding students attitude and performance in the clinical area. She provides support, recognition, and appreciation to nurses who does exemplary nursing care to patients. Nurse manager ensures integration of theory or classroom learning to clinical practice and coordinates with nursing schools/colleges which are affiliated with their hospital/unit.

Interpersonal Relationship

Nurse managers are responsible for nursing personnel. At the same time they maintain a good interpersonal relationship with medical team, members of other health care discipline, social workers, therapists, technicians, pharmacists, and others who participate to patient care. Nurse managers maintain the ward environment, dietary and nutritional services, physical facilities, and supportive services by maintaining good IPR with the concerned departments.

Documentation

Nurse managers maintain adequate and complete records and reports of patients care and reports to the physician as and when needed. After discharge of the patients, she checks the completeness and accuracy of records before it is sent to Hospital Medical Record section.

Research

The nurse manager participates in research work or conducts research, inculcates interest among nurses to read research journal. As a professional, she promotes evidence based practice in clinical setting.

Box 4.1: Research highlights

THE ACTIVITIES OF HOSPITAL NURSING UNIT MANAGERS AND QUALITY PATIENT CARE IN SOUTH AFRICAN HOSPITALS

A cross sectional descriptive study was conducted in 2011 on the *Activities of Hospital nursing unit managers and quality patient care in South African Hospitals* by Susan J Armstrong, Laetitia C. Rispel and Loveday Penn-Kekana to examine the activities of nursing unit managers facilitate the provision of quality patient care.

The study was conducted in six public, three private hospital in two South African states. In each hospital, in selected units 36 nurse managers were the samples. Informed consent from each sample was taken and the unit manager was observed for a period of 2 hours and the activities recorded on a minute-by-minute basis. The activities coded into categories, and analyzed according to the time spent on activities in each category. The observation data were complemented by semi-structured interviews with the unit managers who were asked to recall their activities on the day preceding the interview. The interviews were analyzed using thematic content analysis.

The study observed that nursing unit managers spent 25.8% of their time on direct patient care, 16% on hospital administration, 14% on patient administration, 3.6% on education, 13.4% on support and communication, 3.9% on managing stock and equipment, 11.5% on staff management, and 11.8% on miscellaneous activities. There were also numerous interruptions and distractions. The semi-structured interviews revealed concordance between unit managers' recall of the time spent on patient care, but a marked inflation of their perceived time spent on hospital administration.

The researchers concluded that the unit managers require an enabling practice environment, supportive executive management and continuing professional education to provide high quality patient care.

SUMMARY POINTS

- ✓ Role of nurse administrator in a hospital highlighted in this chapter include ensuring patients' safety and welfare, supervision of care given and supervision of employees, budgeting, policy making, mentoring, coaching, conflict management through effective leadership, public relation, academic role and role in research.
- ✓ As a nurse manager, this chapter focused on the nurse 's responsibility on administrative role, patient safety and care, supervisory role, roles of communicator, educator, maintaining interpersonal relationship, documentation and participating or conducting research.

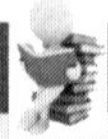

REVIEW QUESTIONS

1. What is the role of nurse administrator in hospital administration?
2. Describe the role of nurse manager in a ward unit.
3. Differentiate nurse administrator vs nurse manager
4. **Write short notes on:**
   a. Patient safety and quality care
   b. Supervisory role of a nurse manager
   c. Interpersonal relationship
   d. Role conflict
   e. Communication skills of nurse administrator.

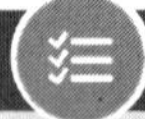

SELECTED READINGS

1. Difference between a nurse administrator vs. nurse manager
   work.chron.com › Business Management › Managing Employees
2. Nurse administrator: Job description, requirements and ...
   study.com/.../Nurse_Administrator_Job_Description_Requirements_
3. Nurse Manager Sample Job Description I Monster.com
   hiring.monster.com/hr/hr-best.../nurse-manager-job-description.aspx
4. Nursing Leadership I Nursing Administration
   www.graduatenursingedu.org/nurse-administrator/
5. Nursing services
   www.aiims.edu/aiims/nursingservices/NURSING%20SERVICES.htm

6. Perceptions of nurse manager responsibilities - Nursing ...
   www.nursingcenter.com/cearticle?tid=1469511
7. Susan J. Armstrong et al. The activities of hospital nursing unit managers and quality of patient ... http://www.globalhealthaction.net/index.php/gha/article/view/26243Global Health Action 2015.
8. The role of a nurse manager | Chron.com
   work.chron.com › Business Management › Managing Employees

UNIT III
FUNCTIONS OF ADMINISTRATION

5

Planning

LEARNING OBJECTIVES

This chapter imparts learning about:

- Concept, Definition, Principles, Goals, Objectives of Planning
- Description of Operational Plan
- Concept of Strategic Planning and Proactive Planning
- Explanation of Organizational Planning
- Managerial Planning
- Philosophy, Mission and Vision of Nursing Service Administration
- Planning for Change
- Planning a New Venture

CONCEPT, DEFINITION, PRINCIPLES, GOALS AND OBJECTIVES OF PLANNING

Introduction

Planning is the first function of nursing service administration that determines the selection of the policies, procedures objectives and program ahead in order to achieve quality patient care outcome. It is a cognitive ability of the administrator characterized by thinking before action taken. Good planning envisages better performance for the future.

Definitions of Planning

According to Alford and Beatt, planning is an organized vision of a person based on intellectual foresight and experience which is required for an intelligent action.

Theo Haimann explains that planning is something that is decided in advance to achieve the organizational goals.

Billy E Goetz views, planning is selecting an activity from many course of action in order to solve a problem.

According to Koontz and O'Donnell, planning is an intellectual process, conscious determination of course of action, the basing of decision on purpose, facts and considered estimates. According to Allen 'a plan is a trap laid to capture the future.' Planning is the process of chalking out the activities that are necessary to achieve the goals of the organization. A plan is nothing but an outline for action that guides the activities needed to achieve the goals of an establishment.

Nature of Planning

From the above definitions one can understand the nature of planning. They are:

- ***Planning is an intellectual process:*** Planning requires intellectual capabilities of contemplating ahead of time for the future development of an organization. It is a method that decides a sequential order of events to be considered.The administrators select and consider various activities including alternative course of actions to achieve the organizational goals.
- ***Planning Contributes to the objectives:*** The main objective of planning is the achievement of goal. The

success of the organization depends upon the nature and feasibility of the objectives formulated during planning phase. When the objectives are unrealistic and impractical, it will lead to organizational failure whereas effective planning contributes to the achievement of organizational goals.

- *Planning is a primary function of management:* Planning is the first and foremost function of management. All the other functions like organization, staffing directing and controlling, follows planning. The success of the organization depends upon the objectives formulated during planning phase.
- *Planning is a continuous process:* Health care delivery system is constantly changing hence planning too is changing and is a dynamic ongoing process. The nurse administrator needs to move with the changes and accordingly the plan needs modification, and revision, as per changes observed in health care system, George R Terry states that it a ongoing, dynamic and continuous process. It involves determining the data to be collected, collection of data and evaluation of selected data in a continuous manner and it also involves scientific investigation and analysis of the best possible alternative courses of action.
- *Planning is a managerial activity:* Planning is the responsibility of every administrator. It depends upon the leadership characteristics of the person who prepares the plans. Plan is very important because from the plan the execution or actions are determined. If the actions is followed without a strong plan the actions may not bring success to the organization.

Principles of Planning

Planning is an ongoing and continuous process. Good planning ensures success of an organization. In order to make a realistic plan, the administrator has to keep in mind the principles of planning. Principles guide the administrator to formulate sound plans. These principles of planning are as follows:

- *Principle of contribution:* Planning cannot be done by one person or administrator. It is an enabling process where the team of experts work together aiming at to achieve the organizational objectives. The accomplishment of the objectives always depends on the soundness of plans and the adequate amount of contribution of establishment/hospital administration towards the same.
- *Principle of sound and consistent premising:* Premises are the assumptions regarding the environmental forces like economic and market conditions, social, political, legal and cultural aspects, competitors actions, etc. These are prevalent during the period of the implementation of plans. Hence, plans are made on the basis of premises, and the future of the establishment depends on the soundness of plans they make so as to face the state of premises.
- *Principle of limiting factors:* The organization requires monitoring all limiting factors such as lack of motivated employees, shortage of trained personnel, shortage of capital funds, government policy of price regulation, etc. and needing to them in an efficient way for successful achievement of goals of the organization.
- *Principle of commitment:* The nurse administrator should be committed to carry out the plan.
- *Principle of coordinated planning:* Since short-term plans are developed from the long-term plans, it should be coordinated with one another.
- *Principle of timing:* The plans should be arranged in a time in sequential order and major and minor plans should be arranged in systematic manner.
- *Principle of efficiency:* All planning incur cost in terms of man, money material and time resources. Effective utilization of resources shows efficiency and effectiveness of implementation of plan. This provides satisfaction to employees and success of the organization.
- *Principle of flexibility:* When we execute the plan unforeseen events could be expected. In order to make up those unexpected conditions, a contingency plan to be developed. Thus planning could be flexible to meet unexpected situation in organization.
- *Principle of navigational change:* There should be periodical review of the plan. Sometimes that may require changes in strategies, objectives, policies and program s of the organization, so as to meet the goals of the organization.
- *Principle of acceptance:* Since the successful implementation of plans requires the willingness, cooperation and efforts from the employees the administrator should that ensure plans are accepted by the employees. Hence plans should be effectively communicated to all in the organization for successful implementation.
- *Principles of team work:* Planning is a team work. The success of the plan based on how the team members work in synchronized manner to bring organizational effectiveness.

Goals and Objectives of Planning

Goals and objectives are vital because they help to formulate the mission and vision into specific measurable targets. Goals and objectives are specific and measurable and help to translate the mission and vision into reality. Planning is one of the most important functions of management. Koontz and O'Donnell, view that without planning administration becomes random in nature and decisions become meaningless.

Goals

Goals are outcome statements to guide implementation of the plan of operation.

- **Objectives** are more detailed explanation than goals and explain how goals will be achieved. Objectives must be specific, measurable, achievable, realistic and time bound activity.

The goals of planning of administration are:

Goal 1: ***Provides a quality service to the population under care.*** To meet this goal the administrators establish the following objectives:

- To coordinate nursing services and standards according to institutional goals.
- To maintain continuous liaison with patients, family and nursing personnel.
- To plan for continuous improvements in nursing service.
- To create a working culture and activities for open accountability.

Goal 2: ***Provides expert administrative service leadership.*** In which the administrators establish the following objectives:

- To identify financial resources and administrative implications of institutional development.
- To estimate and forecast future needs of nursing services.
- To facilitate expert suggestions for improvement within and outside organization.
- To plan effective utilization of available resources for future development.
- To Support and encourage nurses to enhance care through innovative ideas and practices.

Goal 3: ***Ensures to meet the employees and patients needs.*** In which the administrators establish the following objectives:

- To advice and suggest on major initiatives taken by the administration to nursing personnel with other employees.
- To communicate effectively to concern related to patients and nursing personnel.
- To develop and empower nurses.
- To take challenge to solve vital issues affecting patient care.
- To participate, support and encourage in organizational initiatives.
- To make administrative decision promptly.
- To prioritize activities for better patient care outcome.

Goal 4: ***Encourages the ongoing development of staff.***

It is achieved through the following objectives:

- To provide support for staff development program.
- To integrate staff development as a part of nursing.
- To plan, design, implement and evaluate staff development programs.
- To ensure an academic climate and facilitate learning environment in work setting.

Importance and Advantages of Planning in Administration

Reduction of Uncertainty

Planning reduces uncertainty. Changes are inevitable There is a paradigm shift in health care industry, changes in health care technology and government policies and regulations that can bring uncertainties. Good planning can face all challenges.

Better Utilization of Resources

Good planning helps in effective and optimum utilization of available resources such as man, money materials and time in the establishment.

Increases Organizational Effectiveness

Good planning enhances organizational effectiveness by achieving organizational goals. It helps in economy, efficiency and effectiveness of the organization.

Good planning is cost effective in administrative procedure. It minimizes, organizational crises and chaos, and supports the employees.

Concentration on Objectives

All good planning formulated within the jurisdiction of established organizational goals. All the functions in an organization are planned to achieve the organizational objectives.

These help in intra and inter departmental coordination according the plan developed for achieving the goals of the organization. Thus, there is an integration and harmony in the future that is always full of uncertainties. Administration can run successfully if it is able to predict the uncertainties. Some of the uncertainties can be predicted by undertaking systematic forecasting. Thus, planning helps in foreseeing uncertainties.

Reduces the Cost of Performance

Planning ensures in reducing the cost of performance. It includes the selection of only one course of action amongst the different courses of action that would provide the best results at minimum cost. It prevents hesitancy, organizational crises and chaos, and supports the employees.

Makes Control Effective

Planning and control are two sides of a coin. Because it is impossible to control unplanned actions. Planning helps control by establishing and implementing standards of performance.

Encouragement to Innovation

Good planning helps to develop innovative and creative thinking among the administrators. It creates a future oriented attitude the administrators.

Increase in Competitive Strength

Good planning envisages capacity building, innovative work methods brings high and desired quality, the expectations of consumers and involvement of technology. This become a challenge for the organization brings competition in the market.

Delegation is Facilitated

A good plan always ensures delegation of authority to empower the employees to improve their performance.

OPERATIONAL PLANNING

Operational planning is the process of planning strategic goals and objectives to tactical goals and objectives. It describes the development expected activities to be completed within a period of time specifically during the financial year. (The financial year in government set is from first of April to March thirty first of the next year.) An operational plan gives justification of an annual operating budget.

Operational plans chalks out the activities and budgets for each part of the organization for the next 1 – 3 years and implement activities of the organization within the allocated budget and other resources.

Operational planning is a process. It will enlighten the administrator regarding the aims to achieve, what to do, when to do and how it will be achieved. It also focuses whether the objectives are achieved or not.

There are a few benefits of operational planning.

For the Administrator

- To focus on delivering the organization's objectives
- To manage workload better
- To cope with change
- To have confidence
- To give a sense of achievement.

For Senior Managers

- To coordinate between functions of various departments
- To allocate resources to ensure priorities are achieved
- To hold people accountable for progress.

For the Organization

- To develop a shared understanding of priorities
- To promote the organization to stakeholders
- To learn in a more systematic way about what works

Terms Used in Operational Planning

- *Objectives:* These are statements with five characteristics such as Specific, Measurable, Actionable, Realistic Time-framed (SMART). That helps the administrator the ways and means to realize them.
- *Activities:* These are the major tasks that the administrator will identify, select and implement in pursuit of team's objectives.
- *Tasks:* The performance based on the activities accorded to each employee.
- *Resources:* In administration resources are referred as the money, people, time, facilities and equipment required to complete the task of an organizational operation.
- *Outputs:* The outcome of an activity, often measured in volume.
- *Outcomes:* The impact of the activities and the final results they achieve.
- *Performance:* Well defined outcome measures used to track the success of the activities.
- *Targets:* The objectives are expected to be achieved by a time frame.

Approaches to Operational Planning

There are three approaches to operational planning (Mike Hudson 2011)

1. Establish 'departmental' objectives
2. Agree activities
3. Propose timetable, resources

- ***Establish departmental objectives:*** The major tasks involved are to focus on achieving. Strategic plan objectives, and make sure that they are specific, measurable, actionable, and realistic and time bound. They should be 3–6 objectives which are clearly stated.

- *Agree activities:* From the objectives stated, select challenging activities and maintain focus on strategic plan objectives
- *Propose timetable, resources:* The administrator should keep in mind the number of days the employees work and the money incurred for their work. Activities to be prioritized and within the time frame it needs to be completed.

The Role of Nurse Administrator in Operational Planning

- Once all activities are planned, assess overall resource implications
- Identify interdependencies
- Then prioritize, change activities to fit budget guidelines
- Do not change time and financial budgets without changing the activity
- Prepare plan submission in agreed format
- Discuss with colleagues and improve
- Submit draft to line manager
- Revise following robust review with line manager
- Submit final plan
- Support colleagues throughout.

STRATEGIC PLANNING AND PROACTIVE PLANNING

- **Strategy** refers to planning and managing an operation for a particular purpose such as in a war.
- **Strategic planning** is a systematic and planned process developed to support an organization to identify and maintain a maximal alignment with the most important components of the organizational environment.
- It is a complex and ongoing process of organizational change.

Steps in strategic planning (10 steps in strategic planning—Wiki spaces)

The administrator has to follow the following steps in strategic planning:

- *Step 1: Identification of vision and mission:* The administrator establishes the vision and mission of the organization. Vision describes the cause of existence of the organization and mission describes major goals and objectives of the organization. For example in nursing our vision could be nursing to be recognized and respected as one of the premier health care profession and service organization in the world. Whereas the mission describes major goals and performance objectives of the organization. For example, mission defines what you are doing and for the purpose the organization (nursing) exists currently. Each member of the nursing service department should be able to express this mission. For example, our mission is to provide high quality patient care based on our strong commitments to practice, and education.
- *Step 2: Environmental scan:* The administrator collects and analyses data about the organization's economic, social, demographic, political, legal, technological, and international factors. They are the internal and external environmental factors have an impact on planning.
- *Step 3: Gap analysis:* In this step the administrator assesses the existing position and expected future of the organization.
- *Step 4: Benchmarking:* The administrator assesses and compares the organization's operations, practices, and performance against other organization.
- *Step 5: Strategic issues:* Identifies the basic issues and solves those issues in the organization It is basic task of the administrator to achieve its mission and move towards its desired future.
- *Step 6: Strategic programming:* Establish strategic goals (SMART), action plans and specific activities.
- *Step 7: Emergent strategies:* Many times more than the organizational planned strategies there occur un predicted or un expected happenings, strategic plan needs alternative actions to combat those situations.
- *Step 8: Evaluation of strategy:* The success of the plan depends on continuous monitoring of the actions made along with other process.
- *Step 9: Review of the strategic plan:* Based on the evaluations made in step 8 and periodical, review is essential to make necessary changes if needed for the success of the plan.
- *Step 10: Strategic thinking:* It is a cognitive activity of mind to identify and decide various positive options, alternatives and decisions that are effective and suitable for the organization in terms of resources and work environment.

STRATEGIC PLAN AND NURSING SERVICE ADMINISTRATION

The strategic planning process emphasizes creating a vision, and mission of nursing services .The nurse administrator is a visionary she communicates and shares the vision. It should be resonate with all members of nursing and help them to feel proud, excited, motivated and part of something much bigger than themselves.

Understanding the current state of nursing services, and studying the gap analysis based on that current nursing situation, the nurse administrator develops strategic plan that helps to identify the strengths and opportunities and also rectify the gaps of any weaknesses that might exist in nursing services. Once gap analysis is complete, a realistic vision is formulated.

As a next step, the nurse administrator formulates strategic objectives from the strategic plan to realize the vision that is the foundation for developing action plans. The administrator ensures inclusion of as many nurses as possible to provide input and share thoughts about a preferred future in nursing and to make the plan more effective. That will help the administrator to identify issues and solution for the problems and prioritization of tasks. Strategic plan helps the administrator to perform effective administration with minimum input to obtain maximum outcome. Nurses can work with innovative technology, evidence based practices and effective strategic plan to bring better performance in nursing the patients and families.

The creation of a strategic plan allows opportunities for expanding the vision for nursing. A nursing strategic plan can be incorporated in nursing research activities by defining nursing research as a strategic objective. Clinical nurses as bedside scientists elevate the standard nursing profession and the practice by clinical nursing research by identifying issues related to nursing, select alternative courses of action, implement the actions and monitor the effectiveness of particular action or intervention. These become the best practice evidence informed when it is repeated in similar situations. Strategic direction can integrate all parts of the nursing care team, helps to move nurses from reactive response to proactive high performance as nurses, and that may bring patients satisfaction.

PROACTIVE PLANNING

Proactive planning is one of the four approaches of planning that involves planning strategies before the adverse things happen. It is the planning for the future.

Planners actively shape the future, rather than just trying to get ahead of events outside of their control. The predicted changes of the proactive planner are seen not as absolute constraints, but as obstacles that can be addressed and overcome.

The health care delivery system is constantly changing. The influence of change in technology, knowledge explosion and the complex health care poses a great challenge for nurses. Our health consumers are more knowledgeable today than ever before. Hence, it is imperative that the nurse's knowledge, technical competence, interpersonal skills and commitment also need to be improved. Nurses perform varied role at each level of their work environment are constantly in touch with consumers. In this complex health care environment, nurses require to have knowledge and leadership skills of management. A nurse like proactive leaders who had a definite vision of nursing and could motivate fellow nurses to work toward achieving common goals of nursing service department.

ORGANIZATIONAL PLANNING

Definition

It is process of identifying an organization's immediate and long-term objectives, and formulating and monitoring specific strategies to achieve them. It also entails staffing and resource allocation, and is one of the most important responsibilities of a management team.

Steps for Creating an Organizational Plan

The following are the few steps presented for creating an organizational plan

Decide on Categories

In creating categories of work that is done in an organization. For example in hospital set-up, the works may be preventive maintenance week, in-service education for nurses, CME program for doctors, fundraising activity for poor patients out reaching program for geriatric care, etc.

Set Goals

As a second step establish goals for the category of work selected. For example, every year in the month of April an in-service program for nurses will be conducted.

Set Tasks

Following establishing goals the next step is to discuss this matter with all concerned in the hospital (management, doctors and nurses), Discuss each goal and all the tasks that need to be done to achieve that goal. Develop an in-service education program for nurses on leadership training. For example. Identify resources like man, money and materials for training the nurses. Develop a schedule for in-service education program including the tasks involved in this program.

Plan a Schedule

After all the tasks are listed, put them in a sequential order from the first activity to the last activity. For example from the above goal we can plan. Inaugural program that comes first, conducting the teaching sessions and valediction program comes at the end.

Choose Responsibilities

Allocate responsibilities for each task is the next job of the administrator the persons can be selected from nurses or they can voluntarily accept the responsibility. Ensure that the persons who are assigned the task will do it properly the task. For example, the person who assigned to distribute the invitation shall do the work with meticulous care. The task could be further broken down such as purchasing, printing, teaching, accommodating the delegates, food travel and finance, etc.

Support

Identify support, assistance and advice from other agencies individuals or organization to conduct the particular task to achieve the goals.

Evaluation and Follow Through

A follow-up program is required to know whether the tasks are completed and the plan achieved the goals. It can be done by follow-up meetings regularly, mailing feedback and observation in performance behavior who attended the program.

An organizational plan helps the administrator to set priorities in job, ensure the task is done one at a time, stresses team work, make the goals explicit, and brings organizational success.

SOUND ORGANIZATIONAL PLANNING FOR NURSING SERVICES ADMINISTRATION

The nurse administrator should plan and develop the following organizational plans for the smooth running of the nursing services:

- A written statement of the purpose and objectives of the nursing services
- A plan of organization
- Policy and administrative manuals
- Nursing practice manuals
- Nursing service budget
- A master staff planning
- Plans of appraisal of nursing
- Nursing service administrative meetings
- Advisory committees
- Adequate facilities, supplies and equipment and stock book
- Written job descriptions and job specifications
- Personnel records
- Health services
- In-service education of nursing personnel
- Meeting with personnel from other departments.

MANAGERIAL PLANNING

Managerial planning is the process refers to identification of goal, and developing a realistic plan of action, for achieving organizational goals. The basic steps in the managerial planning is defining each task to meet the objectives of the establishment.

Establish Goals

Formulating goals is the fundamental step in management planning of the establishment. It includes the review of each goal, and justification of their selection and the expected outcome written in both quantitative or qualitative terms. An example of a goal is to raise immunization status of under five children 100 percent over a 12 months period.

Identify Resources

Each goal should have man. Money, time and material resources allocated for its completion. For example, a management plan may identify how many registered nurses it will require and how much it will cost to meet the goal of increasing under-fives immunization status by 100% in 12 months period.

Establish Goal-Related Tasks

Each goal should have tasks or projects associated with its achievement. For example, if a goal is to raise the immunization status of under-fives, a manager will need to outline the tasks required to meet that objective. Examples of tasks might include teaching, demonstration and training under supervision developing advanced training and techniques for nursing personnel.

Prioritize Goals and Tasks

Prioritizing goals and tasks is about ordering objectives in terms of their importance. The tasks seems most important will be approached and completed first. For example, if a goal is to increase the immunization status of under-fives 100% and an associated task is to increase the number of registered nurses for home visits.

Create Assignments and Timelines

As the establishment prioritizes projects, it must develop time frame for completing the each tasks and assign individuals to complete them. The capabilities of staff members and the time frame is important in completing the task assigned.

Establish Evaluation Methods

A management planning process should develop evaluation strategies such as who will do? What are the criteria? How it will be done? And how often it should be done, etc. If the evaluation is not satisfactory what will be next course of action should be determined.

Identify Alternative Courses of Action

A management plan should include alternative courses of action that can be incorporated into each segment of the planning process, or for the plan in its entirety.

PHILOSOPHY, MISSION AND VISION OF NURSING SERVICE ADMINISTRATION

Vision

The very essence of administration is that the administrator has a vision. It has got be a vision that the administrator articulate clearly and forcefully on every occasion. Leaders have vision. They share a dream and direction that other people want to share and follow. The leadership vision goes beyond the written organizational mission statement and vision statement. Vision focuses how the organization wants to be perceived in the future – what success looks like. It is an expression of the desired end state. Challenges everyone to reach for something significant – inspires a compelling future and provides a long-term focus for the entire organization.

The vision of nursing administration permeates the work place and is manifested in actions, beliefs, values and goals of the organization. Vision describes as what is nursing want to become? It should be resonate with all members of nursing and help them to feel proud, excited, motivated and part of something much bigger than themselves.

Example: Our vision – Nursing to be recognized and respected as one of the premier health care profession and service organization in the world.

MISSION

Mission is that defines what you are doing and for the purpose the organization (Nursing) exists currently. Each member of the organization should be able to express this mission.

Example: Our mission is, we want to be the best health care service organization in the world.

VALUES

Values shape one's own action. Active participation in organization with certain personal values: such as competency, integrity, respect, commitment, dedication, dignity, collaborativeness, innovativeness, compassion, assertiveness, etc.

Example: Our values focus on preserving and improving human health. We are committed to the highest standards of ethics and integrity. We are dedicated to the highest level of scientific excellence and commitment. Our ability to excel depend on the integrity, knowledge, skill, attitude and teamwork of nursing.

PLANNING FOR CHANGE

Change is inevitable. There are many factors influence organizational change Leadership skills are required to ensure that the change we are going through is important for organization. The administrator can find from the work force that what type of change is required for the future for better performance. Earlier days the change was brought from top to bottom but it does not work as per the evidences.

- **Planned change** is intended, purposeful attempt or proactive plan by an individual (nurse administrator/ change agent) or group to create something new. It is a well-planned, initiated and coordinated, change require well-developed leadership skills. The administrator should be a visionary with expert planning skills required dealing with change. An organization functions effectively with the vision that guides the organization than a mission.
- **Unplanned change** occurs without any control or effort.
- **Covert change** that occurs without awareness, we do not know they are happening.
- **Overt change** that occurs with awareness, we know they are happening.
- **Developmental or maturational change** that is the organizational development. Change agent is a person skilled in the theory and implementation of planned change, referred as 'change facilitator,' usually an outsider of the organization.

LEWIN'S MODEL OF CHANGE

- Kurt Lewin (1951) identified three phases that the change agent must initiate before a planned change can occur A successful change involves three elements:
  1. ***Unfreezing:*** Occurs when the change agent convinces members of the group to change.
  2. ***Movement:*** The change agent identifies plans, and implements appropriate strategies, ensuring that driving forces exceed restraining forces.

Box 5.1: Sample of mission, vision, and philosophy of nursing service administration

Mission, Vision, and Philosophy of Nursing Service Administration

Our mission is to provide high quality patient care based on our strong commitments to service, education, research, and administration.

Vision

our goal is to be an outstanding institution among academic and health care health facilities. We are building on our traditional missions of patient care, education and research; providing the best practices evidence informed in nursing; with the available resources to succeed in a changing environment; and working collaboratively as partners with our professional colleagues, and individuals, communities and organizations we serve.

Philosophy of nursing service administration

Nursing is an art and a science dedicated to improving the physical and psychological well-being of patients. The department of nursing services and patient care supports the practice of nursing within the service, education, and research and Mission of the Kerala University of health sciences in order to benefit patients, the people of Thrissur and neighborhood. We are committed to excellence in service, education, informatics, research, and administration.

We provide care to patients and their families in a respectful, and caring manner. We deliver care which is appropriate, effective, efficient, and aimed toward specific outcomes to facilitate care delivery and to achieve desired patient outcomes, we foster positive working relationships among nurses and with other members of the health care team. We reach out to our community network and integrated delivery system by responding to service needs and contributing to the education and community oriented research the Westfort community health centre at Mundur which is coming up is an example for achieving this Mission.

We provide education that empowers patients, families, and nurses to make decisions about health care. We promote a learning environment for staff. Our staff participates in all aspects of education, including professional development; role modeling professional behavior; sharing expertise with colleagues; and assisting patients and families in understanding their health status, their care, and choices that affect their health. We value academic education, and we support staff members who seek advanced education. Our vision to signing a MOU with foreign nursing universities and hospitals may enhance interactive relationships with the nursing personnel to enhance clinical practice and education. We support the development of efficient electronic systems that enhance communication among staff and facilitate the flow of patient information throughout the hospital system.

We improve the quality of care by assuring that patients and families receive nursing care which has been demonstrated by research to improve outcomes. We are committed to an environment which fosters scientific inquiry, critical thinking, and adoption of innovations. Research is an integral component of nursing practice and clinical decision-making to achieve our goals, clinical practice and institutional/departmental research are found very beneficial Nursing service administration works to create an environment which promotes and, supports participative management, and fosters innovation. Nurses provide quality, cost-effective care in an environment where they are recognized for excellence in clinical practice and achievements in education, informatics, and research.

(Printed with kind permission of Shri K M Mohandas, Managing Director, Westfort Hospital Group, Thrissur from Personnel Policies, 2005)

The administrator sets goals, target dates to implement the change gradually.

3. *Refreezing stage:* The nurse administrator (change agent) is in stabilizing the system change. Change agent is being supportive, helping people adapt, and employees are helped to achieve the goals. Nurse administrators as change agents who facilitates and perceives for a clear need for the employees involvement in the organization and motivate them through rewards and incentives.

- **Driving forces for change** are useful for economic gain, improve situation, takes challenge that brings future impact, development, approval, improved relationships.
- **Restraining forces for change** occur when employees perceive the need for safety in work environment, inadequate time to complete the task, lack of energy and feels loss of freedom and negative past experience. Resistance to change is a part of change process. Resistance may be caused by anxiety or fear, fear a loss of status, power, control, job, lack of trust, etc. There are false belief about the change due to inadequate information.

Change Occurs in Sequential Order

In change process it is a fact that there is a problem exists and we need to diagnose that problem. Then we need to assess the people in the organization who have the capacity to change and also the administrators motivation, attitude and resources to motivate the employees. As a next step the administrator as a change agent implements the change and monitors and maintains when the change is initiated. The process concludes by maintaining helping relationship with the employees.

The Following are Some of the Elements in the Process of Planned Change

Building a relationship with employer and employee, diagnosing the existing problem that needs to be addressed, gathering resources to bring change, selecting a solution for the problem identified, once it is selected and ensuring acceptance from the members and implementing change and continuing relationship with members.

The Following Factors Should be Kept in Mind While Implementing Change

- There must be relevant cause to implement change.
- All changes to be well planned and should be implemented gradually.
- While planning for a change, the individuals who will be affected due to change, should be definitely involved in planning process.
- Those members wants to bring change and believe that the change is good for the future and the members who believe that to include the best from the past and present in bringing change to be closely work together in the process. They may not resist for the change.
- It is necessary for the change agent that she should communicate the needs and rationale for bringing change and ensure that the members understand it.
- Ensures adequate time for bringing change.
- Ensures clarification of doubts if any among members.

It is difficult to accept and cope with the change. The change agent needs to support and help the members to cope-up with the change implemented.

Managing Change

The nurse administrator to keep the following things in managing change. Nurse administrator initiates and influences direction of change in an organization. Through planned communication, the members who are accepting change implements the plan of actions. Through informal communication the actions are clarified by members from the nurse administrators. Nurse administrators monitors the action of change by the members. The members communicate about the change through informal discussion and narration to the administrator. Nurse administrators need to adopt change to solve problems related to nursing services, change to make innovative models of nursing care for better patient care outcome and change to minimize excessive workload that in turn will bring organizational effectiveness development.

PLANNING A NEW VENTURE

What is Venture?

It is nothing but a risky start-up of an establishment/ company. Venture planning is a personal assessment of feelings and the feasibility of a venture. The Venture Feasibility process examines the key factors in any venture.

Meaning of Venture

It refers managerial plans that give an opportunity or chance to set up a new establishment based on innovative concepts It is developed on customer focused ideas or technology. It is a process composed of various phases.

Process of Venture Planning

- Identify the project and define the complete nature of the project. Confirm whether this venture brings new initiatives.
- Analyze the feasibility of the venture by doing a feasibility study.
- Identify financial and other resources feasibility to initiate the venture. Consider for sponsorship from agencies.
- Planning for physical and infrastructure facilities.
- Analyze any legal or ethical implication for the venture.
- Develop operational plan.
- Implement the new venture.
- Evaluate and monitor the progress made.

The Following are the Key Factors to be Considered in Venture Concept Planning

- The administrator should concentrate on one venture at a time in one establishment.
- Identify the scope for a venture plan and study how to utilize that opportunity.
- Categorize three concepts such as good, bad and likely for each venture concept.
- Identify the type, model, implementation method and outcome of the venture. The success of each factor depends on the approach and style of administrator who plans and implement the venture.

Emerging Venture Areas in Nursing that Needs Planning

There often occurs a crisis situation in the health care industry when nurses try to defend existing models of practice instead of embracing innovative changes. In order to gain successful planning of good ventures, we should examine the traditional models of nursing care such as institution based care, process oriented care, procedure driven practices, care based on mechanical and manual intervention, treatment based care and reflection and reflective practice model of care.

Role of Nurse Administrator

- The nurse administrator needs to know the plans and programs of the health facility of other departments in which personnel contribute to the joint effort of providing health care services.
- Should be a participatory, voting member of all committees of the institution including those dealing with budgeting, planning, credentialing, auditing, utilization, infection control, patient care improvement, library or any other committees concerned with nursing services, nursing activities and nursing personnel.
- Should develop a marketing operational plan based on the overall view of the agency problems and activities.
- Marketing plan should include gathering and analysis of data related to product or service.
- Operational plan consists of pinpointing possible strengths, weaknesses, problems and opportunities.
- Before launching a venture, a control plan is made to measure performance of implementation of venture within a time frame.

Practical Day-to-Day Planning Actions to the Nurse Administrator Include the Following

- At the beginning of each day make a list of actions to be accomplished for the day.
- Plan ahead for meetings.
- Identify developing problems.
- Review the operational and management plan.
- Review the appropriate portions of the division operational and management plan.
- Plan for discussion of ideas and suggest similar practical planning actions to other nurse managers.

SUMMARY POINTS

✓ Planning is an important administrative function. It is an intellectual process of thinking in advance. It is a process of deciding the future on the series of events to follow. Planning is a process where a number of steps are to be taken to decide the future course of action. Managers or executives have to consider various courses of actions to achieve the desired goals, go in details of the pros and cons of every course of action and then finally decide what course of action may suit them best.

✓ Operational planning is the process of planning strategic goals and objectives to tactical goals and objectives. It describes milestones, conditions for success and explains how, or what portion of, a strategic plan will be put into operation during a given operational period. An operational plan is the basis for, and justification of an annual operating budget request. Operational plans should establish the activities and budgets for each part of the organization for the next 1–3 years. They link the strategic plan with the activities the organization will deliver and the resources required to deliver them. Operational planning is a process. It will enlighten the administrator regarding the aims to achieve, what to do, when to do and how it will be achieved. It also focuses whether the objectives are achieved or not.

✓ Strategic planning is a formal process designed to help an organization identify and maintain an optimal alignment with the most important elements of the environment within which the organization resides. It is a complex and ongoing process of organizational change. Whereas proactive planning is one of the four approaches of planning that involves designing a desired future and then inventing ways to create that future state. Nurses work at each level of the health care system, have varied role, and are constantly in contact with people. Dealing with this dynamism and responsibility requires nurses to have knowledge and skills of management. It becomes apparent that the leadership needed to get work done through people is increasingly important for nurses to exercise their professional performance.

✓ Organizational planning is the process of identifying an organization's immediate and long-term objectives, and formulating and monitoring specific strategies to achieve them. It also entails staffing and resource allocation, and is one of the most important function of administration. An organizational plan helps the administrator to set priorities for work, make sure tasks get done on time, focus on one thing at a time, share work among staff, board members and volunteers, make goals clear to funders, get a handle on big projects by breaking them down into smaller tasks and see the big picture of what the organization is doing.

- ✓ Managerial/management planning is the process of assessing an organization's goals and creating a realistic, detailed plan of action for meeting those goals. The basic steps in the management planning process involve outlines of each task the establishment must accomplish to meet its overall objectives.
- ✓ The philosophy, vision, mission and values of an organization focuses how the organization wants to be perceived in the future—what success looks like. It is an expression of the desired end state. Challenges everyone to reach for something significant that inspires a compelling future and provides a long-term focus for the entire organization. It also emphasizes the commitment required for nurses to serve the humanity.
- ✓ Planned change is intended, purposeful attempt or proactive plan by an individual (nurse administrator/ change agent) or group to create something new. Well thought out, deliberate, initiated and coordinated, plan require well developed leadership. The administrator requires visions and expert planning skills. Vision is the future goal, An organization will function effectively with the vision that guides it, different than a mission. Whereas an unplanned change occurs without any control or effort.
- ✓ Venture planning is built upon customer driven ideas or technology. Venture planning does not require detailed funding, source analysis, professional opinions, entity formation or detailed market analysis.

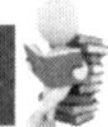

REVIEW QUESTIONS

1. Define Planning. Describe the principles, goals and objectives of planning in nursing service administration.
2. Enumerate the purposes of operational planning. Discuss the role of nurse administrator in operational planning.
3. Differentiate strategic and proactive planning. Discuss the steps involved in strategic planning.
4. What is organizational planning? Explain the steps involved in organizational planning.
5. Outline the philosophy, Vision Mission statement and values of nursing service administration.
6. Write short notes on:
    a. Managerial plan
    b. Organizational planning in nursing service administration
    c. Levin's theory of change
    d. Venture planning
    e. Change management
    f. Strategic plan in nursing service administration.

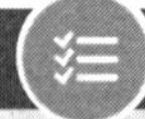

SELECTED READINGS

1. All About Strategic Planning - Management Library
managementhelp.org/strategicplanning/index.htm
2. Approaches to Planning (Reactive, Inactive, Preactive ...
www.entarga.com/stratplan/approaches.htm
3. Change Management - Mind Tools
www.mindtools.com/pages/article/newPPM_87.htm
4. Managerial Planning and Goal Setting – SlideShare
www.slideshare.net/.../managerial-planning-and-goal-setting
5. Operational planning - Wikipedia, the free...
en.wikipedia.org/wiki/Operational_planning...
6. Operational planning: the Purpose of an ...
www.leoisaac.com/operations/top025.htm
7. Planning for a venture – SlideShare
www.slideshare.net/bivinjose/planning-for-a-venture

8. Planning for a venture 1. Bivin Jose Department of Psychiatric Nursing MB CN, Kothamangalam 2
9. Planning for Change - Changing Minds changingminds.org › Disciplines › Change Management
10. Planning Principles and Practices [PDF, 208KB] -... www.vtpi.org/planning.pdf
11. Planning the New Venture – Springer
    www.springer.com/cda/content/document/cda_download...
12. Seven Principles of Planning By John C. Maxwell
    www.teamexpansion.org/.../Seven_Principles_of_Planning.pdf
13. Strategic Planning Facilitator | Working Strategic Planning ...
    strategicplanning.com
14. What exactly is change management?
    www.planningchange.com
15. What Is Proactive Planning? | eHow www.ehow.com › ... ›

6

Innovations in Nursing Service Administration

LEARNING OBJECTIVES

This chapter imparts learning about:

- Program Evaluation and Review Technique (PERT)
- Critical Path Method (CPM)
- Gantt chart
- Management by Objectives (MBO)

PROGRAM EVALUATION AND REVIEW TECHNIQUE (PERT)

Introduction

Program (project) Evaluation and Review Technique (PERT) is a managerial tool. It is used with the aims of scheduling, organizing, and coordinating work related activities in an establishment. It systematically analyses the data related to the tasks and the time required to complete each task in a given project. PERT also facilitates decision making in terms of reduction of the time and cost required to complete a project.

The following steps are used in PERT planning:

- Identify the activities (tasks) that need to be performed. The manager identifies the activities or the tasks and calculates the time needed to complete each task in the project. The tasks are defined in advance and the time required from the beginning to the competition of each task is assessed. These are referred as milestone or events. If the task is not completed in the planned period a provision of extension period is also determined.
- The second step is determination of each task to be done in a sequential order.
- After each task is defined, the manager constructs a network diagram. Using the activity sequence information, a network diagram is drawn showing the sequence of the serial and parallel activities. Each activity represents a node in the network, and the arrows represent the relation between activities.
- The final step is to estimate the time required for each activity in terms of weeks as unit of time for activity. For each activity, three time estimates such as optimistic time, most likely time and pessimistic time are usually expressed.
  - **Optimistic time** is referred as the shortest time in which the activity can be completed.
  - **Most likely time** is referred as the completion time having the highest probability.
  - **Pessimistic time** is referred as the longest time that an activity might require.

Advantages of PERT

- PERT (Program Evaluation and Review Technique) forces the managers to plan, which helps them see to work together for the project.

- Each subordinate is responsible to plan and complete the tasks that is assigned.
- It concentrates on difficult situation that may need rectification.
- It makes possible a kind of forward-looking control as there is a time limit.
- The network system with its subsystems enable managers to obtain reports and compel the subordinate for completion of task in time.
- The project is completed on the determined time.
- The critical path activities influence the completion time.
- Activity start and end in determined date.

Disadvantages of PERT

- More emphasis on activity and time is given in PERT method. Sometimes it lacks scheduling.
- It does not care for cost incurred in the project. However, it concentrate more on time.

Application of PERT in Nursing Service Administration

- The nurse administrator should have a good understanding of the project to be undertaken
- She should be aware of managerial tools and techniques
- Understanding of concept of PERT form
- She should develop a project plan and determine relevant list of all activities
- She should be able to choose the most appropriate scheduling method and select appropriate team to perform project tasks in systematic manner
- She designs PERT network related to all activities
- She calculates the time schedule for each activity
- After estimation of time schedule of each activity, she determines the critical path
- Assesses PERT chart as the program progress

PERT sequence diagram for the project Neonatal Intensive Care Unit (NICU) in a hospital (Fig. 6.1).

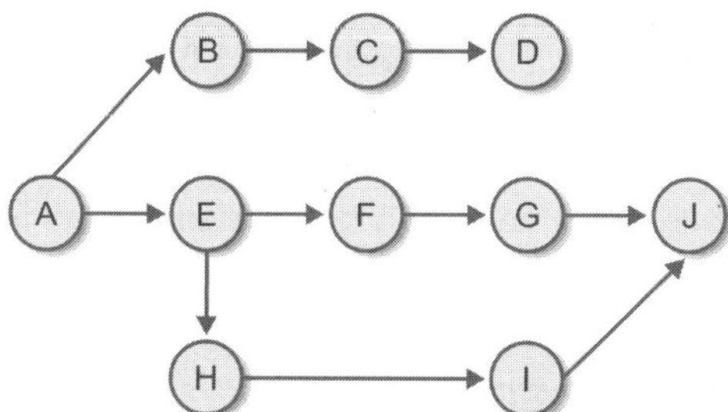

Fig. 6.1: PERT sequence diagram

A. Finalization of plan for setting up of an NICU in the hospital
B. Planning for infrastructure and training of NICU nurse
C. Prepare the articles required for NICU and put them for tender notice
D. Finalize the tender
E. Order for the materials
F. Prepare budget, both capital and operating
G. Floor plan for NICU and estimate cost
H. Call work contractors to start the work
I. Get materials and trained personnel
J. Start project.

CRITICAL PATH METHOD (CPM)

It is a mathematical algorithm for scheduling a set of project activities, sequential tasks upon which the project completion time and date depends. It helps the nurse administrator in making decisions regarding resource allocation.It also helps the nurse administrator to utilize available resources appropriately and in an effective way. It is beneficial for the administrator to prioritize activity to be carried out first to minimize the total costs of the project during the period the project established.

Benefits

To Nursing Staff

- It is a documentation tool
- Nurse is accountable for every action
- It enhances nurse's empowerment
- Improves quality patient care outcome
- Enhances nurse-patient-physician interaction
- Avoids omissions and repetition
- Brings better quality care.

To Patients

- Enhances patient empowerment
- Reduces patient's hospital stay
- Decreases hospital infection and other complications improves standards of patients care.

Need for CPM in Nursing

a. To combat with increasing competitions in medical and nursing field
b. To enhance cost effectiveness in quality nursing care
c. Effective utilization of available resources
d. To enhance economy, efficiency and effectiveness in achieving patient care outcome.

Goals of CPM in Nursing Service Administration

1. Selecting the best practice evidence informed for care
2. Define a standard for expected duration of patient stay in health care setting
3. Examining and assessing the time spent by various cadre of health personnel in the process of patient care
4. Developing a goal plan for each day for each cadre of nurses in overall care process
5. Providing a framework for data collection on time spent on care process by nurses
6. Enhancing patients satisfaction with the care by educating and involving patient and family during implementation of care process.

Sample Format for CPM

- Outline the patient care process based on time matrix (e.g. am care and pm care)
- List the components of care in one column and time in the other column
- Give specific activities for each day of hospitalized patient
- Mark transition point of patient's progress
- Layout a coordinated map of each staff activities to achieve the transition in the most effective way as possible.

GANTT CHART

Henry L Gantt developed this chart. It exhibits a well-developed schedule that communicates the employee to see the tasks assigned to him or her.

Advantages

- This chart shows actual and planned progress of the task done
- It indicates the details of the project, resource allocation and how far the tasks has been completed
- It helps the administrator to begin the work in time, be on the tract without concentrating on other tasks and report the project
- This chart is helpful to know what is completed and what should have been done at a point of time
- Shows action plan when there is slackness in the task done.

Below presented is a sample chart (Fig. 6.2) showing the work plan for 2 years for PhD scholar in nursing developed by the author.

Strengths

1. The administrator can develop and maintain the chart easily.
2. The administrator can understand at a glance as the status of work being done
3. It can be utilized as reporting tool in administration
4. It can be easily interpreted.

Weakness

1. Concentrates on project management only
2. Provides little information on display chart
3. All activities planned shows the work load as equal
4. It limits the magnitude behind the schedule condition in the display.

The organization has a clear understanding of the aims or objectives as well as awareness of their own roles and responsibilities in achieving those aims.

MANAGEMENT BY OBJECTIVES (MBO)

What is Management by Objectives?

Management by objectives (MBO) is a orderly and systematic approach that helps the management to utilize available resources to achieve desirable goals in an effective manner. Since, each employee is aware of his/her assignment and its objectives, it increases organizational performance. In this technique, the, employees are given strong input to identify their objectives, and time plan for completion. This technique provides a feedback from employees time to time as the work is progressed.

In 1954, Peter Drucker in his book 'on The Practice of Management the concept of MBO was emphasized'.

Concept of MBO

MBO is an approach of management that respects on the participation of subordinates, allowing them to make decision and participate in decision making process. Traditionally, the top level management team formulated goals and objectives of the organization before giving instructions down to middle management, who then communicated that information on to the lowest level employees. It was a method that did little to encourage participation or cooperation from the lowel group of employees of the organization.

Whereas MBO ensures that everyone is included in the decisions process, from the top, all the way down to the lowest employee level.

Principles of MBO

MBO ensures that all the employees of the organization has an explicit comprehension about the aims, objectives,

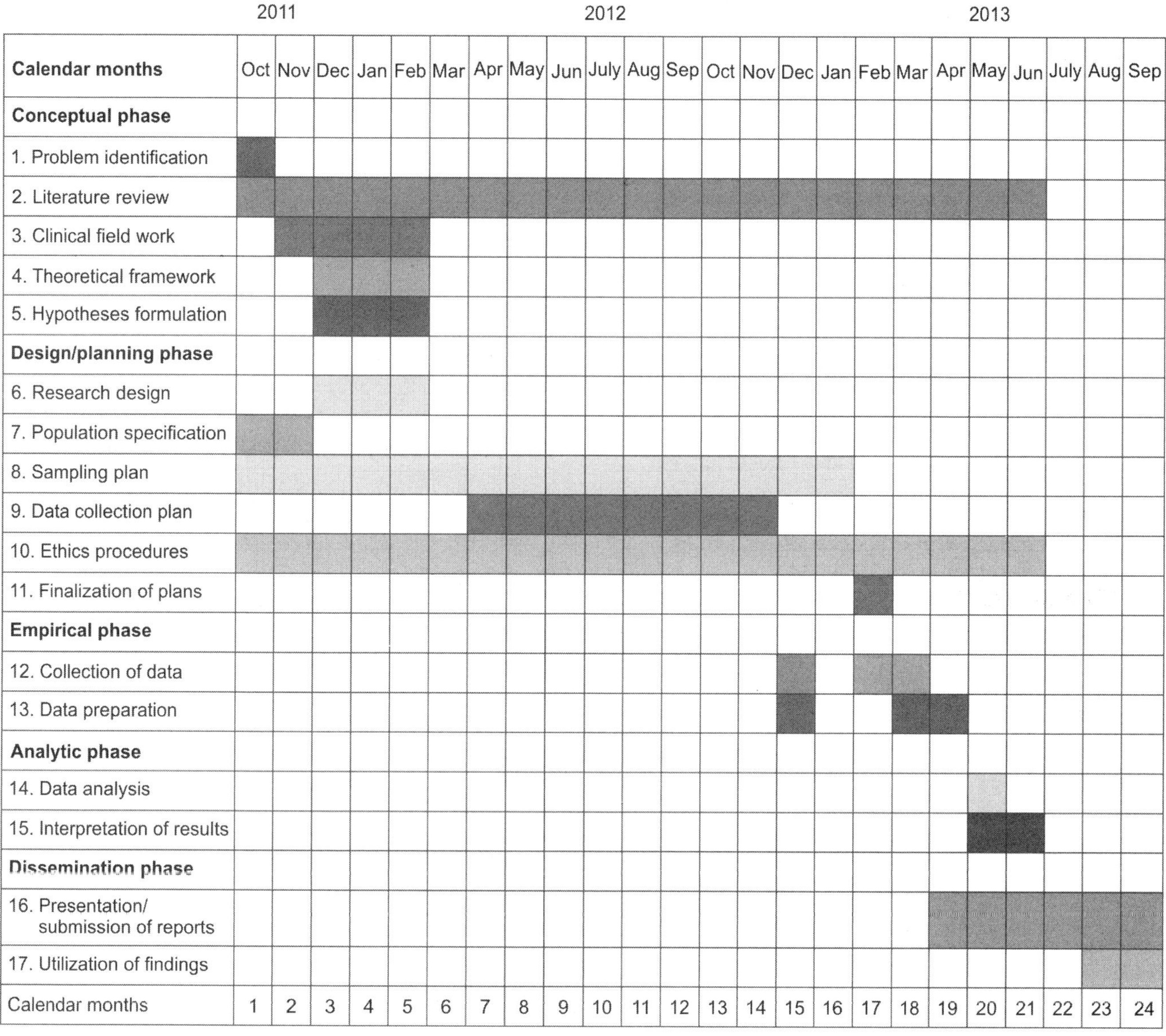

Work plan

	2011								2012										2013					
Calendar months	Oct	Nov	Dec	Jan	Feb	Mar	Apr	May	Jun	July	Aug	Sep	Oct	Nov	Dec	Jan	Feb	Mar	Apr	May	Jun	July	Aug	Sep
Conceptual phase																								
1. Problem identification																								
2. Literature review																								
3. Clinical field work																								
4. Theoretical framework																								
5. Hypotheses formulation																								
Design/planning phase																								
6. Research design																								
7. Population specification																								
8. Sampling plan																								
9. Data collection plan																								
10. Ethics procedures																								
11. Finalization of plans																								
Empirical phase																								
12. Collection of data																								
13. Data preparation																								
Analytic phase																								
14. Data analysis																								
15. Interpretation of results																								
Dissemination phase																								
16. Presentation/ submission of reports																								
17. Utilization of findings																								
Calendar months	1	2	3	4	5	6	7	8	9	10	11	12	13	14	15	16	17	18	19	20	21	22	23	24

Fig. 6.2: Work plan for a PhD scholar

roles and functions of each employee in achieving the organizational goals of that organization. It is one of the approaches that the management and employees are empowered in their task and responsibilities that in turn bring organizational effectiveness.

Setting Objectives

In MBO systems, at each level of organization aims, objectives and targets are clearly written and given to employees. This ensures each employee about the organizational objectives, the role and responsibilities of each employee in helping the organization to achieve the objectives laid down. The objectives formulated are precise, small and measurable. The management knows the tasks to be done to meet each specific objective and control all the performance of employees in the organization.

The evaluation of MBO system helps the administrators to measure the performance of each employee, as well as management, marketing strategies, human resource organization financial resources, physical resources production, and profit requirements.

Balancing between Management and Empowering Employees

In order to establish balance between management and employees, MBO system establishes specific objectives, develops teams, motivates and empowers employee and management, ensures effective communication, conducts performance appraisal periodically and facilitates for personal and professional development.

MBO Strategies

- The managers and the employees formulate objectives together for the organization. These are mutually set and agreed upon by managers and employees.
- All individuals including the managers in the organization are assigned objectives and specific tasks related to the objectives that should be achieved within a specific time period.
- To ensure achievement of objectives, performance appraisal of employees are conducted periodically.
- To encourage and motivate employees, rewards and incentives are facilitated to employees who showed better performance and achieved the objectives.

Stages of MBO

1. Establish and define the overall objectives of the organization
2. Analyze management tasks and develop written job specifications, which allocate responsibilities and decisions to individual managers
3. Establish performance standards and communicate to employees
4. Agree and set specific objectives with employees and managers
5. Assign each employee targets with corporate objectives
6. Establish a management information system to monitor achievements against objectives.

According to Peter Drucker, the five steps of MBO process are:

1. Review of organizational objectives
2. Establishing employees objectives
3. Monitor the progress
4. Evaluation of performance
5. Rewarding the achievers.

Advantages and Disadvantages of MBO

Advantages

- In order to achieve organizational goals, MBO focuses on the various specific tasks for employees and managers.
- MBO process facilitates and ensures employee's commitment to attaining organizational goals.

Disadvantages

- It is time consuming to develop objectives that provides less time to managers and employees to complete their tasks.
- The volume of paper work increases in the organization because of the detailed written goals, ways and means of communication and an elaborate performance appraisal of all employees in the organization.

SUMMARY POINTS

- ✓ In nursing service administration, the nurse administrator uses modern techniques for effective administration. Few of them are Program Evaluation and Review Technique (PERT), Critical Path Method (CPM), Gannt chart and Management by Objectives (MBO).
- ✓ Program (project) Evaluation and Review Technique (PERT) is a managerial tool. It is used with the aims of scheduling, organizing, and coordinating work related activities in an establishment. It systematically analyzes the data related to the tasks and the time required to complete each task in a given project. PERT also facilitates decision making in terms of reduction of the time and cost required to complete a project.
- ✓ Critical Path Method (CPM) is a mathematical algorithm for scheduling a set of project activities, sequential tasks upon which the project completion date depends. It helps the nurse administrator in making resource allocation decisions. It also helps the nurse administrator 's ability to use resources in an efficient way by providing a strategy for determining which activity can be expedited to minimize the total project costs during the life of the project.
- ✓ Gannt chart demonstrates highly developed schedule that allows one to visualize multiple tasks that has to be done within a time frame.
- ✓ Management by Objectives (MBO) is an orderly and systematic approach that helps the management to utilize available resources to achieve desirable goals in an effective manner. Since each employee is aware of his/her assignment and its objectives, it increases organizational performance. In this technique, employees are given strong input to identify their objectives, time plan for completion. This technique provides a feedback from employees time to time as the work is progressed.

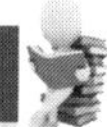

REVIEW QUESTIONS

1. List the modern techniques used in administration. Discuss any one of them in detail with advantages.
2. Define PERT. Describe the steps of PERT while establishing an ICU in a hospital setup with graphical representation.
3. What is Management by Objectives? Discuss the principles of MBO.
4. Write short notes on:
   a. Gannt chart
   b. Use of Critical Path Method in nursing service administration
   c. Stages of MBO
   d. Application of PERT in Nursing service administration.

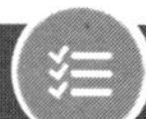

SELECTED READINGS

1. Critical Path Analysis and PERT Charts - Mind Tools.
   https://www.mindtools.com/critpath.html
2. http://www.managementstudyguide.com/management-by-objectives.htm
3. http://www.netmba.com/operations/project/cpm/
4. http://www.netmba.com/operations/project/pert/
5. Management By objective MBO: Developing Plans Principles...
   http://www.zeepedia.com/read.php%3Fmanagement_by_objective_mbo_developing_plans_principles_of_management%26b%3D54%26c%3D24
6. Management By Objectives (MBO) - Peter Drucker MBO http://kalyan city.blogspot.com/2010/06/management-by-objectives-mbo-peter.html 12 June 2010 ...
7. Management by Objectives (MBO) Definition I Investopedia
   http://www.investopedia.com/terms/m/management-by-objectives.asp
8. PERT Chart – Net MBA.
9. Program evaluation and review technique - Wikipedia, the free...
   https://en.wikipedia.org/wiki/Program_evaluation_and_review_technique
10. Program Evaluation and Review Technique (PERT) - Encyclopedia...
   http://www.inc.com/encyclopedia/program-evaluation-and-review-technique-pert.html
11. What is a Gantt chart? Gantt Chart Information, history and Software.
   http://www.gantt.com/
12. What is Critical Path Method (CPM)? - Definition from WhatIs.com.
   http://whatis.techtarget.com/definition/critical-path-method-CPM
13. What is Management by Objectives (MBO)?
   http://study.com/academy/lesson/what-is-management-by-objectives-mbo-definition-advantages-disadvantages.html 25 Apr 2015.
14. What is PERT chart (Program Evaluation Review Technique..)
   http://searchsoftwarequality.techtarget.com/definition/PERT-chart

UNIT IV
ORGANIZATION

7

Organizational Structure

LEARNING OBJECTIVES

This chapter imparts learning about:

- Concept, Definition, Principles, Goals, Objectives of Organization
- Organizational Structure
- Organizational Chart–Advantages and Disadvantages

CONCEPT, DEFINITION, PRINCIPLES, GOALS, OBJECTIVES OF ORGANIZATION

Concept of Organization

Organization is the quality of being orderly, systematic, and efficient. Organization is the systematic, and orderly process of identifying people, and grouping the work to be performed, specifying the work, defining and delegating the responsibility with authority to the personnel and establishing interpersonal relationships for the purpose of coordination of work so as to get the work done together effectively in accomplishing the objectives of the organization/institution/enterprise.

Organization is social units (or human groupings) deliberately constructed and reconstructed to seek specific goals.

Definition of Organization

It is defined as a group of people who work together in an organized way for a shared purpose. Organization is the act or process of putting the different parts of something in a certain order so that they can be found or used easily. It is the act or process of planning and arranging the different parts of an event or activity.

Organization refers to the structure of relationships among position jobs, which is created to achieve certain objective and control the activities of man with a mechanism.

Types of Organization

- Organizations functioning with the objective of economic profit are private organization like corporate hospitals, private hospitals or other business organization.
- Organization working under the Government sector at various level like public health centers, government hospitals, or health education bureau.
- Non-governmental Organizations (NGO) functioning at voluntary or service sector provides humanitarian services which are financed by private citizens like lions club, rotary club, etc.

Principles of Organization

Principles are guidelines that direct an individual to make decisions and act accordingly. If the organization has certain principles that helps and guides the administrators or managers to make organizational decisions and act according to the decision taken in order to achieve organizational goals.

The following are some of the principles of organization can be used by a manager.

Principle of Specialization

The organizational tasks are divided among the employees according to their qualification, experiences and the area of specialization This in turn enhances the quality of activities of employees of organization. According to the principle, division of work and according to specialization can result in effective function of organization.

Principle of Functional Definition

In order to function effectively, each employee should know his/her responsibilities, authority and accountability in an organization. This principle facilitates clearly defined job, job responsibility and authority of each employee and manager that ensures duties responsibilities and relationship of all personnel working within the department and outside the department. This brings effective coordination thereby organization can function effectively. For example, the broad functions of nurse administrator are planning, organization, staffing, coordinating, controlling and budgeting for nursing care. She has the authority and responsibility relationships in these areas and the overall accountability lies on her.

Principle of Span of Control/Supervision

Span of control means a span of supervision that denotes the number of subordinates/employees who can be supervised and controlled effectively by a single administrator/manager. Based on this principle, the manager makes a decision about the number of employees could be supervised or controlled by him/her. There are two types of decision. The manager can take one is wide span of control and the other is narrow span of control.

Wide Span of Control

When a manager can supervise and control a large number of employees effectively in an organization at a time is termed as **wide span of control**.

The main characteristics of wide span of control are:

- Decreases overhead cost of supervision
- Facilitates favorable response from the employees
- Provides for better communication
- Ensures better supervision
- Provides better co-ordination
- It is suitable for repetitive jobs.

Narrow Span of Control

When a manager can supervise and control a small number of employees effectively in an organization at a time is narrow span of control. According to this approach, supervisory work and authority is divided amongst many personnel and a manager doesn't supervise and control a large group of employees under him.

The characteristics are:

- The managers in the smaller group need ability to supervise and control
- Coordination is difficult because of many smaller groups
- Communication gaps may arise
- Messages can be misinterpreted
- Specialization work can be achieved.

Factors influencing span of control

- *Managerial abilities:* Wide span of control is possible in an organization when managers are skilled, capable, qualified and experienced in supervision and control.
- *Competence of subordinates:* Wide span of control is possible where the employees in an organization are capable and competent and seek managers' advice for solving problems if any.
- *Nature of work:* When the work is specialized, highly skillful needs mental and intellectual ability, narrow span of control is desirable. Whereas unskilled repetitive job requires less supervision and wide span of control.
- *Delegation of authority:* Wide span of control is suitable and the supervisors can manage and control large number of sub-ordinates at one time when the work is delegated to lower level of employees who do the work in an efficient manner.
- *Degree of decentralization:* In decentralization, authority is shared by many employees and managers at different levels. This ensures direct personal communication, and coordination between managers and employees. In such cases, wide span again helps for effective organization.
- *Principle of scalar chain:* In scalar chain principle, authority which flows from top manager to employees working at the bottom. Since authority is flowing, wastages of resources are minimized, communication is affected, overlapping of work, is minimized it clarifies the authority positions to managers at all level and that facilitates effective organization.
- *Principle of unity of command:* This implies one employee-one superior relationship. Every employee is accountable to one manager at one time. This helps

in ensuring better communication, good feedback and prompt response from the employee. This principle facilitates effective utilization of resources which helps in effective organization.

Authority Flows from Top to Bottom

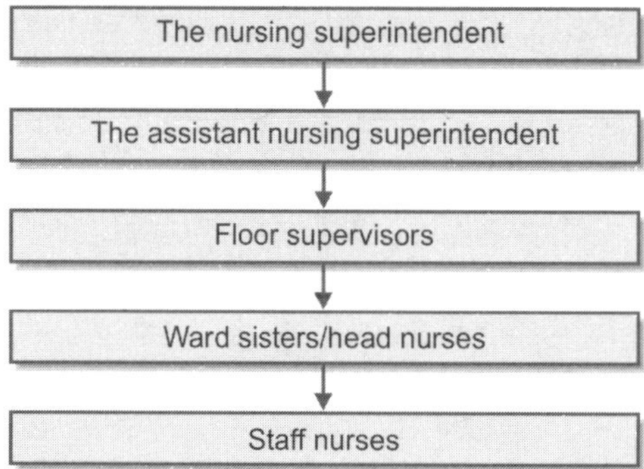

Fig. 7.1: Organization of hospital nursing

According to the above diagram (Fig. 7.1), the nursing superintendent has the highest level of authority. This authority is shared by the assistant nursing superintendent who shares his authority with the floor supervisors, then head nurses to staff nurses. From this chain of hierarchy, the official chain of communication becomes clear which is helpful in achievement of results and which provides stability to a concern. This scalar chain of command always flow from top to bottom and it defines the authority positions of different managers at different levels.

Goals and Objectives of Organization

Goals: Goal provides the foundation for evaluation. Goals are outcome statements that define what an organization is trying to accomplish, both practically and organizationally. Goals are usually a collection of related programs, a reflection of major actions of the organization, and provide rallying points for nurse administrators. For example, by 2015, we want to bring down maternal mortality rate to 109 per lakh live births; this example is Millennium development goal (MDG) five which has some targets and activities.

Objectives: Objectives are very precise, time-based, measurable actions that support the completion of a goal. Objectives typically must

1. Be related directly to the goal,
2. Be clear, concise, and understandable,
3. Be stated in terms of results,
4. Begin with an action verb,
5. Specify a date for accomplishment, and
6. Be measurable

To achieve the above MDG 5, we need to put objectives such as registration of pregnant mothers before 16 weeks 60% and after 16 weeks 40% to be done by midwives, minimum 4 visits to be completed by a skilled birth attendant from registration to delivery of the mother, etc. It can be measured and the outcome is observed during childbirth. Objectives are set by the organization and the achievement is measured periodically to know the effect of the activities by midwives in maternal care.

Objectives can be established for short-term and long-term depending on the goals of the organization.

ORGANIZATIONAL STRUCTURE

It is the arrangement of authority, communications, rights and duties of employees in an organization from top level to bottom level stated as hierarchical organization. Organizational structure ensures the assignments of the roles, power and responsibilities and their coordination and control between the different levels of management.

An organizational structure depends on the organization's objectives and plans of operation. In a centralized structure, the decision-making power and tight control over departments and divisions are vested in top level manager. Whereas in a decentralized structure of organization, the decision-making power is distributed and the departments and divisions may have different degrees of independence.

An organizational chart clearly exhibits the organizational structure.

An organizational chart is a diagram that shows the structure of an organization and the relationships and relative ranks of its parts and positions/jobs.

ORGANIZATIONAL CHART

Organizational chart is a good tool to exhibit the organizational structure. It is visual communication of information which is more effective to understand by each employee in an organization.

Purposes of Organizational Chart

- Organizational chart helps to build and design the organizational structure to meet the institutional (hospital, nursing services) objectives.
- Organizational chart can guide the nurses and other employees to know their channel of communications and responsibilities.
- Organizational chart help to divide the functions of various departments in nursing service administration.

- It also shows the staff and line relationship (Fig. 7.3) between the organization's staff members.
- With organizational chart, it is easy to find whether the employee's workload is too heavy.
- It is easy to find whether the unrelated persons undertake the work of several loose, no relationship.
- Find out whether an employee is incompetent in this work at important positions.
- Make everyone clear within their organizations and improve employee performance.
- Other departments are also able to understand and enhance the coordination of the organization.
- It is easy to see the promotion channels open.
- Some managers can use the organizational chart tool to analysis budget, design work team and generate reports.
- Organizational chart often outlines the employee's tasks and by which the nurse administrator is responsible for overseeing each employee.

Advantages of Organizational Chart

1. It is an administration tool to communicate with nurses about their position in hospital, nursing services and their relationship with other employees/ nurses.
2. It shows the line and staff relationship of the nurses in a hospital.
3. It serves as a valuable guide to the new nurses to understand the hierarchy and relationship of each employee in the organization.
4. It provides a framework of personnel classification.

Disadvantages of Organizational Chart

1. An organizational chart shows only display the formal relationship of the employees and does not depict the informal relationship within the organization that may influence the organizational decision-making.
2. Though the organizational chart shows the lines of authority, but it fails to show how much authority, responsibility and what extent the nurse is accountable for the task being given to her or him.
3. Administration is ongoing and dynamic. The organizational chart is not flexible in structure.
4. It is rigid in nature of organizational relationship.
5. Defective organizational chart may cause confusion, misunderstanding among nurses, superiority and inferiority tendencies causing organizational conflicts.

Example of organization structure of state government hospital (Fig. 7.2).

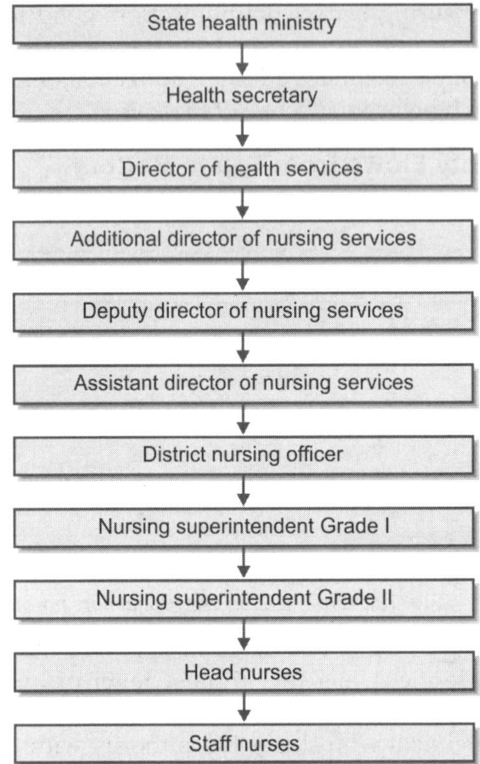

Fig. 7.2: Example of organization structure of Government hospital

ORGANIZATIONAL CHART OF THE NURSING SERVICE DEPARTMENT

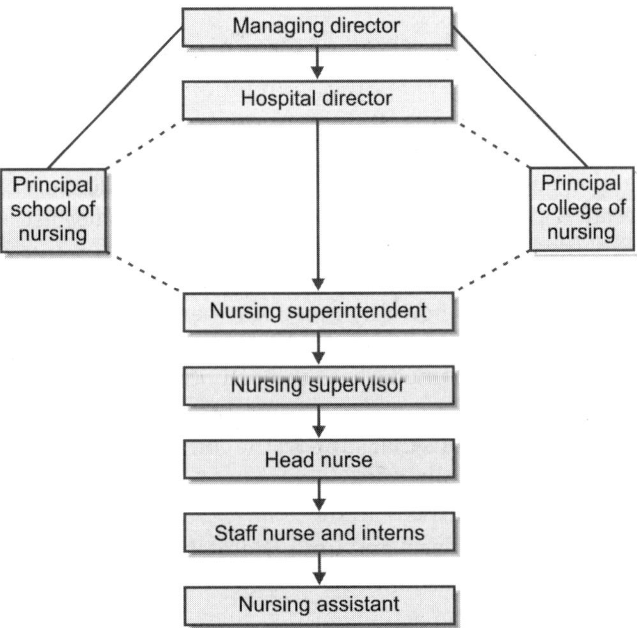

Fig. 7.3: Staff and line relationship in nursing service department

Note: Straight line donotes line relationship and dotted lines denotes staff relationship)

SUMMARY POINTS

- ✓ Organization is the important function of nursing service administration. It is the synchronization of people together to achieve the objectives of nursing services of the hospital. Organization is the process of identifying and grouping the work to be performed, specifying the work, defining and delegating the responsibility with authority to the personnel and establishing interpersonal relationship for the purpose of co-ordination of work, so as to get the work done together effectively, and in accomplishing the objectives of the institution.
- ✓ The organization is guided by certain principles like principle of specialization, functional definition, span of control, scalar chain and unity of command.
- ✓ The main objectives of nursing service organization is to provide quality patient care with best available resources.
- ✓ Organization structure is the hierarchical arrangement of lines of authority, communications, rights and duties of an organization. Organizational structure determines how the roles, power and responsibilities are assigned, controlled, and coordinated, and how information flows between the different levels of management.
- ✓ Organizational chart is an administrative tool to communicate nurses about their position in hospital nursing services and their relationship with other employees/nurses. It shows the line and staff relationship of the nurses in a hospital. Functional relationship lies in between staff and line and the authority is vested on functional manager who is an expert in that particular field.

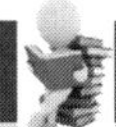

REVIEW QUESTIONS

1. Define organization. Enlist the goals and objectives of organization.
2. Enumerate the principles of organization and apply the same in nursing service administration.
3. Define organizational chart. Explain its advantages and disadvantages.
4. Draw an organizational chart of the hospital from where you had your clinical experience.
5. **Write short notes on:**
   a. Unity of command
   b. Objectives of nursing service organization
   c. Purposes of organization chart
   d. Organizational structure
   e. Concept of organization.

SELECTED READINGS

1. 10 Principles of Organization Design - Strategy Business
   http://www.strategy-business.com/article/00318%3Fgko%3Dc7329 23 Mar 2015 ..
2. Organizational chart - Wikipedia, the free encyclopedia
   https://en.wikipedia.org/wiki/Organizational_chart
3. Organizational structure - Wikipedia, the free encyclopedia
   https://en.wikipedia.org/wiki/Organizational_structure.
4. Principles of Organizing - Management Study Guide
   http://www.managementstudyguide.com/organizing_principles.htm
5. The Concept of Organization - JStor
   http://www.jstor.org/stable/2016073
6. What is an organization? definition and meaning
   http://www.businessdictionary.com/definition/organization.html

8

Organizational Process

LEARNING OBJECTIVES

This chapter imparts learning about:

- Definition of Organizational Process
- Basic Elements of Formal and Informal Organizational Structure
- Centralization and Decentralization of Organization
- Delegation-Authority, Responsibility and Accountability
- Division of Services and Departmentalization

DEFINITION OF ORGANIZATIONAL PROCESS

It is the process of determining the activities to be performed, arranging these activities to administrative units, as well as assigning managerial authority and responsibilities to people employed in the organization.

Types of Organizational Structure

There are two types of organizational structure. They are formal and informal organization.

FORMAL ORGANIZATION

The following are the basic elements of formal organizational structure:

- Centralization and decentralization
- Delegation of authority
- Span of control (supervision)
- Division of service
- Departmentalization.

Centralization vs Decentralization

In centralization structure of the organization, all the decisions, policy making and actions are performed by the top level management.

Advantages of Centralization

- The top level manager is entrusted with power and prestige in centralized structure.
- Centralized organization ensures policies and practices promoted in an uniform manner.
- In this type of structure, there is no possibility of duplication of function.
- There is no need to exercise extensive controlling measures to employees.

Disadvantages of Centralization

- In a hospital set up, the middle managers and the frontline workers like staff nurses are neglected because their functions are taken away by the top level management. This causes demotivation among head nurses and staff nurses.

- The nursing supervisor's functions become liaison between the staff nurses and nursing superintendent. The nursing supervisor may not function as a manager.

Decentralization

In this structure of organization, the authority is delegated to the lower level of employees in a planned and systematic manner. It helps in empowering lower level of employees in their assigned functions.

Advantages of Decentralization

- In a hospital setting, it ensures increased morale and good interpersonal relationship among nursing personnel.
- In this structure, it relieves the top level management from the burden of the daily administration, long range planning, policy development and system integration.
- Since the lower level personnel are responsible to execute any plan, it helps them to make decisions close to action.
- It helps the young managers to develop managerial functions and leadership.
- It enhances nurses' enthusiasm and coordination in work setting.
- In this type of organization, the nursing personnel execute the task in an increasing speed as they need not to wait for the decision from the top level and avoids delay in decision-making.
- This structure enhances inter and intradepartmental coordination among nursing services.

Disadvantages of Decentralization

- Top-level management may perceive that decentralization interfere their status in the organization and internally they may not like it.
- This structure may not allow effective utilization of personnel with high qualification and expertise.
- Decentralization requires more managers at the lower level when the number of staff are large. It increases the organizational budget.
- There is a possibility of overlapping and duplication of services.
- It may result in lowering the standards of organizational decisions that may result in lack of uniformity in care.

Delegation

Definition

Delegation is a managerial task. It refers to assigning tasks from the higher level executive to the lower level employees. For example, the superintendent of nursing assigns tasks to staff nurses and gives authority to achieve the task done. Thus delegation flows from the top level management to bottom level.

Delegation Process

It involves:

- The allocation of duties to employees
- The delegation of authority
- The assignment of responsibility
- Creation of accountability, i.e. subordinates must be held answerable to carry out their tasks properly.

Factors that determine as to how much authority to be delegated

- *Organization's size:* When the organization is large and complex, there is an increased need of delegation from the higher authority to subordinates.
- *Importance of duty or decision:* It is to remember that the more important the task is and decision is that needs to be delegated more.
- *Task complexity:* When the task is a more complex one, there is a need for delegation of the task with authority.
- *Organizational culture:* The organizational morale will come down when the top-level manager does not believe or have confidence in the abilities of the subordinate and that will lead to inadequate delegation.
- *Qualities of subordinates:* Successful delegation is influenced by subordinates' skills, abilities and motivation to accept authority and shows responsibility to accomplish the tasks assigned and act on it.

Principles of Delegation

- Delegation of authority and responsibility to be given in a balancing manner. Responsibility without authority is not effective.
- Authority and responsibility should be in equal proportion.
- Financial power is not delegated to subordinate.
- Authority to take disciplinary action by subordinate to employee is not delegated.
- Policy-making power also is not delegated.

Barriers to Successful Delegation

We may categorize the barriers with reference to:
- Administrator
- Subordinate.

Barriers in relation to administrator

- The nurse administrator fails to delegate because she does not possess delegation ability to her subordinates.
- She does not have confidence in her subordinates that they will perform the given assignment.
- Not able to control the subordinate is another cause of failure of delegation.
- The nurse administrator refuses to delegate because she feels better if the task is done by her.
- Does not want to share the knowledge, information and skill as the nurse administrator feel insecure with subordinates, as the subordinates may outshine her.
- Does not want to take risk because the subordinates may do wrong things or wrong decision or they are not capable to use the authority given.

Barriers in relation to subordinates

- The subordinates may not accept the delegated task because they believe that decision-making is a tough work and it is better to avoid them.
- Subordinate tend to fear for criticism and mistakes done by them.
- The delegation may be incomplete such as lack of information, training and resources.
- The subordinates may refuse because the delegation may bring overload in their job.
- Another reason is there is no possibility of getting incentives if delegation is accepted.

Authority

Authority is a person who by the virtue of his position and power has the right to take final decision for the organization and take action or command actions from other personnel in a downward direction.

Types of Authority

- *Ultimate authority:* It is a right of a person or agency to take final decision. It deals with the original source from which one derives the right to take actions. Thus, in the health sector, the Ministry of Health becomes ultimate authority.
- *Legal authority:* Refers to a person who is legally permitted by the virtue of the position to take an action; For example, a hospital director delegates to director of nursing service to act on behalf of the nursing service department.
- *Technical authority:* It refers to a person who is a recognized expert in a particular field but it has nothing to do with the position. For example, an automobile engineer in the organization is an expert authority in transport and ambulance related activities.
- *Operational authority:* It is a giving authority to a person to assure certain responsibilities. For example, the nursing superintendent delegates responsibility to assistant nursing superintendent in her leave period.

Responsibility

Refers to the person when he has accepted the assignment, he is answerable to or responsible to complete the job.

Accountability

When a task is given to a person from the higher level to the employee, the employee is responsible to do the task.But the superior or who has given the responsibility is accountable where the employee does the job good or bad. Accountability moves in an upward direction.

Organizational Relationship

There are three types of organizational relationships:
1. The line relation
2. The staff relation
3. The functional relation

The Line Relation (Organization)

It is one of the important organizational relationships. Line relationship is a framework that depicts the employer-employee relationship in a hierarchical manner. It has command over the personnel. The employer has every right to give orders and demand accountability. Each employee in the organization knows his position in the organization as whom he is responsible to and what he is responsible for. It is depicted by a solid line in the organizational chart. It represent a structure in a direct vertical relationship through which authority flows from top to bottom. The authority is highest at the top and lowers down at each level of hierarchy. The line authority enhances the channel of communication, coordination and accountability in an organization.

Advantages of line organization

- This structure of organization is easy to develop and is easily understood by employees in the organization.
- It ensures scalar principle of the organization by facilitating unity of command.
- This type of organization identifies the authority and responsibility relationship and the employees comprehend the boundary of their job.

- Since each employee knows to whom she or he is responsible, this line organization enhances good discipline in the setting.
- This organizational structure defines authority in each level that enable prompt decision-making by the authority at each level.

Disadvantages of line organization

- In a complex/large organization, the superiors are overloaded with responsibilities, it is difficult for the supervisor to pay individual attention to each employee.
- The overall decision-making authority is placed at the top level. When that authority is incapable in his activities, the organization may not be successful.
- Since the concentration of authority is at the top level, the employees at the bottom level has no voice and upward communication is hampered. Even if the wrong decision is taken by the top management, the bottom employees has to accept the wrong things to implement.

Staff Relation in Organization

In staff relationship framework, the personnel function is to advise, assist and support the personnel of line relation in order to achieve better performance. It has no commanding over any person. The staff are considered as experts or specialized in that area of organization, it is depicted by a dotted line in the organizational chart (refer Fig. 7.3 in Chapter 7). For example, Indian Nursing Council (INC) has a staff relationship in all colleges of nursing.

Functional Organization

Functional authority occupies position in the midway between staff and line relation. In this structure, the organizational activities are assigned to different functional units like transportation or vehicle maintenance, finance, marketing, stores and supplies, public relation, etc. The incharge of the unit will be an expert or specialist. He is called functional manager who has the authority over his functions. Functional managers exist in large or complex organization where expert knowledge is required.

Span of Control or Span of Supervision

It means a supervisor can supervise number of subordinates effectively in an organization at a time.

Dimensions of Span of Control

There are two dimensions of span of control that can be implemented in an organization:

Narrow span of control

In this control, the manager supervises a smaller number of subordinates.

Advantages of narrow span of control

- In this dimension of control, a close monitoring of the subordinates is possible.
- It facilitates fast communication between subordinates and superiors.

Disadvantages of narrow span of control

- Since the subordinates are few in number, the superiors likely to be too much attached in subordinates' work.
- It requires many levels of management.
- It incurs more budgets because of too many levels in an organization.

Wide span of control

In this control, the manager supervises a large number of subordinates.

Advantages of wide span of control

- In this dimension, a large number of subordinates are to be delegated and to be supervised.
- Wide span of control needs definite policies for monitoring and supervising subordinates.
- It is imperative that the subordinates to be carefully selected to get the work done.

Disadvantages of wide span of control

- The supervisors are overloaded to take more decision to the organization.
- There is a possibility of loss of control to supervise a large number of subordinates.
- The supervisors to be carefully selected to achieve quality control.

Factors Determining Span of Control

The following factors are to be considered in determining span of control:

- The degree to which the supervisor and the subordinates are competent. More the supervisor and subordinates are competent, a wide span of control is possible.
- The interaction between the unit supervisor and subordinates decides the span of control.
- The extent of duties and responsibilities of top level manager and lower level managers.
- The type of activities both similar and dissimilar being supervised by the supervisor.
- The emerging problems of a new unit.
- Policies, standardized procedures and plan of work are available in the unit.

- The physical layout of the organization.
- The stability and complexity of the work.

Division of Work

Division of work refers distribution of large number of tasks to be assigned among many number of subordinates.

Advantage

It helps the subordinates to become master a task with a maximum skill, and a minimum time and effort.

Disadvantages

Division of work makes different, narrow tasks, which need effective managerial supervision and coordination. Another disadvantage is that it creates more human problems, fatigue and stress, and which in turns results in inadequate quantity and quality of work, increased absenteeism and higher turnover of employees.

Departmentalization

It is referred as grouping of various activities into small administrative units.

Types of Departmentalization

Departmentalization can be grouped and implemented through one or more of the following types:

- *Departmentation by services:* Activities are grouped according to similarities of skills needed to accomplish the goal, i.e. medical, surgical and pediatric units. It is simple and commonly used.
- *Departmentation by time:* Activities that need coverage twenty four hours a day, seven days a week (e.g. acute care settings), or activities coverage for 8–12 hours a day for 5–6 days a week (e.g. preventive services) at the most.
- *Departmentation by degree of acuteness of illness of the patients:* Example progressive patient care (PPC), i.e. intensive care unit, intermediate care unit, self-care unit, long-term care unit, and home care unit.
- *Departmentation by function:* This method is referred as according to function, and resources one unit manager is given authority to supervise and implement the tasks, e.g. laundry, pharmacy, dietary services.
- *Departmentation by location:* Activities that are used with wide geographic activities in a given location are grouped and assigned to a manager, i.e. inpatient department, outpatient department, and administrative department.
- *Departmentation by patient:* This is done when service is important and the welfare of the patient is of primary interest, i.e. gender based, (Male/female units) age specific units (geriatric, pediatric units) economic status (paying wards, free general wards), etc.

INFORMAL ORGANIZATION

An **informal organization** is the social and practical structure of the organization, as opposed to the formal structure of an organization. It establishes to work in concurrence with the formal organizational structure, parallel with it, or against it.

Concepts and Structure

In the **formal organization,** the structure and operation is typically set forth in the official documents, rules, and procedures of the organization (like a corporation's articles of incorporation and bylaws). The roles, authority and responsibilities of each member of the organization are clearly defined. For example, in nursing service administration th role and functions of each cadre of nurses are well defined and stated in a written form.

In an **informal organization**, it structured around the sum total of social norms, relationships, and interactions that affect how an organization works. While a formal organization is cold and impersonal, an informal organization is intensely personal. It is all about social interactions and relationships between the members. Members of an informal organization can certainly hold offices and have formal duties, but they also bring their own values, personal interests and assumptions into the equation of how they act. Members develop friendships, alliances, enemies, trusted sources of information, and preferences on how tasks should be performed.

Table 8.1: The difference between formal and informal organization structure

Formal organization	Informal organization
Structured	Evolving constantly
Top to bottom authority	Grass roots
Follow vision and mission	Dynamic and responsive
Static	Excellent motivation of employee
Planned assignment	Requires inside knowledge to be seen
Treat people like an employee	Treats people individual like
Hierarchical	Coherent by trust and reciprocity
Top level management decides	Collective decision-making

Advantages of Informal Organization

- Informal organization cannot work alone, it has to work with formal structure.
- Lighten the management workload.

- Fill gaps in management abilities.
- Employees may experience psychological stress, tension, and emotional distress with management and with other employees' in formal organization. Whereas the informal group ensures a means for relieving these emotional and psychological problems by allowing an employee to discuss them among his group friends openly and freely.
- Encourages improved management practice and understanding and dealing with the environmental crisis.

Disadvantages of Informal Organization

Informal organizations also possess the following potential disadvantages and problems that require careful management attention.

- Resistance to change
- Role conflict
- Rumor
- Conformity
- Benefits of the informal organization.

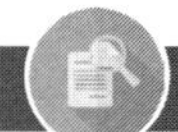

SUMMARY POINTS

- ✓ Organization process is the process of determining the activities to be performed by nursing personnel, arranging these activities to administrative units, as well as assigning managerial authority and responsibilities to people employed in the organization at each level.
- ✓ There are two types of organizational structure. They are formal and informal organization. The nurse administrator should know the basic elements of formal organizational process such as centralization and decentralization, delegation of authority, span of control (supervision), division of service and departmentalization.
- ✓ Centralized organizational structures rely on one individual to make decisions and provide direction for the institution. The nurse administrator uses this structure because she/he is responsible for nursing aspects of the hospital.
- ✓ Decentralized organizational structures often have several individuals responsible for making decisions. Decentralized organizations rely on a team environment at different levels. Individuals at each level in the hospital may have some autonomy to make some decision. For example, in functional type of structure, the transport manager, store and purchase, manager may make decision for their department.
- ✓ Delegation is the assignment of authority and responsibility to another person to carry out specific activities. The nurse administrator who delegates the work to her head nurses remains accountable for the outcome of the delegated work. Delegation provides a means for increasing productivities and empowers a nurse to make decisions. Delegation includes three components—authority, responsibility and accountability.
- ✓ Authority is the kind of right and power through which it guides and directs the actions of others so that the organizational goals can be achieved. It is also related with decision-making. It is vested in particular position, not to the person because authority is given by an institution and therefore it is legal.
- ✓ Responsibility is when an authentic body of an organization is top level management, (the nurse administrator) direct the nurses. Departmental managers and other personnel take the direction from top level management to perform the task. Authority is necessary to perform the work; only authority is not provided to the people but obligation is also provided. So, the obligation to perform the duties and task is known as ***responsibility***.
- ✓ Nurses (subordinates) receive the authority from top level of the organization and they also receive the command and direction to perform the work. In other words, they are authorized and responsible for a specific function. Sometimes the task may not be performed effectively. The nurse must report to the nurse administrator about the assigned task. She must answer his/her performance which is known as ***accountability***.
- ✓ Line and staff relations are names given to different types of functions in organizations. A 'line function' is one that directly advances an organization in its core work. This always a hierarchy that flows from top to bottom. A 'staff function' supports the organization with specialized advisory and support functions. For example, human resources, accounting, public relations and the legal department are generally considered to be staff functions.
- ✓ Span of management is also known as *span of control, span of supervision, span of authority* and *span of responsibility*. It indicates the number for people directly managed effectively by a single person.

- ✓ A sound organization depends upon the effective performance of work by the executives. So, the executives should neither be overloaded nor be idle. For example, for a clinical instructor in nursing can supervise 10 nursing students.
- ✓ Formal structure, through departmentalization and work division, provides a framework for defining managerial authority, responsibility and accountability. It should not be flexible, it is channeled individual and group efforts.It has well-defined jobs. Formal organization always have well-definds authority/ responsibility.
- ✓ Whereas in informal structure is generally social, with blurred or shifting lines of authority and accountability. It also has its own channels of communication, which may distribute information more broadly and rapidly than the formal communication system. It is flexible, loosely organized ill-defined informal organization structure, communication networks ('grapevine'), and relationships (behaviors and norms) do not necessarily follow those of the formal organization.

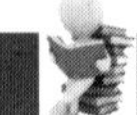

REVIEW QUESTIONS

1. Define organization process. Describe centralization and decentralization structure with their advantages and disadvantages.
2. Define delegation. What are the barriers in delegation specific to nursing service administration?
3. Differentiate staff and line structure in organization with their advantages and disadvantages.
4. Describe the basic elements of formal structure of an organization.
5. Differentiate formal and informal type of organization.
6. Write short notes on:
   a. Functional relation in an organization
   b. Span of control
   c. Authority and responsibility
   d. Departmentalization
   e. Division of work.

SELECTED READINGS

1. Centralized and decentralized structure. http://smallbusiness.chron.com/centralized-vs-decentralized-organizational-structure-2785.html.
2. Centralized Vs. Decentralized Organizational Design I Chron.com.
3. Delegation - definition of delegation by The Free Dictionary. http://www.thefreedictionary.com/delegation.
4. Delegation I Definition of delegation by Merriam-Webster. http://www.merriam-webster.com/dictionary/delegation.
5. Distinguish Difference Between Formal and Informal Organisation. http://kalyan-city.blogspot.in/2011/07/distinguish-difference-between-formal.html 29 Jul 2011.
6. Formal and Informal Organization: Features, Advantages and Disadvantages http://www.yourarticlelibrary.com/organization/formal-and-informal-organization-features-advantages-and-disadvantages/8654/.
7. http://smallbusiness.chron.com/centralized-vs-decentralized-organizational-design-11476.html.
8. Organizational Process. Definition ttp://chrguibert.free.fr/cmmi12/cmmi-acq/text/pa-opd.php.
9. Span of control - Wikipedia, the free encyclopedia. https://en.wikipedia.org/wiki/Span_of_control.
10. Span of Control in Management: Definition, Disadvantages and Advantages. http://study.com/academy/lesson/span-of-control-in-management-definition-disadvantages-advantages.html 29 Nov 2014.

9

Organizational Theories

LEARNING OBJECTIVES

This chapter imparts learning about:
- Concept of Organizational Theories
- Organizational Effectiveness
- Organizational Climate
- Organizational Culture

CONCEPT OF ORGANIZATIONAL THEORIES

An organization is a group of individuals working together in a harmonious manner under a hierarchy of management to achieve the organizational goals. It is a synchronization of all available resources focusing on the improvement of the functioning of an establishment.

A study on the organizational structure is referred as organizational theory. It has theoretical concepts to comprehend what the structure is, the function of the structure that helps in prediction and control of organizational productivity.

There are **four** major contributing theories of organizations and management, namely:
- Classical Theory.
- Human relations theory
- Contingency/decision theory
- Modern systems theory

These are already discussed in Chapter 3.

ORGANIZATIONAL EFFECTIVENESS

Organizational effectiveness refers to the functions and efficiency of the members of the organization who are able to achieve the organizational objectives or in other words the organization that brings positive outcome or an organization that is productive to achieve its goals. It is the concept of how effective an organization in achieving the outcomes that the organization intends to produce. It directly concerned with talent management, leadership development, organization design and structure, design of evaluation, implementation of change and transformation, deploying smart processes and smart technology to manage the establishment's human capital and the development of the broader human resources.

In order to achieve organizational effectiveness, each member in the organization works with understanding the goals and with minimum input to get maximum outcome. When the members in the organization works efficiently and increases the productivity to achieve the desired goals is termed as **organizational effectiveness**. The desired outcome will be based on the goals of the organization, which could be, for example, bringing quality patient care outcome by efficient and effective nursing care.

Yankey and McClellan (2003) described organizational effectiveness. It is the degree to which an organization has achieved the desired goals and objectives and the quality of the performance of its members. Malik et al. (2011) referred organizational effectiveness as a concept of how far the organization is able and effective in achieving what it wants to achieve.

They referred that organizational effectiveness is an abstract concept because it is difficult to evaluate it. However, organizational effectiveness, could be measured by efficiency of management, performance of employees and their competencies, number of people served, types and sizes of population served, etc.

An organization, if it operates efficiently, will produce better outcome. The organization is said to be desirably effective when it demonstrates potentials for its managerial leadership, decision-making capability, quality human work process within the system, organizational structure, and culture. It adopts and ensures an ongoing and dynamic work environment. Continuous evaluation and improving organizational effectiveness and efficiency is one of the plans of operation for the success and growth and development of organization.

If we want to know the organizational effectiveness, we need to have definite criteria to evaluate the goals and objectives. The criteria differs from establishment to establishment. However, the employees may be in a right position to assess the effectiveness through self-assessment of their performance to achieve the goals of the organization.

Determinants of Organizational Effectiveness

Various factors are responsible for organizational effectiveness. According to a study conducted by Watana Vinitwatanakhun Thailand (1998), out of the eight factors such as environment, technology, leadership style, culture, strategic planning, human resource development, structural design, and power control studied, only four factors such as leadership style, technology, strategic planning, and human resource development were significantly explained and predicted organizational effectiveness. In addition, it was found that leadership style is the best predictor of the perceived organizational effectiveness, because of the importance of effective leadership in all kinds of group action in the organizations.

- ***Leadership style:*** Various studies have shown that both transformational and transactional leadership in nursing had shown better effectiveness in nursing administration bringing quality patient care outcome and nurses satisfaction. Effective leaders influence nurses to work towards achieving the goal.
- ***Policies, procedures and standards:*** Organization effectiveness depends upon the vision, mission statement, values, various strategies to achieve goals, and objectives of the nursing service department. Apart from the policies and procedures, hospital and nursing units must have standards according to the services provided. These standards acts as guidelines for nurses to work and also help the nurse administrator can do performance appraisal according to the standards.
- ***Decision-making and effective communication:*** Decision-making based on evidences influence nurses positively. It is said that 99% of friction in organization is caused by defective communication. When there is an effective communication from both upward and from downward, nurses feel a sense of empowerment and security and that brings organizational effectiveness.
- ***Human resource development:*** Human resources (HR) is a cross-functional process in the organization. HR collects feedback, ideas, internal knowledge about processes and best practices. HR role is to work with the feedback and to share the responsibility for the organizational effectiveness. The organizational effectiveness is crucial for the success of the modern organization. The effectiveness has a enormous impact on the profitability of the organization and allows higher investments or better development opportunities for employees. HR has to challenge the effectiveness of the organization (and has to share the responsibility for the improvement). For example, when the nurse administrator has to develop her nurses in terms of knowledge, and nursing competencies including unit management and better performance the nurse administrator needs to provide incentives, and safe work environment, staff welfare and guidance for the effectiveness of administration.
- ***Work environment:*** A positive work environment makes nurses/employees feel good about coming to work, and this provides the motivation to sustain them throughout the day. Ward policies, nursing standards, sufficient equipment and supplies, autonomy, supervision, work schedule and unbiased appraisal of nurses influence organizational effectiveness.
- ***Organizational structure:*** Compared to the functional system, the relationship between employees and their superiors in organization process is drastically different. The superiors' role is mainly to direct their staff in the right direction and act as their coach. Workers increasingly make independent decisions on how to reach the set objectives. The process organization requires that:
  1. Workers and superiors have better co-operation skills.

2. Superiors are capable of creating a goal-directed atmosphere.
3. The remuneration system must provide sufficient incentive to facilitate total management success.
4. Goals are established and indicators devised to support patient care services.
5. The efficiency of operations is measured and reported and rewarded.
6. Responsibilities and authorizations are in balance.

The organization effectiveness also influenced by the staffing structure in quality (qualification, experience, and specialization) and quantity according to norms and standards recommended by regulatory bodies.

- *Technology:* Technology has a positive influence on nursing. Health information technology (HIT) enhances the knowledge and the quality of nursing records reports and improve positive attitudes towards care given. It helps to reduce medication administration errors. Today nurses are in a position to design and implement health information technology in nursing.Various studies have observed that effective leadership in HIT processes, can improve positive influences on nurse satisfaction and patient care. Effective nursing leadership can positively influence the effective development, dissemination, and use of HIT.
- *Performance of nurses:* Professional knowledge, attitude and professional competencies influence the standard of nursing in a hospital. Periodical in-service education, skill training, leadership management and good work culture enhances empowerment and motivates nurses to work and influence organizational effectiveness.

The Role of Nurse Administrator in Facilitating Organizational Effectiveness

- *Assessment:* The nurse administrator collects comprehensive data pertinent to the trends and issues-related nursing by SWOT analysis (Strengths, Weaknesses, Opportunities and Threats).
- *Identifies issues, problems or trends:* The nurse administrator analyzes the assessment data to determine the issues, problems or trends. Analyzes the future needs of nursing by analyzing the gap between strengths and weakness. She or he also identifies the culture of the organization and the strengths and weaknesses in the current competencies of the key personnel in organization.
- *Outcomes identification:* The nurse administrator determines the outcome expected and plans for individualized care according to the situation by describing competence needed in nursing for the future.
- *Planning:* The nurse administrator makes strategic plans that defines strategies and alternatives to achieve expected outcomes.
- *Implementation:* The nurse administrator implements the identified plan.
    1. Develops philosophy of nursing services, vision, mission and values of nursing to all nursing personnel.
    2. Establishes organization chart and maintains effective communication.
    3. Explains job responsibilities to nursing personnel.
    4. Delegates and supervises
    5. Makes prompt decision whenever warranted
    6. Maintains effective communication
- *Coordinates* all activities by administrative leadership
- *Health promotion, health teaching and education:* The nurse administrator develops plans to ensure health promotion, health teaching, and the provision of other educational services and resources for better patient care outcomes.
- *Consultation:* Provides consultation to influence the identified plan, enhance the abilities of nursing personnel and others.
- *Evaluation:* The nurse administrator evaluates progress towards attainment of outcomes. Periodical performance appraisal for nurses' development conducted
- *Mentoring and coaching:* is provided as needed by the nurses according to performance appraisal.

ORGANIZATIONAL CLIMATE

Organizational climate is defined as how members of an organization experience the culture of an organization. The climate of an organization is subject to change frequently and can be shaped by the upper management of an organization. If culture represents the personality of the organization, climate is the organization's mood. Organizational climate is much easier to experience and measure than organizational culture and also much easier to change.

When the employees demonstrate high morale and are able to complete the assigned tasks within the prescribed time in an effective manner results in an effective organizational climate

Organizational climate refers to member perceptions of organizational features like decision making, leadership, and norms about work. Whereas organizational culture refers more broadly to the norms, values, beliefs, and assumptions shared by members of an organization or a distinctive subculture within an organization

Factors Influencing Organizational Climate and the Role of Nurse Administrator

Research studies in health care, along with findings from other industries, studied to a wide range of organizational conditions and work processes that may shape the performance of health care practitioners and provider organizations. Despite of the difficulty in implementing far-reaching organizational change, some health providers have succeeded in restructuring their organizations in ways that promote quality health care. Within this growing body of evidence, researchers have sought to understand the influence of organizational climate on health care quality. Various studies show that there many factors that affects organizational climate in nursing services.

Few of them are explained below:

- *Staffing-resource adequacy:* Human resource is the backbone of any organization. The number of nursing personnel in quality and quantity , their individual perception about nursing service administration, values and commitments to serve the patients, social support system, life stressors and their coping strategies, job demands and work related competencies (Knowledge, attitudes and skills)influence organizational climate.
- *Nurse administrator's ability and leadership:* The nurse administrator is the father figure in administration of nursing. Values, vision and support for safety of nurses , conflict management ability, decision making power, supervisory responsibility influence organizational climate.
- *Nurse–physician relations:* A good interpersonal relation with members of the health team, patients and family members , group behavior among nurses and collaborative care affect organizational climate.
- *Nurse participation in hospital affairs:* At each level of nursing , the participation in planning, implementation and evaluation for patient care, policy-making and implementation influence organizational climate.
- *Organizational and structural characteristics:* Health care facilities, infrastructure of the establishment, management structure, accreditation/magnet status of the hospital, organizational stability of the hospital, quality and patient safety as benchmark of care (patient-centered care) good environmental condition, communication and technology and measures to prevent occupational hazards strengthen organizational climate can influence organizational climate
- *Work design:* It includes staffing and scheduling. It facilitates nursing care rendered by trained and qualified nursing personnel round the clock, nurse patient ratio as per recommended norms shift work, overtime, patient population, demographic characteristics etc. that affect organizational climate.
- *Working condition:* Nurses are motivated to work in a safe work environment where they can exercise autonomy. Other factors like salary benefits, opportunities for career development, respect and dignity, managerial support, nursing leadership role and support affect organizational climate.

Impact of good organizational climate in nursing administration

For hospital management, good organizational climate enhances level of performance of nurses/employees and increases the level of quality care outcome. At nurses level, it promotes health and safety among nurses, job satisfaction and helps in retention of nurses. At patients level, it enhances positive health outcome, patient safety, patient's satisfaction and quality care:

ORGANIZATIONAL CULTURE

Organizational culture is referred as the values and attitudes of the members of an organization that influence to the development of an unique social and psychological work setting of an organization. Organizational culture is the embodiments of the values, beliefs and principles of members of the organization, management style, and culture of the country. Culture includes the organization's vision, values, norms, systems, symbols, language, assumptions, beliefs, and habits. (Needle (2004)

According to Ravasi and Schultz (2006), organizational culture is a set of shared beliefs that guide to define desired behavior for its members at various situations. Each member in the organization perceives the same belief, attitude and pattern of behavior and feel they belong to that particular organization. Thus, organizational culture influences the collective behavior and interaction of its members with each other, with clients, and with society.

Organizational culture is a system of shared beliefs and values, that control behavior of its members in an organization that have a definite impact on organizational culture. Each organization has its own dress code, and desired performance level and maintains an unique culture, which provides guidelines and framework for the behavior of the members of the organization.

Organizational culture is composed of seven characteristics that range in priority from high to low as described below.

Characteristics of Organizational Culture and Role of Nurse Administrator

- *Innovation (risk orientation):* Each innovation is expected to face some kind of risk. The organization which maintains high organizational culture encourages its members to innovate things in their job performance to bring quality outcome. Thus encouraging risk taking behavior is unique to organization culture. For example, in nursing the administrators must encourage and support nurses and unit managers to bring innovative models to improve quality patient care outcome and improve organizational effectiveness.
- *Attention to detail (precision orientation):* This is a unique characteristic of organizational culture that advocate their employees/nurses to function with accuracy or precision and meticulous care at work settings. Nursing is a human engineering and one cannot function with trial and error. The nurse should be competent in her performance that should be evidence-based, and the patients should be satisfied. That in turn brings high morale among nurses.
- *Emphasis on outcome (achievement orientation):* Some organization give more stress on achieving good result as an organizational value. The nurse administrator/ nurse manager directs the nurse about the outcome of nursing care and support them with protocol and standards according to service given.
- *Emphasis on people (fairness orientation):* The organization that gives more importance to human values and healthy environment contributes to high organizational culture. The nurse administrator treat each nurse with pride, dignity and respect that develops a sense of belongingness of nurses in the organization and it is easy to follow the vision and mission of nursing administration and brings a positive organizational culture.
- *Teamwork (collaboration orientation):* Good organizational climate values team work and team achievements. Nursing care is a team work. Nurses work with interdisciplinary team for better patient care out outcome. Nurses who work for patients as a team tend to have a positive collaboration and relationship with their coworkers, members of the interdisciplinary team and managers that influence organizational culture.
- *Assertiveness (competitive orientation):* Assertiveness is one of the qualities of employer and employee that contributes a positive organizational culture. Nurses should keep in mind that they provide the highest quality of care to all patients and proud to say that they belong to the profession that has high ideals, values and commitments. This characteristic influence organizational culture.
- *Stability (rule orientation):* Rule-oriented, predictable, and bureaucratic values are observed in certain organization. These characteristics promotes stability of the organization and enhances positive outcome and desirable organizational climate.

SUMMARY POINTS

- ✓ An organization is a collection of people working together under a division of labor and a hierarchy of authority to achieve a common goal.
- ✓ Organizational theory is the process of creating knowledge to understand organizational structure so that we can predict and control organizational effectiveness or productivity by designing organizations.
- ✓ An organization, if it operates efficiently, will produce better outcome. Highly effective organizations exhibit strengths across five areas: Leadership, decision-making and structure, people, work processes and systems, and culture. For an organization to achieve and sustain success, it needs to adapt to its dynamic environment.
- ✓ Organizational effectiveness is the extent to which an organization has met its stated goals and objectives and how well it performed in the process.
- ✓ The organizational climate within an organization is extremely positive as evidenced by high employee morale and the willingness of its workers to complete tasks in a timely and efficient manner.
- ✓ Organizational culture is a system of shared assumptions, values, and beliefs, which governs how people behave in organizations. These shared values have a strong influence on the people in the organization and dictate how they dress, act, and perform their jobs.

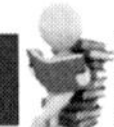

REVIEW QUESTIONS

1. Define organization. Describe human relation theory in detatil.
2. Define organizational effectiveness. Describe determinants of organizational effectiveness with example from nursing administration.
3. Describe the role of nurse administrator in enhancing organization climate in hospital nursing administration.
4. Differentiate organization climate and culture. As a nurse administrator, how will you promote organizational culture in your work setting.
5. **Write short notes on:**
   a. Characteristics of organizational culture
   b. Impact of organizational culture in nursing
   c. Organizational climate
   d. Organizational theory.

SELECTED READINGS

1. Factors Affecting Organizational Effectiveness... - AU Journal
   http://www.journal.au.edu/au_techno/2002/apr2002/article8.pdf
2. Factors Influencing organizational effectiveness
   http://onlinelibrary.wiley.com/doi/10.1111/j.1744-6570.1953.tb01031.x/pdf
3. Factors Influencing Organizational Effectiveness.
   http://onlinelibrary.wiley.com/doi/10.1111/j.1744-570.1955.tb01214.x/pdf
4. Mohamed Tariq et al . Connotation of organizational effectiveness and factors affects it. Int. J og Behavioral Sciences; Vol2:9 sept 2012
5. Nursing Administration Scope & Standards of Practice | Texas ...
   http://txsno.org/standards/nursing_administration_scope_standards_of_practice
6. Organization climate - Wikipedia, the free encyclopedia
   https://en.wikipedia.org/wiki/Organisation_climate.
7. Organizational climate and hospital nurses' job satisfaction, burnout ...
   http://repository.upenn.edu/dissertations/AAI3165703/
8. Organizational Climate and Intensive Care Unit Nurses ... – Medscape
   http://www.medscape.com/viewarticle/540188
9. Organizational Climate and Nurse Health Outcomes in ...
   http://citeseerx.ist.psu.edu/viewdoc/download?doi=10.1.1.410.9853&rep=rep1&type=pdf.
10. Organizational Climate: Definition, Factors & Impacts on Culture ...
    http://study.com/academy/lesson/organizational-climate
11. Organizational culture - Wikipedia, the free encyclopedia
    https://en.wikipedia.org/wiki/organizational_culture.
12. Organizational Effectiveness - The Bridgespan Group
    http://www.bridgespan.org/Publications and Tools/Organizational Effectiveness.aspx. Publications and Tools >
13. Organizational theories. http://www.fao.org/docrep/w7503e/w7503e03.htm
14. Organizational theory - Create Advantage
    http://www.createadvantage.com/glossary/organizational-theory.
15. The Nature of Organizational Theory - Home - KSU Faculty Member ...
    http://faculty.ksu.edu.sa/Hanan_Alkorashy/Nursing%2520management%2520489NUR/3._The_Nature_of_Organizational_Theory.pdf

16. What is organisational effectiveness? How an organisation could achive it?
http://www.researchgate.net/post/What_is_organisational_effectiveness_How_an_organisation_could_achieve_it. 5 May 2014 ...
17. What is organizational climate? Definition and meaning
http://www.businessdictionary.com/definition/organizational-climate.html
18. What is Organizational Culture? - Definition ** Characteristics ...
http://study.com/academy/lesson/what-is-organizational-culture-definition-characteristics.html.

10

Organizing Nursing Services and Patient Care

LEARNING OBJECTIVES

This chapter imparts learning about:

- Patient Classification System
- Methods of Patient Assignment–Advantages and Disadvantages
- Primary Nursing Care
- Planning and Organizing: Hospital, Unit and Ancillary Services

PATIENT CLASSIFICATION SYSTEM (PCS)

Today nurse administrators are facing lot of health care issues such as acute shortage of nurses in hospitals, high rocketing health care cost, need for decreasing length of hospital stay, quality and patient safety, consumerism and lack of resources for nursing care. These issues are affecting patients, families and nurses also. The management is constantly seeking reduction of health care cost at the same time intends to bring high-quality patient care.

Concept of PCS

PCS is an administrative tool that aims to provide quality patient care and the degree of nursing care requirements.The patient classification system (PCS), is referred as patient acuity system. Thus, PCS is used to assist nurse administrators to determine workload of nurses and staffing needs.

Purposes of PCS

- To provide quality and safe patient care.
- PCS helps to decide the nursing hours required for each category of patients that will help to bring best possible patient care outcome as per norms recommended by the health facility.
- Enhances staff satisfaction through a stress-free work environment. Determine the number and category of nurses (skill mix) needed for providing quality patient care.
- Monitors changes in patient demographics and care needs.
- Provides information on each patient care unit that directs and supports staffing decision-making.
- Ensures that quality of nursing care is provided in a safe environment.
- Assesses the level and support services required for each category of patient.
- Enhances staff satisfaction through a stress-free work environment.
- The PCS data generated is used to improve patient satisfaction by providing required time to the patient according to his/her needs and enhances staff satisfaction by determining staffing needs and thus decreasing workload.
- Monitors the provision of quality nursing care according to international standards in a safe work environment.

Types of PCS

There are different kinds of PCS used in administration, but the three most commonly used types are:

1. *Descriptive system:* This is a purely subjective system wherein the nurse selects which category the patient is best suited.
2. *Checklist system:* Another subjective system, wherein the patient is assigned to a numerical value based on the level of activity in specific categories. The numerical values are added up to give the nurse an overall rating.
3. *Time standards system*: This is another method where the nurse assigns a time value based on the various activities needed to be completed for the patient. This time value is sum up and converted to an acuity level. Among these three, the most commonly used is the descriptive kind of PCS. These are subdivided into four classifications namely:

- **Self-care/minimal care:** The first classification of patients who are recovering and normally requires only diagnostic studies, minimal therapy, less frequent observations, and daily care for minor conditions For example patient waiting for elective surgery.
- **Moderate care:** The patient in this category is moderately ill or under the recovery stage from a serious illness or operation. They require nursing supervision or assistance that is related to ambulating and caring for their own hygiene.
- **Maximum care:** Patient needs close attention and complete care all through the shift. The nurses initiate, supervise and perform most of the patient's activities.
- **Intensive care:** The last category or classification, wherein the patients are acutely ill and high level of nurse dependency is required. Intensive therapy and/or intensive nursing care is needed because of the unstable condition of the patient. Frequent evaluation, observation, monitoring and adjustment of therapy is also required. A patient in these levels includes those in critical conditions or in life and death situations.

But whatever PCS is used, this will be applied to forecast staffing needs within each department. Nurses should be informed of the patient care ratios that are relevant to each department and should understand how to predict the staffing needs.

Diagnosis-Related Group (DRG) Patient Classification

The DRG system was created in 1983 to cut costs for medicare patients. The DRG system is a patient classification system that groups patients with similar diagnoses and/or procedures into the same category because the cost of care depends on the materials and procedures incurred to patients according to the diagnosis. For example, a patient with a fracture would be grouped to the Musculoskeletal Major Diagnostic Category. At this point, the patient is considered a medical DRG. If the patient has a surgical procedure, then the patient is grouped to a surgical DRG. The other factors that influence DRG assignment is age of the patient, any complication/morbidities, and discharge status. Thus patient's principal diagnosis and the procedures that they are treated with during hospital admission are used to select the group in the DRG classification that most appropriately describes the overall type of care that has been delivered.

Diagnosis-related groups (DRG) are a system classifying in-hospital patient cases into categories with similar resource use. The grouping is based on diagnoses, procedures performed, age, sex and status at discharge. The group selected is associated with a typical cost. Specifically, DRG funding requires the use of a cost weighting that is applied by the funding agency to determine the actual amount that should be paid to an institution for treating a patient with a particular DRG.

Purposes of DRG Method of Patient Classification System

- DRGs are used for reimbursement in the prospective payment system of Medicaid health care insurance systems.
- DRGs are designed to support the calculation of reimbursement.

Types

- *Self-care/minimal care:* The first classification of patients who are normal and mostly ambulatory and able to manage their care means the basic care. They are self-dependent and help themselves without nurses support. These category of patients require minimum nursing care hours. They require less observation, and monitoring.
- *Moderate care:* The patients are moderately ill in this category and waiting for recovery. These type of patients are guided and supported by nurses for early ambulation and self-care.
- *Maximum care:* Patients need maximum nursing care hours and medical supervision in this group in all shifts. They need constant monitoring, supervision and evaluation.

METHODS OF PATIENT ASSIGNMENT: ADVANTAGES AND DISADVANTAGES

One of the important functions of the head nurse who is the incharge of the unit is responsible for organizing the activities of staff nurses and other members of the ward to enhance quality of patient care for patients admitted in that unit. She is the frontline manager responsible to establish effective relationships and collaboration between the activities to be performed in that unit.

Definition of Assignment

Assignment is defined as a written document of assigning of tasks to render patient care for a group of patients by trained nursing personnel working in that ward.

Purposes of Assignment

- To distribute the work to be done for patient care to the nursing staff.
- To ensure the cooperation of the nursing personnel by knowing and accepting of the work to be done.

Principles of Personnel Assignment

Personnel assignment should be done by the head nurse or nurse incharge for each individual nurse assigned in that unit.

Assignments should be based on:

- Nursing hours required for each patient and type of care required.
- The staff nurses' qualification, experience and competencies, and interest.
- According to the job description provided to her during her induction period by the nurse administrator.
- The head nurse plans the assignments daily, weekly, and revised if necessary to ensure continuity of care.
- The head nurse plans assignment to staff nurses keeping in mind all the direct, indirect and unit activities.
- The head nurse also keeps in mind that the task assigned is balanced among all nursing staff.
- She ensures that the same task is not given to more than one nurse.

What are the Characteristics of Effective Assignment?

The assignment should be:

- Simple
- Easy to comprehend
- Clear and definite
- Written
- Signed by the head nurse
- Planned and communicated in advance.

Steps Involved in Organizing Patient Care

The head nurse carries out the following duties and responsibilities through applying the following five steps:

Planning

It is a process of forecasting the needs of patient and determines what tasks should be done, when, how, where, by whom (nurse) and to whom (patient).

Assigning

Delegating tasks of patient care and nursing activities that are written in the assignment sheet by the head nurse/ nurse incharge.

Leading

In this step, the head nurse implement the plan by communicating the tasks, motivation, supervision and coordination of activities, by making patients round, evaluating performance and conducting patient care and nursing care conferences.

Evaluating

The head nurse reviews nursing performance, patient progress and compare with the task given and written nursing care plan developed by the individual nurse.

Reporting

The head nurse prepares a nursing unit report in the report book in each shift which includes patient's needs,and problem when taken over from the previous shift nurse, medication and treatment given, diet, special observations, census, (admission, discharge, transfer in, transfer out, death) and general condition of the patient by bed, and handing over the report with patient to the next shift nurse.

Methods of Assignment

There are several methods of patient care assignment practiced in hospital. In general, there are two main classification:

- Traditional methods
- Advanced method.

Traditional Methods Include

- Case method
- Functional method
- Team method
- Modular nursing
- Primary nursing method.

Advance Method

Case management.

CASE METHOD (PATIENT METHOD OF ASSIGNMENT)

It is one of the oldest methods of organizing patient care. It means the assignment of one or more patients to a particular nurse for a specific period of time. (Fig. 10.1) She is responsible for the complete care including assessing vital signs, general nursing measures, treatment, medication administration nourishments and imparting health education, etc. Nurses assume total responsibility for meeting all the needs of assigned patients. When she goes off duty, another nurse takes over the patients/ patients. This method is widely used in hospitals and in nursing homes, private duty nurses, and specialty units such as ICU, ICU, etc.

Advantages

- This method ensures comprehensive care by meeting total needs of patients.
- More individualized nursing care is facilitated.
- Continuity of care can be facilitated.
- Patient/nurse interaction and rapport can be developed.
- Patient and family feel more safe and develop trust in nurse.
- Equal workload for nurses is possible.
- The nurse exercise a high degree of autonomy in care.
- The nurses are very clear about the line of authority and their accountability are clear.
- Patient receives unfragmented and total care
- Better patient education.
- Enhances patient satisfaction.
- Enhances nurse's satisfaction.

Disadvantages

- Many patients do not require the inherent care.
- Qualified nurses are always not available.
- Not cost-effective.

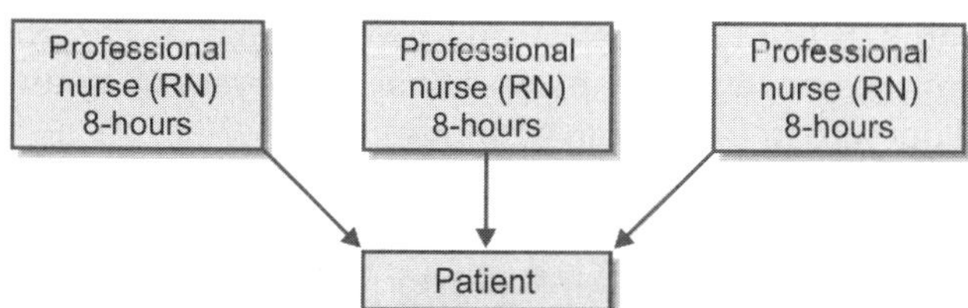

Fig. 10.1: Patient care method (case method) of assignment model (registered nurse organizes and performs all care to patient)

FUNCTIONAL METHOD OF PATIENT ASSIGNMENT

The functional method of delivering nursing care originated as a result of World War II. In 1950s, when few registered nurses and some practical nurses were available in many countries, most of the patient care was rendered by nurse's aides. Whereas the registered nurses were utilized with administrative and non-nursing responsibilities. Nurse's aides were assigned the majority of patient care. Unskilled workers were trained and assigned to complete certain tasks. For example, checking blood pressure changing linen, bathing patients, etc.

In this method, specific functions like giving medication or treatment to all patients were carried out by one nurse whereas the other nurse is assigned to take care of specimen collection and diet distribution. This method is usually practiced when there is shortage of nurses in the day or evening/night shift (Fig. 10.2).

Advantages of Functional Method of Assignment

- Nurse can become skilled in performing one particular assigned task.
- The best care can be given with available nurses with efficiency.
- Less equipment is needed as one nurse handles one type of task.
- This method saves time of nurses.
- Potential for development of technical skills.
- There is an improvement in nursing care.
- It is easy to organize the work of the unit and the nurses.
- Tasks are completed quickly.
- Useful in emergency situations.

Disadvantages

- Patient care become monotonous and mechanical.
- It may reduce the continuity of care.

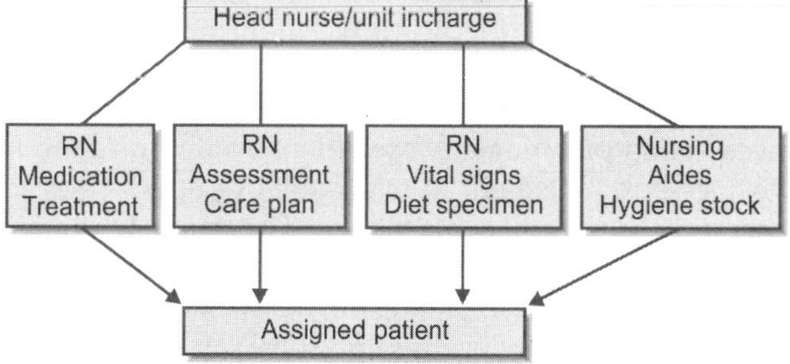

Fig. 10.2: Functional method of assignment model

- Staff may become demotivated because of one type of work for all patients.
- Work may become become unchallenged.
- The staff nurse are accountable for the task.
- Lack of feeling of security among patients.
- Only parts of the nursing care plan are known to personnel.
- Patient care may be given part by part by nurses.
- Patient may be disturbed and confused with many care providers.

TEAM METHOD OF PATIENT ASSIGNMENT

It is a method of nursing assignment that comprises of all personnel involvement in care of patients. This method utilizes all professionals, technical and nursing aids into small teams efficiently and effectively for patient care. The unit incharge becomes head of all teams who through the direct supervision, guidance, and teaching of professional nurses enhances patient care outcome. The fundamental aim of this method is to improve nursing services by utilizing the knowledge and skills of all professional nurses and supervise the work of auxiliary staff (Fig. 10.3). Thus in turn enhances in-patient and nurses satisfaction. Nursing aides collaborate in providing care to a group of patients under the direction of a professional nurse. Team nursing is based on the philosophy that supports the achievement of goals through group intervention.

How does Team Method of Assignment Work?

One registered nurse in the team is appointed by the head nurse to serve as a team leader. The team members commonly consist of at least one professional nurse, one technical nurse, nursing students (If a nursing school is attached to the hospital) and nursing aides. All team members receive reports about their patients' care needs from the team leader or team member from the previous shift. Each ward or nursing units may have two to three teams.

The main functions of team leader include administration of medications, monitors parenteral fluid therapy for all patients assigned to the team and supervision of any other intensive therapy. Team method needs good planning and execution. Communication is very essential element in team nursing, it is achieved through the team conferences. The team leader is responsible for knowing the condition and needs of all assigned patients. Depending on the workload, assisting the members and giving direct personal care to the patient which is determined by the team leader. The team leader usually assigns a professional nurse to care for the most seriously ill patients, to ensure informed observation and skilled interventions and the technical nurse to bath, feed, and move and change dressings for patients. Aides are assigned to make beds, assist ambulatory patients with bathing and grooming, back care, month care, testing urine and performing simple nursing care procedures.

Advantages

- High-quality comprehensive care is possible by team nursing by utilizing all members in the team.
- Team members actively participate in decision-making for care and imparts their own expertise in improving patient care.

Disadvantages

- When the team assignment changes every day, it affects the continuity of care.
- Team nursing fails when the team leader have inadequate leadership skills.
- It becomes difficult for the team leader to assign the patient during changing team membership.

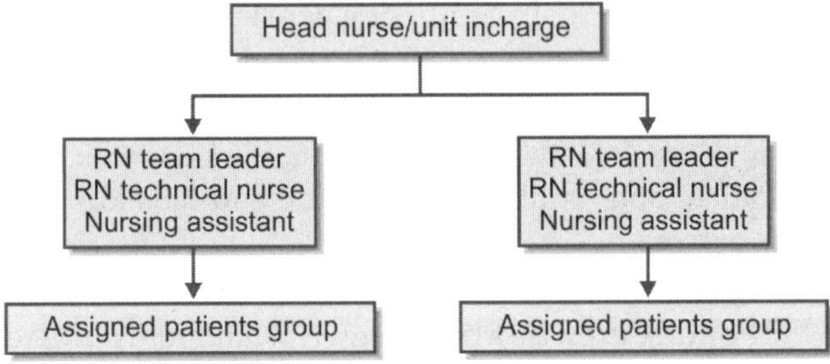

Fig. 10.3: Team method of assignment

MODULAR METHOD OF NURSING

In Modular nursing assignment, technical and nurse aides, as well as professional nurses are involved. In each module, two or three persons are assigned and, the professional nurse becomes responsible for the care of assigned patients (Fig. 10.4). The non-professional nurses are guided and trained by the professional nurse. Modular nursing is similar to team nursing because under the leadership of one professional nurse, the professional and non-professional employees work and cooperate in caring the patients.

Modular nursing is sometimes considered as similar to primary nursing because each group of nursing personnel are responsible for the care of the patients in their caseload from admission to discharge, following discharge and during subsequent admissions to the health facility.

Advantages

- Continuity of care is improved.
- Professional nurse becomes more responsible and engaged in planning, coordinating and collaborating care.
- Since the group works cohesively in one unit geographic closeness and efficient communication. is more possible.
- Develop leadership skills among professional nurses.
- Nurses identify more opportunities to learn and to teach.
- Patients fees secure as they are well aware of the nurses under whom they are cared.
- The professional nurse directs and guides for all patient care.
- Between professional and non-professional nurses the barriers are reduced.
- Everyone in the module has the opportunity to develop, contribute and execute to the care plan.

Disadvantages

- This assignment reduces cost effectiveness.
- Modular team members tends to change and that makes nursing care difficult.
- All personnel in the module needs to have effective skills and knowledge, i.e. communication, leadership.
- Since the modular leader is responsible and accountable for care given there is less individual member's responsibility and independence regarding nursing practice.

PRIMARY NURSING METHOD OF PATIENT ASSIGNMENT

In the early 1970, Primary nursing was evolved in some hospitals initiated by professional nurses. In primary nursing, the patient is the central focus (Fig. 10.5) not the task rendered. It is a well-planned, comprehensive, collaborative and coordinated nursing process that maintains continuity of care facilitated to meet the total needs of each patient.

The basic concept of primary nursing are:

- ***Patient assessment*** is made by a primary nurse, who plans the care that needs to be given by secondary or associate nurse when the primary nurse is off duty. The 24 hours responsibility for care is put into practice through the primary nurse's written directive on a preplanned communication assignment.
- ***Complete communication*** among nursing staff regarding the daily patient care by reporting method in oral and written way of communication.
- ***Discharge planning:*** The primary nurse ensures that discharge planning includes teaching, family involvement and providing appropriate references. That is the special feature of primary nursing.

How is Primary Nursing Method of Assignment Implemented?

- ***The head nurse:*** Assigns primary nurse to patients by assessing the skills of the nurse to the needs of the patients. She ensures proper scheduling for all shifts so that if primary nurse takes off in the unit an associate nurse is available for care. The head nurse also guides, counsels and evaluates care given. Sometimes she may also assign herself to patients either as a primary nurse or associate nurse.
- ***Primary nurse:*** who is professional staff nurse performs the following functions:
  - Conducts an admission assessment of patient
  - Develops, plans, implements, and revise the nursing care plan
  - Directs care in her absence to associate nurse
  - Collaborates with physicians and families
  - Makes referrals when needed
  - Teaches health concepts according to the need of the patient.
  - Makes discharge plans and interprets to patient
- ***Associate nurse*** is professional staff nurse or may be technical nurse. In the absence of the primary care nurse, associate nurse take care of the patients

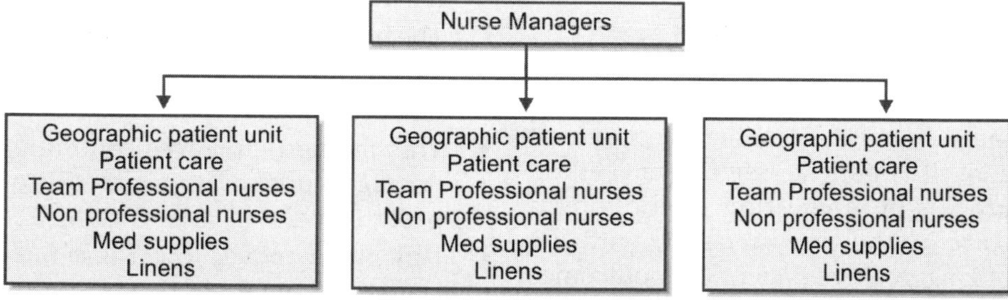

Fig. 10.4: Modular Method

according to the nursing care plan developed by the primary care nurse.

- *Technical nurse* carries out the nursing functions as assigned and directed by the primary or associate nurses in giving the care.
- *Nurse aides* carries out activities that are mostly non-nursing functions away from the direct care of patients like messengers or transporters.

Advantages

- Decreases the number of errors due to inadequate communication.
- This method enhances quality patient care outcome.
- Increases good interpersonal relationship among the team and with the patients.
- Professional nurses perceive this type of assignment more challenging and rewarding.
- Enhances job satisfaction among nurses and satisfaction of care among patients.
- As a result of good performance, nurses perceive good patient care outcome.

Disadvantages

- This type of assignment causes isolation of nurses from other nurses.
- It may be expensive.
- Nurse's expertise rendered to a limited number of patients.
- With the permission of primary nurse only the nursing care plan can be changed.

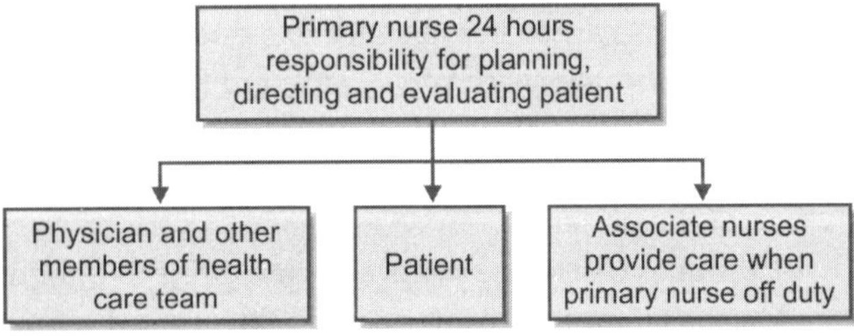

Fig. 10.5: Primary nursing

ADVANCE METHODS OR ALTERNATIVE METHODS OF PATIENT ASSIGNMENT

Case Management

One of the advanced methods of patient assignment is case management. It is patient assignment method described as a process of monitoring an individual patient's health care by the case manager, with the objective of optimizing positive patient care outcomes and cost-effectiveness. In order to become a case manager, she or he should be a graduate professional nurse or advanced level prepared nurse practitioner. The case manager role warrants not only advanced nursing skills but also advanced managerial and communication skills.

Case management is the coordination and collaboration of services rendered on behalf of an individual patient who is considered a case in different settings such as health care.

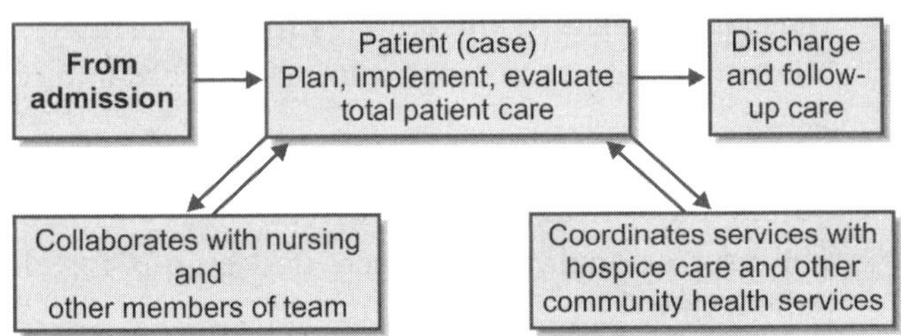

Fig 10.6: Nursing case management model

Responsibilities of a Case Manager

- The case manager may take over the patient from admission/the diagnostic phase throughout hospitalization, rehabilitation and back to home for follow-up care (Fig. 10.6).
- Case manager has responsibility and authority for planning, implementing, coordinating and evaluating patient care throughout the period of illness, sometimes movement from one unit to another (such as patient admission in emergency room, pediatric intensive care unit (PICU), pediatric surgical unit, observation unit, etc.)
- The case manager plans for care in advance. Through this plan, she/he assists with decision-making and helps to ensure that the patient receives care that will achieve the most positive outcomes in the most effective manner. This process helps to eliminate delays in progress.

Advantages of Case Management Method of Assignment

(a) For the patient:

- A standard or expected nursing care is achieved for the patient.
- The hospital length of stay of the patient is reduced.
- Using the minimal resources, maximal health care outcome is achieved.
- This method enhances continuity of patient care through collaborative practice of diverse health professionals.
- Patients are moved towards self-care, independence is fostered where indicated.

(b) For the nurse:

- This method facilitates for nurse's professional development and job satisfaction.
- Facilitates the transfer of knowledge of expert clinical staff to novice staff.

Disadvantages

- Discomfort to patients as they are followed up from admission to home care.
- Continuity of care is difficult as case managers may not always available.
- Long-term nurse-patient relationship are difficult to arrange.

PLANNING AND ORGANIZING HOSPITAL, HOSPITAL UNIT AND ANCILLARY SERVICES

Planning and Organizing Hospital

One of the important functions of nurse administrator is planning. While planning for hospital and hospital units, the nurse administrator must ensure whether the community needs a hospital or not. The need for a hospital can be estimated by two ways:

1. *Analytical method*: Data to be collected through survey, e.g. distributing questionnaire, taking feedback and analysis of data.
2. ***Estimation method:*** Planning is forecasting about and organizing the activities required to achieve a desired goal. When one plans for a hospital, he/she must be very sure about the expected outcome, expected activities, rationale to build a hospital, the site of hospital, time plan and the personnel responsible to complete the project.

The administrator must make sure that community interest is more than that of individual interest, preventive services are more beneficial over curative services. Since, the weaker section of the population is deprived of quality care services, the nurse administrator to prioritize for rendering services to rural population than urban.

What are the Data Required to Plan a Hospital?

- Demographic details of the community such as population, sex and age ratio and social status of the community.
- Educational level of the community served.
- Geographic data rural or urban community including morbidity and mortality status.
- Need and demand for health facility.
- Details of existing health care facilities.
- Financial feasibility to establish and run a hospital.

What are the Basic Needs to be Met by the Hospital?

- Hospital must meet the needs of the patients.
- The size and proportion of the hospital should be planned within the budget of the agency.
- Must have sound and safe architectural plan.
- Ensures economic viability.
- Maintains effective community orientation.
- Provides quality patient care.
- Facilitates research/innovation.

Basic Principles of Planning a Hospital

- Protection from unwanted and unnecessary noise and other disturbances in order to help speedy recovery of the patient admitted.
- Separation of dissimilar activities and control.
- The nurses' station should be planned in such a way to enable proper monitoring of visitors entering and leaving the ward.
- Infants and children should be protected from theft and infection, etc.
- All the departments of a hospital must be properly integrated to one another.
- Selection of site to be appropriate.
- Needs of the community to be identified and established.
- Ease of accessibility for patients and family.
- Range of services offered as per need.
- Availability of specialists throughout 24 hours a day and 7 days a week.
- Availability of technology.
- Study of existing hospital for getting an idea if any in neighborhood.
- Requirements of staff and services to be planned in advance and trained for special units.

Bed Planning and Financing

Number of beds can be calculated with the following formula:

Bed: Population = A × S × 100/365 × PO

A = Number of inpatient admissions/1000 population/year

S = Average length of stay

PO = Percentage occupancy.

- ***Planning of finances-once the number of beds are calculated:*** Identify funds required for constructing, furnishing and equipping the hospital. Various revenue generation process to be tapped such as bed charges, charges for diagnostic and treatment modalities. Planning for operating funds to be decided to pay salaries, loans and interest, supplies and other maintenance expenses.

Planning a Hospital Project in Stages

- ***Stage A functional content:*** The administrator proposes a brief–project team for assessment of functional content and is submitted to the owners (Government, private organization, etc.) for approval. The hospital site is appraised for floor areas, building space and the draft of master plan is prepared. With the help of financial experts, estimation of cost for each phase of construction is determined. Appraisal of work by owners is done.
- ***Stage B operational policies:*** In the next phase, plans are developed for operational policies, such as policies for departmental and inter-related activities, departmental and hospital policies, development control plan and budget cost. Periodical informal discussion with the agency also decided to appraise the progress of the work.
- ***Stage C schedules of accommodation, sketches, final cost estimate:*** Plans for accommodation, sketch drawing, equipment estimates, cost revenue and staffing estimates is to be prepared for final cost approval.
- ***Stage D Detail design working drawings, tender action:*** In this phase, drawing of the plan (blue print) is prepared, completed and decided for calling tenders.
- ***Stage E Contract and construction:*** Tenders are opened and assessed of tenders contract for work is given and construction completed and verified.
- ***Stage F commissioning:*** When the work is completed, employees are appointed. Equipment and supplies are assembled and tested for their functioning after installation.

Equipment Planning

- ***Built-in equipment*** include counters and cabinets in laboratory, pharmacy and other parts of the hospital, elevators, incinerators, coolers, fixed sterilizing equipment, etc .While planning itself these responsibilities included in the construction contract and to be carried out by the architect.
- ***Depreciable equipment*** includes equipment that has a life of five years or more and is not purchased through construction contracts. These are large pieces of furniture which have a relatively fixed location and are capable of being moved. For example, diagnostic and therapeutic equipment, laboratory instruments, office furniture, etc.
- ***Non-depreciable equipment*** are small items with a low unit cost and life span of less than five years. These are generally under the control of the hospital store and are bought through other than construction contracts. They include kitchen utensils, surgical instruments linen, waste baskets, stationaries, etc.

Hospital Noise Control Planning

Hospital administrators have a great responsibility to provide a noise free environment to patients and staff in hospital. Patient comfort, employee satisfaction and environmental concerns are always at the forefront in the continuous design and maintenance of a wide array of systems that keeps a medical facility running efficiently.

PLANNING INTENSIVE CRITICAL CARE UNIT (ICU) IN A HOSPITAL

The location of intensive critical care unit (ICU) should be on the ground floor. It should have a convenient access to operation theater, emergency unit and easy accessibility to wards. This unit constitutes of patient area, staff area, support area.

Four Basic Requirements of an ICU

1. Provision for monitoring the patients' directly by doctors and nurses.
2. Provision for continuous physiological monitoring.
3. Adequate space required for efficient use of routine and emergency diagnostic procedures and interventions.
4. Both manual and electronic documentation facilities to record patient's health status.

Design and Layout of ICU

When design and layout of ICU is to be planned, the integration and smooth functioning of, the patient area, the staff area and the support area to be considered. Per patient or per bed 350–500 Sq ft area is required that comprises circulation area, nursing station and sanitary and ancillary services (areas).

Ancillary and Support Services

- Preferably this area should be centrally air conditioned.
- With regards to light in ICU, it is preferred for subdued illumination for the patient bed with capacity for increasing it in case of need.
- For patient bed, proper light to be facilitated. Main light at the bed head should be fitted with dimmer switch.

- A high intensity emergency light or spot focusing light should also be provided to do procedures at the time of emergency.
- Facility to be made to have an emergency buzzer switch connected to central buzzer and location panel at central nursing station.
- Multiple electrical gadgets required to meet all the above.
- In ICU, a standby generator is required when there is a fluctuation of electric supply or no supply to avoid delay in treatment.
- For diagnostic support, there should be round the clock access to laboratory services.
- Radiology imaging should be accessible to ICU.
- Physiotherapy department near to ICU may help the patient for rehabilitation.
- Equipment maintenance to be done periodically. preventive maintenance is good for efficiency, effectiveness and economy of equipment material management.
- There should be proper visitor lounge with basic facilities.
- The temperature of the ICU to be maintained as per norm.

Organization of ICU services

- **Intensive care** is defined as the provision of advanced life support with modern technological equipment that are mostly available in tertiary care facilities for a variety of adult and pediatric patients. The patients require constant and close medical and nursing monitoring. There is guideline available to care for such patients in hospital policy manual and this manual is given to ICU nurses and doctors.
- **ICU planning committee:** The members of the ICU planning committee include medical superintendent, nursing superintendent, Head of the department, Anesthetist CPWD Architect, surgeon, neurosurgeon, physician, and pediatrician and other members as per policy manual.
- **Decision-making:** The planning committee is responsible to make policy decision regarding critical care needs of the hospital. Type and size of the ICU, appointment of ICU incharge. Appointment of ICU matron, planning, designing and physical facilities. Guidelines, policies and procedure in ICU functioning and patient evaluation. Pre-requisite training is very necessary for nursing and medical and supportive staff prior to placement in ICU. Beds, ICU equipment and supplies are procured in advance. Protocols for monitoring and life support techniques to be established before commissioning and opening of ICU.

Designing ICU

There are various types of design utilized structuring ICU such as:

- Circular placement of beds with central nursing station
- Rectangular with central monitoring system.
- Semi-circular with monitoring station at the front
- L shaped ICU with central nursing station. The lay-out design depends on the availability of space and number of beds planned for ICU.

Physical Facilities Needed in ICU

For effective functioning of ICU, the following physical facilities are suggested in ICU:

- Patient area, (Patient bed space and equipment) as already mentioned above.
- Broad corridor at entrance to carry patients in stretcher.
- Separate toilet facilities to be provided for male and female.
- There should be a reception counter, to receive patients, visitors and families.
- ICU needs to maintain free from infection, therefore a changing room, shoes, gown and mask to be facilitated for doctors and nurses.
- Entrance double door swinging 5′ – 6′ width to carry patients in trolly/wheelchair.
- There must be telephone, facilities.
- A visitors lounge 2 sq ft/ visitor to be provided.
- There should be snack bar or coffee shop.
- Nursing monitoring station with all facilities including toilet facilities.
- Hand washing facilities with plenty of water availability is a must in ICU.
- Wall mounted call bell system is required for emergency situation.

Bed Space

Sufficient bed space is required for each bed for free movement of the nurse/doctor and keeping ventilator, monitoring system and other equipments. They are required for each bed 100–120 sq ft in open ICU and 140–180 sq ft in cubicle. Minimum of 15 sq ft of clean area to be planned Head wall space 1–2 ft and space between two beds 5–8 ft is recommended. The cubicles must have glass partitions or transparent curtains for clear observation from nursing/monitoring station.

Bed Head Fixtures and Call Bell System

High intensity spotlight connected to generator is advisable for wall panels and call button near the bed is mandatory. Sufficient electric sockets to be made for plugging. Wall suction tubes and piped oxygen supply. Small wash basin is necessary with continuous water supply. No extension wire to be used. Equipments with CV stabilizer/UPS to be installed.

- *Equipment:* Ventilators, fluids stand defibrillator, pulse oximeters monitor and minor procedure trolley infusion pump and dialysis machine and other equipment as needed.
- *Nursing station:* Central monitoring system counter, must have the facilities like keeping case records and essential drugs. Complete visibility of all patients needs to be ensured. Two way communication/ intercom system to be available.
- *Facilities in ICU:* The ICU requires the following facilities such as auxiliary area, medication and nursing area, isolation room/area, pantry, clean and dirty utility room, doctor's duty room, dressing room, store room, equipment maintenance and nurses changing area.

Staff Required Per Shift

- *Nursing staff:* Ideally 1:1 ratio during day and 1:2 during night. Broadly 4–5 nurses per bed including reliever is recommended. One assistant matron for administration of the unit or specialized unit incharge to be posted.
- *Medical staff:* One physician per 5 beds round the clock, consultant ICU to be available on routine and on call—one senior resident and two junior resident per shift is recommended.
- *Technical staff:*
  - Respiratory therapist: One
  - Physiotherapist: One
  - ICU technician: One
  - Lab oratory technician: One
  - OT assistant: One
  - Safety officer: One per shift is recommended
- *Ancillary staff:*
  - Receptionist: One
  - Ward boy: four
  - Stretcher bearers: two
  - Sweepers: Two per shift is recommended

Quality assurance in ICU to be maintained with the objectives.

- To enhance high standard of care, keeping in mind hygiene and cleanliness throughout care.
- To prevent hospital acquired infection.
- To ensure proper treatment.
- To ensure hospital waste management.
- To monitor daily maintenance/checking of vital equipments/inventory.
- To prioritize on patient comfort and safety.
- To conduct exit interview of patients and relatives so as to appraise the standard and quality of care given.

SUMMARY POINTS

- ✓ The patient classification system (PCS) is a method that arranges the patients in groups according to the amount and complexity of their nursing care needs. It serves as an administrative device to evaluate patient needs, nurses' interventions, and the competency required in meeting those needs of patients. It is patient-acuity systems, used for managing and planning the allocation of nursing staff according to the nursing care needs. This is a managerial tool to assist nurse administrators to calculate workload requirements and staffing needs.
- ✓ One of the important activities of the head nurse who is at the first-line management position of nursing service department is organizing the activities of the staff nurses and other members in the ward to make a pattern to meet patient needs.
- ✓ Traditionally, patient care assignment, functional method of assignments, team method, modular method and primary nursing care model were used and still these methods are used in our country according to the availability of staff nurses. Modern approach to patient care delivery system is case management model in which a professional registered nurse take care of the patient from admission to resolution of illness by collaborating with members of the health care team and coordinating with community health care agencies. All methods have their own advantages and disadvantages.
- ✓ Primary nursing is done by professional nurses. It is a comprehensive, continuous and coordinated nursing process for meeting the total needs of each patient based on the philosophy of that patient, instead tasks. It is a holistic approach model of care.

✓ The nurse administrator plays an important role in planning a hospital or hospital units. She is the right person to advise the planning committee regarding the infrastructure required for total patient care especially the layout of wards, nursing station, facilities for patients and nurses, equipment and supplies for nursing care staffing structure and policies. Therefore, she must possess a good knowledge on hospital planning.

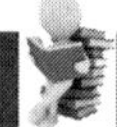

REVIEW QUESTIONS

1. Define patient classification system (PCS). Differentiate functional and team method of patient assignment.
2. Enlist the purposes of patient classification system. Discuss any one of the common types of patient classification in detail.
3. Describe various patient classification methods with their advantages and disadvantages.
4. Describe the role of nurse administrator in planning an intensive care unit in a hospital.
5. Write short notes on the following:
   a. DRG classification of patient care
   b. Modular method of assignment
   c. Case management
   d. Planning a hospital
   e. Equipment and supplies for intensive care unit.

SELECTED READINGS

1. Case management - Wikipedia, the free encyclopedia.
   https://en.wikipedia.org/wiki/case_management.
2. Definition and Philosophy of Case Management I CCMC
   http://ccmcertification.org/about-us/about-case management/definition-and-philosophy-case management.
3. Diagnosis Related Groups (DRGs)
   http://www.powershow.com/view/3c554d-ZjJhY/Diagnosis_Related_Groups_DRGs
4. From the staff development bookshelf: Patient classification systems to coordinate patient care. Staff Development Weekly: *Insight on Evidence-Based Practice in Education,* April 20, 2012.
5. Hospital Administration Made Easy. http//hospiad.blogspot.com
6. Patient Care Delivery System - Home - KSU Faculty Member websites
   http://faculty.ksu.edu.sa/hanan_alkorashy/nursing management 489nur/10.
7. Patient Classification Systems Address Nurse Staffing Balance.
   http://healthleadersmedia.com/technology

11

Power and Politics in an Organization

LEARNING OBJECTIVES

This chapter imparts learning about:

- Concept of Power and Politics
- Types of Power Used in Nursing Administration
- Factors Contributing to Political Behavior in Nursing
- Role of Nurse Administrator in Power and Politics

CONCEPT OF POWER

When an individual uses his ability to achieve his goal in a manner in which he desires from other individuals or his subordinates is referred as power. French and Raven (1962) state the fundamental principle of power is control over the behavior of their employees by the virtue of the position in an organization, the administrator derive power called position power and from individual capability when derive power is called personal power. The more the employees are dependent, the administrator exercises more power on them. Therefore, it is sometimes mentioned that power of dependency, leadership and power are related to each other in the context of an organization. Leaders utilize power to achieve goals of the group. Power does not take interest in goal achievement. Leadership emphasizes the influence of followers that is downward in nature whereas power emphasizes the top and lateral influence in an establishment.

Various Types of Power Used in Nursing Service Administration

- *Formal power:* It is vested on the position that an individual occupies in an establishment. This individual has the formal authority to get the work done or reward the other individuals by the virtue of his or her formal power in hierarchy. For example, a nursing administrator may transfer, or demote a staff nurse who does not perform her task as the administrator wants. Formal power is described in subsections as Coercive power, Reward power, *Coercive power:* In this power, the administrator uses threat or develops fear among the subordinates. That creates frustration among the subordinates. This power is used by any individual who occupies a higher position in an organization, has the power to dismiss, suspend, or demote another person.
  - *Reward power:* It is the power utilized as just reverse of coercive power. It is an ability of the administrator to use rewards to control the subordinate. Many administrators use this power to enhance quality patient care and morale of the employee. In nursing, some of the rewards given to nurses are promotion, increment, sponsorship for higher studies, etc.
- *Informal power:* This power is personal power based on the intelligence and expertize in the work setting and does not care for the position in an organization.

- *Expert power:* It is the capability to control a subordinate by the knowledge, attitude, experience and expertize in the field of working among administrator that the subordinate does not possess. A staff nurse obeys the ward sister because the ward sister knows better about what to do and how to do than the staff nurse in a particular situation.
- *Referent power:* Many a times, the subordinates appreciate or like the working of their supervisor or administrator. These subordinates want to imitate or want to become like their supervisor. Thus, referent power is the ability to control subordinate's because the subordinate wants to be like the supervisor having the power.
- *Charismatic power:* It is like the referent power. It develops in an individual from his/her personality, interpersonal and leadership style. The subordinates follow the administrator or leader because they can express, involve and participate with such type of administrator or leader in all organizational activities.

  Dependency is the key component to power. There are three factors that are responsible for dependency:
  - *Importance:* When a matter is more important, it creates more dependency.
  - *Scarcity:* When a resource material is scarce, it creates more dependency.
  - *Non-substitutability:* When a thing has no practical substitute, the dependency on that thing increases.

Power Tactics

Today, nurse administrators are facing a great challenge to achieve the desired goal using their power. The most common methods to maintain relationship with employees (Kipnis et. al, 1984) are:

- *Reason:* The administrators utilize facts and figures to present his/her ideas in logical manner.
- *Friendliness:* Sometime the administrators use, flattery, goodwill, humble behavior and demonstrate friendliness to subordinates.
- *Coalition:* It is a method or technique to get the cooperation of other individuals in the establishments.
- *Bargaining:* To prevent negative aspects or complicating the event in the organization negotiation can be used.
- *Assertiveness:* It is technique to get the work completed by a forceful approach.
- *Higher authority:* It refers to obtain facilities and cooperation from the top level of individuals in the organization.
- *Sanctions:* In power tactics, rewards and punishments are introduced in the organization.
- *Empowerment:* The process by which the administrators give subordinates the power and the power to make decisions affecting their work and themselves, this is called empowerment. The organizational structure where decentralization is found, employees empowerment also seen. Employees' empowerment helps in making fast decision and getting the work done effectively.
- **Changing position power** requires employees training in use of empowered position correctly. They also should clearly know the authority, responsibility and accountability process. When power is given to subordinate, without clear-cut understanding of a position they tend to misuse the power and it may be detrimental to organization.

POLITICS

Politics is the manner by which people use their power in the organization. The administrator uses politics in an organization to overcome employees deficiencies and inadequacies; to cope with emerging trends and changes and to improve staff morale. There are many reasons for demonstrating political behavior in an organization. Some of them are scarcity of resources non-programmed decisions, ambiguous goals of the organization, technological changes, greed of power, stagnation on career, and other psychological factors.

Legitimate Political Behavior

Legitimate political behavior is common politics we experience in all organization like complaining to supervisor, groupism, etc. This type of behavior breaks the norms and values of the organization, for example damaging the property of the work setting, or speaking against the organization. A literature review on organizational politics observed that there are two philosophies describe about organizational politics: The first philosophy is based on Machiavelli's philosophy that means politics are originated in terms of self-interest of the administrator and they use non-authorized means to achieve the goals. The second philosophy believes politics as an essential function that originates from the differences in the self-interests of individuals in an organization.

Factors Contributing to Political Behavior

- *Individual factors:* Political behavior of an individual is based on his personality traits, his needs and other factors. Employees who demonstrates high self-monitors, have an internal control. These individuals are predicted for political behavior. The individuals who demonstrates the high self-monitor character is liable to be skilled in political behavior than the low self-monitor individuals.

- *Organizational factors:* Organizational cultures are basic for affecting political behavior. The organization where the employees perceive low trust, unclear performance, unsatisfactory evaluation system, high pressure for performance, demonstrate a high degree of political behavior.

ROLE OF NURSE ADMINISTRATOR TO DEAL WITH THE EFFECTS OF POLITICS IN ORGANIZATION

The nurse administrators may take the following three plan of operations to manage politics in an organization:

1. Avoid the situation, stick on to the rules and policies of the organization action and risk taking
2. Redirect accountability and responsibility to employees
3. Defend their turf.

- *Avoidance:* It is a very common strategy taken by administrators. They avoid the situation and strictly adhere to the rules, policies, and procedures and show no deviations or exceptions.
- *Redirecting responsibility:* It is another strategy where the administrator uses tactics when there is a problem that affects his/her reputation and he/ she may likely to protect herself. Since, the administrator is very sensitive to politics, the responsibility is redirected to employees.
- *Defending turf:* It results from the competition of each department in the organization. The organization is a collection of competing interests held by various departments and groups. As each group tries to increase its influence, it starts to encroach on the activities of other groups.

Nursing research has been able to demonstrate the relationship between the first two components and empowerment; yet there remains a need for research to examine the power that exists in relationships. Nursing research from a relational theory perspective may help to make nurses' power more explicit and more visible and politics play an important role in administration.

SUMMARY POINTS

- ✓ Power is the ability of individuals or groups to make their own concerns or interests even where others resist. Power sometimes involves the direct use of force, but is almost always also accompanied by the development of ideas whereas politics is a process involving the exercise of control, constraint and coercion in society.
- ✓ Power may arise from three components: A workplace that has the requisite structures that promote empowerment; a psychological belief in one's ability to be empowered; and acknowledgement that there is power in the relationships and caring that nurses provide. The nurse administrator has a role in bringing power and politics for positive patient care outcome and staff management.
- ✓ Politics is the manner by which people use their power in the organization.
- ✓ The administrator uses politics in an organization to overcome employees deficiencies and inadequacies; to cope with emerging trends and changes and to improve staff morale.
- ✓ There are many reasons for demonstrating political behavior in an organization. Some of them are scarcity of resources. non-programmed decisions, ambiguous goals of the organization, technological changes, greed of power, stagnation on career, and other psychological factors.

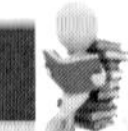

REVIEW QUESTIONS

1. Differentiate power and politics.
2. Discuss various types of power used in nursing service administration.
3. Define empowerment. Write a paragraph on empowered nursing service administrator.
4. Discuss factors influencing political behavior in administration.
5. Discuss the role of nurse administrator to deal with the effects of politicking.
6. Write short notes on the following:
    a. Expert power
    b. Coercive power

c. Referent power
d. Power tactics
e. Assertiveness
f. Legitimate political behavior.

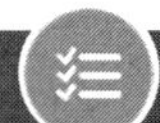

SELECTED READINGS

1. Perceptions of organizational politics
GR Ferris, KM Kacmar - Journal of management, 1992 - jom.sagepub.com
2. Power and politics in organizations - SlideShare http://www.slideshare.net/mdfaizan/power-politics-in-organizations 10 Jul 2011 ...
3. Power and politics - SlideShare http://www.slideshare.net/TasneemKanchwala/power-and-politics-10250528 21 Nov 2011 ...
4. Power to Influence Patient Care - American Nurses Association
http://www.nursingworld.org/MainMenuCategories/ANAMarketplace/ANAPeriodicals/OJIN/TableofContents/Volume122007/No1Jan07/tpc32ntr16088.html 31 Jan 2007 ...
5. Power, Politics, and Nursing in the United Kingdom http://ppn.sagepub.com/content/3/2/108.short
6. Power</i> of Professional Nursing Practice – An Essential Element ...
http://www.nursingworld.org/MainMenuCategories/ANAMarketplace/ANAPeriodicals/OJIN/TableofContents/Volume122007/No1Jan07/tpc32_316092.html 31 Jan 2007
7. The Role of Nurses in Politics and Health Policy | NurseTogether.com
http://www.nursetogether.com/role-nurses-poPlitics-and-health-policy 28 May 2012.

UNIT V
STAFFING

12

Staffing and Scheduling

LEARNING OBJECTIVES

This chapter imparts learning about:

- Concept, Definition, Philosophy of Staffing and Scheduling
- Staffing Norms: Staff Inspection Unit (SIU), Bajaj Committee, High Power Committee, Indian Nursing Council (INC)
- Estimation of Nursing Staff Requirement: Activity Analysis
- Research Highlights

INTRODUCTION

Quality patient care is very much depends upon the number of health care professional available to provide care. Like money and materials; human resource is an important component that determines the organizational success. It is the responsibility of the nurse administrator to estimate staffing and scheduling in Nursing service administration.

CONCEPT, DEFINITION, PHILOSOPHY OF STAFFING AND SCHEDULING

Concept of Staffing

Staffing is the series of activities of providing nursing personnel in quality and quantity for effective nursing care. Quality includes qualification and experience of nursing personnel and quantity means the number of nurses required as per statutory norms. The series of activities include recruiting, selecting, placing in right position, and retaining nursing personnel to achieve positive impacts on the organizations effectiveness. McFarland explains that staffing is a managerial function to recruit, select and develop staff as capable persons to build an organization.

The term 'Staffing' denotes to the recruitment, selection, development, training and compensation of the nursing personnel. Staffing, like all other managerial functions, is the duty which the high level executives perform at all times. According to_Koontz, O'Donnell and Heinz Weihrich, staffing is a management function in the organization structure through identifying staffing requirements, and utilize them effectively that include, recruitment, selection, placement, promotion, appraisal, compensation, and training of needed employees.

Staffing also interpreted as Human Resource Management (HRM). HRM is the management process of combining various activities that are designed to enhance the effectiveness of the manpower in an organization in the achievement of organizational goals. Human Resource Management (HRM) may be defined as the function of planning for human resource needs, recruitment, selection, development, compensation and evaluation of performance to fill those needs.

Staffing ensures that the organization has the required number of people and the needed kind of people at the right places, at the desired time, and that they are skilful to do the services. Importance of stalling helps in identifying and getting the right personnel who for higher performances, by putting their effort for various jobs. Staffing ensures the continuous survival helps in the growth of the establishment through the succession planning for managers.

Definitions of Staffing

Staffing is an important function of the management. Staffing is a task of managing the activities in an organization; the management is in a position to know the manpower requirements of the establishment at different levels and take necessary steps for recruitment, selection, training and placement of employees.

Staffing is a continuous process because existing employees may leave the organization and new employees may join it. Therefore, any type of organization has to recruit additional managerial and operative force to meet the growing requirements of the enterprise.

According to Koontz and O'Donnell staffing involves manning the organization structure through proper and effective selection, appraisal and development of personnel to fill the roles designed into the structure.

According to Theo Heimann, staffing is concerned with the placement, growth and development of all those members of the organization whose function is to get the things done through the efforts of other individuals.

Purposes of Staffing

- To estimate the type and amount of service needed by the hospital patients.
- To decide the categories of nursing personnel that have the knowledge and skill to perform needed services for patients.
- To forecast the number of personnel in each job category that will be needed to meet anticipated service demands of the health facility.
- To plan and obtain, budgeted positions for the number in each job category needed to service.
- To recruit nursing personnel to fill available positions.
- To select and to appoint nursing personnel from suitable applicants.
- To plan scheduling nurses for each shift for complete coverage of care of patients.
- To assign responsibilities for client services.
- To ensure efficient performance of planning, organizing, directing.
- To facilitate effective use of controlling functions of management.
- To motivate and develop nurses for better performance.
- To determine maximum utilization, assess training needs and forecast future needs of nurses.

Philosophy of Staffing

The nurse administrators believe that:

- Qualified and experienced nursing personnel with adequate knowledge, attitude and clinical practice skill enhance quality patient care outcome.
- Professional nurses are competent to ensure quality and safety care to the completely and partially dependent patients because their health needs and problems are complex in nature. The professional nurses are prepared to provide comprehensive nursing care including rehabilitative care.

Nurse administrators accept the fact that:

- Professional and technical nurses need to update their knowledge through continuing education periodically.
- Periodical criterion-based performance appraisal of nursing personnel is important to improve the knowledge and skills of nurses.

Nurse administrators recognize that:

- Estimation of staff requirement should be based on work load of nurses, job analysis and periodical studies done on nursing care hours required by different categories of patients
- Master staffing plan and policies to implement the plan in all units should be developed centrally by the nursing service department of the hospital.
- Staffing process completes only when scheduling of nurses for each shift is determined.
- Rewards and incentives for exemplary nursing services motivates nurses to improve their work

Scheduling

- Scheduling is one of the staffing function of the administrator It is planned in advance keeping in mind the holidays, days off and night offs nurses who are on leave, emergencies in hospital, etc. In some places it is called duty roaster.
- Nurses are the vital workforce in healthcare delivery system. They are very important workforce in the hospital establishment providing round the clock services, whereas physicians have separate system of work. The working shift pattern vary from hospital

to hospital. A three shift pattern is followed in most of the hospitals in the country, depending upon the number of nurses for patient care and, availability of transportation for nurses specially during odd hours the scheduling may differ. In some states in some of the hospitals nurses prefer two shifts and they are compensated with additional days off and nights off. The nurse administrator has a great responsibility in planning and scheduling duty hours for nurses without interfering the quality of care and nurses' morale.

Definition of Scheduling

- It is an activity of the nurse administrator to assign an appropriate number nursing personnel to the each service unit/ward for 24 × 7 days of care. She/he has to determine when an activity should start or end, depending on its hours of the shift e.g. 8 hours shift, and availability of other nurses like technical nurses for each day.
- It is planned for a time period mostly weekly and monthly. It comprises of assigning hours of work, place of work and responsible role for a period of week or month. Many times the work place remains the same but the shift changes.

The functions of Nurse Administrator in Scheduling

- Scheduling plan or duty roaster to be planned in advance
- Distribution of nursing personnel should be balanced as per nursing care hours required by patient
- List the nursing units and determine the maximum and minimum work load of each unit
- Make a list of nursing personnel according to their cadre, position, qualification, experience and specialization
- Determine the number of nursing personnel required for each unit in total and shift wise allocation
- Consider holidays, leave application of nursing staff, any special program planned in hospital etc.
- Refer Personnel manual for eligibility for days off, nights off nd compensatory off. Per week
- Allocate number of nurses for all units and communicate in written to all unit managers or head nurses to prepare shift schedule.

Role of Unit Managers or Head Nurses While Preparing Schedule Plan

- Study types of patients with degree of illness including, admission days, discharging days and operation days
- Study nursing care hours required in morning, evening and night
- Plan weekly schedule
- Plan should be flexible for meeting any emergencies
- Refer leave plan if any during that week given by nurses
- If possible, respect the shift preference by nurses
- Plan for 8 hours duty or as the policy of the hospital
- Provision for days off and extra off particularly in 12 hours shift
- Communicate to each staff nurse, get their signature and file it. Put a copy of the schedule in ward bulletin board.

Box 12.1: Sample of philosophy of staffing as a function of nursing service administration

The nursing service administration believes that:

- Nursing personnel working in the hospitals are our most valuable assets. To foster a quality work environment and maximum patient care outcome, the nursing service department estimates the staff requirements in quality and quantity and utilize them by effective personnel policies.
- The hospitals provides a quality HR services to attract, develop, motivate educate , empower and retain nurses with a supportive work environment for the purpose of enhancing quality care to patients collaborating nursing service department.

The nursing service administration accepts the fact that

- The nurses of today are the leaders of nursing tomorrow. Keeping in mind the nursing service department provides leadership development along with periodical continuing education program for nurses time to time to enhance their professional knowledge, attitude and competency.
- Nurses caring very critically ill patients may experience stress and less coping situation. and other nursing related issues. The nursing service department provides confidential assessment, counseling and crisis intervention management as and when needed to nursing personnel.

The nursing service administration recognizes that

- Facilitating job satisfaction among nurses is the key to patient safety and quality care. The nursing service administration emphasizes creating and fostering a positive work environment for nurses and patients that attracts and inspires excellence in care
- Rewards and incentives for exemplary nursing services motivate nurses to improve their work. For the purpose of boosting the morale of nurses and organizational effectiveness nursing personnel are appreciated with rewards, sponsorship for higher studies, increment and promotional services.

Table 12.1 Example of a schedule plan from Mon-Sun day 2nd Jan to 8th Jan 2015

Nurses	Mon Jan 2, 2015	Tue Jan 3, 2015	Wed Jan 4, 2015	Thurs Jan 5, 2015	Fri Jan 6, 2015	Sat Jan 7, 2015	Sun Jan 8, 2015
A	7–11 12–4	7–12 4–7	7–7	12–7	7–11 12–4	7–12 4–7	Off
B	Off	7–7	12–7	7–11 12–4	7–12 4–7	7–11 12–4	7–12 4–7
C	7–7	Off	7–11 12–4	7–12 4–7	7–11 12–4	7–12 4–7	12–7
D	12–7	7–12 4–7	Off	7–11 12–4	7–12 4–7	7–7	7–12 4–7
E	7–11 12–4	7–12 4–7	7–11 12–4	Off	12–7	7–11 12–4	7–7
Beds	25	24	25	25	24	24	25

Signature of Head Nurse

Fig Sample schedule format for 25 bedded ward with 5 staff nurses, and 1 Head nurse. Head nurse does general duty and evening duty alternate days and takes off on Sundays. 7–7 = night shift, 7–4 afternoon shift, 7–12 and 4–7 evening shift

STAFFING NORMS: STAFF INSPECTION UNIT (SIU), BAJAJ COMMITTEE, HIGH POWER COMMITTEE, INDIAN NURSING COUNCIL (INC)

Staffing norms are standards that direct, guide, regulate and control the number of employees needed in an organization. As a nurse administrator when she/he plans for staffing must know norms for staffing as recommended by various health committees. This chapter highlights norms recommended for staffing in hospitals by Indian Nursing Council, (INC). Bajaj committee, High power committee and Staff Inspection Unit (SIU).

Staffing Norms Recommended by Indian Nursing Council

- Chief Nursing Officer ....1 per 500 beds
- Nursing Superintendent......................1 for 400 beds
- Deputy Nursing Superintendent............1 for 300 beds
- Assistant Nursing Superintendent...............1 (for every 200 beds)
- Ward sister..1 (for 25 30 beds)
- Staff nurse..........................1:3 Beds (Teaching hospital) 1:5 Beds (non-teaching Hospital)
- Staff Nurse for ICU/CCU..1:1

Staffing Norms for Group-D Employees

- Bed ratio Hospital Attendant................1 per 10 beds
- Sanitation Attendant...............................1 per 10 beds
- Security Guard.......................................1 per 15 beds

Staffing Norms for Hospital Laboratory Services

- One laboratory personnel (inclusive of supervisory staff) should perform 8000—10000 tests per annum.
- Laboratories where automation introduced in the laboratory work, the manpower requirement 1 for 20000 tests per person per annum.
- Ratio of supervisor for technical staff....................1:4
- Ratio of technical staff for lab attendant................1:3

Staffing Norms for Blood Bank

- One blood bank technician for every 8000–10000 investigations per annum.
- One technician for every 15000—20000 preparations per annum for component preparations.

Staffing Norms for Radio Imaging Department

- A radiographer should be able to do 12–15 cases in an hour.
- For every four radiographers there should be 1 technical assistant.
- One technical supervisor is required for 8 radiographers to supervise and perform radiography related functions.

Staffing Norms for Electrocardiogram (ECG) Technicians

- One technician and one machine for every 50 ECGs done daily in the OPD.
- One technician and one machine for ECGs in each 20 hour shift for in patient.

Staffing Norms for CSSD

- Staffing norms for CSSD for 750—1000 bedded hospital
- CSSD Supervisor/Manager..1
- Superintendent/Asstt. Supervisor 1
- CSSD Asstt. Grade-I/ Sr.CSSD Operators 6
- CSSD Asstt. Grade-II/ Jr.CSSD Operators 6
- CSSD Attendants...30

Staffing Norms for Laundry Personnel

- Staffing norms for laundry department for 750—1000 bedded hospital
- Laundry Manager/Supervisor..................................1
- Asstt. Laundry Supervisor...3
- Laundry Clerk/LDC..2
- Laundry Operator..30
- Laundry Attendant 1
- Laundry Mechanic...2
- One laundry operator .... for 30 beds

- Average laundry load .... 3–4 kg of soiled linen per patient.
- Operation theater laundry load .... 7–8 kg of linen per operation

Staffing Norms for Dietary Department

- Staffing Norms for Dietary Department for 750–1000 bedded hospital
- Chief Dietician... 1
- Asstt. Dietician 3
- Technical Dietician (Jr. Dietician)............................ 2
- Clerk (LDC)... 2
- Store Keeper.. 1
- Steward/Floor Supervisor... 2
- Head Cook 4
- Cook.. 16
- Cook Aid/Helper... 16
- Bearer.. 24

STAFFING NORMS BY STAFF INSPECTION UNIT (SIU)

The Staff Inspection Unit (SIU) was established in the year 1964 by the Government of India with the objectives of achieving economy in the staffing of Government organizations in accordance with administrative efficiency and developing performance standards and work norms for employees. With regards to nursing, SIU calculated the required nursing personnel and other staff based on the workload observed in service units and wards

- Chief Nursing officer........................... 1 for 500 beds
- Nursing superindent........................... 1 for 250 beds
- Deputy Nursing superindent.............. 1 for 5–7 ANS
- Assistant Nursing superindent...........1 for 4 head nurses
- Ward sister .... 1 for 3–6 staff nurses SIU Recommended 45% of Additional Staff to Make up Leave, Holidays, Days off

SIU recommended the following nurse patient ratio:

- General ward 1:6
- Special wards... 1:4
- Nursery.. 1:2
- Intensive care Units 1:1
- Labor Room ....1:1 per Table
- Operation Theater (Major O T) 1:2 per table (Minor O T) 1-:1 per table
- Casualty.. 1:1
- Gynecology, OBG.. 1:1
- Outpatient department for 100 patients............1 Staff nurse
- 120–220 patients ....2 Staff nurses
- 221–320 patients ....3 Staff nurses
- 321–420 patients .... 4 Staff nurses

OP Departments

- Blood bank, Eye, ENT .... 1 staff nurse each
- Pediatrics, immunization.............. 2 staff nurse each

Staff nurse is recommended in the following departments:

- Preanesthetic room 1
- Cardio lab...1
- Biochemistry lab...1
- Vaccination antirabies 1
- Medical 1
- Dental..1
- Central sample collection...1
- Orthopedic 1
- Psychiatry..1
- X-Ray 2
- Skin..2
- Chemotherapy..2
- Burns...2
- Microbiology 2

SIU also recommended 10% additional staff to make up leave, holidays and weekly off.

STAFFING NORMS BY HIGH POWER COMMITTEE ON NURSING AND NURSING PROFESSION (1987–1989)

This committee was established by the Government of India in July 1987, under the chairmanship of Ms, Sarojini Varadappan Dr Jyothi, former vice-chancellor of SNDT Women University, Mrs Rajkumari Sood, Nursing Advisor to Union Government as the member secretary and CPB Kurup, Principal, Government College of Nursing, Bangalore and the then President, TNAI also one of the prominent members of this committee. The main objectives were:

- To review the existing working conditions of nurses with particular reference to the standards of the nursing care services rendered both in the rural and urban areas.
- To assess and recommend the staffing norms necessary for providing best possible nursing care in both in the hospitals and community.
- To focus and suggest the training needs of nursing, midwifery personnel to meet the nursing manpower requirements at all levels of health services and the education.

- To clarify the role of nursing personnel in the health care delivery system including their interaction with other members of the health team at every level of health service management.
- To examine the need for organized nursing services at the national, state, district and local levels with particular reference to the need for planning service with the overall care system of the country at the respective levels.
- To look into all other aspects, the Committee will hold consultations with the State governments.

Recommendations of high power committee in public health nursing

Appointment of ANM/LHV/HS/PHC

- 1 ANM for 2500 population (2 per subcenter).
- 1 ANM for 1500 population in hilly areas.
- 1 health supervisor for 7500 population (for 3 ANMs).
- 1 public health nurse for 1 PHC (30,000 population and 4 health supervisor).
- Two district PHN officers in each district.
- Simplification of documentation system.
- Adequate provision of supplies, drugs, etc. is to be made.
- Gazette rank for the post of PHN and above grade.
- Specific standing orders be made available to ANM/LHV/HS. (See chapter 2 for further information)

STAFFING NORMS BY BAJAJ COMMITTEE, 1986

Recommendations of appointment of nurses as follows:

- 1 staff outpatient nurse/100 outpatients.
- 1 staff nurse/10 hospital beds + 30% extra as leave reserve.
- 1 ward sister/25 beds + 30% extra as leave reserve.
- 1 nursing superintendent for hospital with 200 beds or more.
- 1 deputy nursing superintendent for hospital with 300 beds or more.
- In rural areas, establish a 'Community Health Center' for every 100,000 population.
- Establish 'Educational Commission for Health Services' on the lines of the university Grants Commission. (For further information refer chapter 2)

ESTIMATION OF NURSING STAFF REQUIREMENT: ACTIVITY ANALYSIS

Staffing is one of the major functions of nursing service administration and it is also problems of any nursing organization of any health care facility.

Nurse staffing is an orderly and systematic process based on sound principle applied to assess the number and kind of nursing personnel required to provide the nursing care as per staffing norms of nursing practice to a group of patients.

Thus staffing is determining how many nurses with type of qualification and experience/skills are needed in a nursing unit and make them available for 24 × 7 days. Staffing also determines what type of activity or task to be done by the nursing personnel posted in that unit and the time period they will work in that unit.

Staffing and Scheduling

Staffing and scheduling goes hand in hand. Staffing a part of organizing and establishing the framework within which the services will be rendered, whereas scheduling is an important component of planning. As explained above the concept of good staffing decides the acceptable number of nursing personnel to provide a desired level of care to meet the demands of patients care. The number of nursing personnel is determined by the increasing or decreasing demands of patient care.

Sometimes the nurse administrator accomplishes staffing and allocation by taking staff from one ward to another or by posting extra nurses on relieving duty.

What is Allocation?

Allocation is appropriate selection of nursing personnel in the department according to their qualifications and experience/capabilities to provide best possible nursing care to their patients. Allocation provides information to adjust the scheduled staff to meet the daily workload demand of each unit. Allocation is a beneficial process because it is concerned with the balancing of nurses to fluctuation of workload among similar nursing units through reallocation.

Objective of Allocations

- To assign working days and days off to nursing staff according to personnel policy so that the patients receive quality care
- To avoid over staffing or under staffing in a unit
- To facilitate desirable distribution of days off for nursing personnel.

Criteria for Allocation

- *Coverage of nurses in all units*
- ***Quality:*** 24 hours patients are supervised by professional nurses
- ***Stability:*** Consistent with leave and rotation policy
- ***Flexibility:*** Meet the needs of emergency of nursing staff
- ***Objectivity:*** allocation must be unbiased.

Allocation Procedure

Some administrators believe that nurses will be allocated by patient classification system. But this method does not give clear picture of nursing care hours required by each patient.

- Another approach is to calculate the workload and hours required to give nursing care to patients in that unit
- Various methods are adopted to categorize the patients and to calculate the nursing care hours required per shift/per day by each category of patients
- A study conducted by College of Nursing. Delhi and TNAI classified patients under 3 major categories.
  a. Completely dependent
  b. Partially dependent
  c. Ambulatory
- Goddard classified the patient's dependency under 5 categories:
  a. Totally ambulant
  b. Partially bed fast
  c. Bed fast but not helpless
  d. Partially helpless
  e. Totally helpless
- EA Schemed classified patients under 4 categories

a *A patient who needs minimal amount of nursing care* that is 2.8 nursing hours per 24 hours

b *A patient who needs average amount of nursing care* that is an average of 4.3 nursing hours in average within 24 hours

c *A patient who needs above average amount of nursing care* that is an average of 5.6 nursing hour in 24 hours

d *A patient who needs maximum amount of nursing care* that is an average of 8.6 nursing hours in 24 hours.

According to the study conducted by College of Nursing, Delhi, the nursing hours needed per category of patients assessed for 24 hours.

- Total number of patients 30
- Completely dependent Patients 5
- Partially dependent patients 15
- Ambulatory patients 10

Table 12.2: Nursing hours care required by each category of patient in each shift N = 30

Category of patient	Morning shift	Evening shift	Night shift	Total
Completely dependent	3.27 hrs	2.50 hrs	1.47 hrs	7.24 hrs
Partially dependent	1.62 hrs	0.91 hrs	0.55 hrs	3.08 hrs
Ambulatory	1.20 hrs	0.70 hrs	0.17 hrs	2.67 hrs
Total	6.09 hrs	4.11 hrs	2.10 hrs	12.29 hrs

Table 12.3: Workload for 30 patients in 24 hours N = 30

Category of patient	Total patients	Daily average time per patient in 24 hours	Calculation per category of patient	Total hours
Completely dependent	5	7.24	5 × 7.24	36.20
Partially dependent	15	3,08	15 × 3.08	46.20
Ambulatory	10	2.07	10 × 2.07	20.70
Total				103. 10 hrs

Calculation of number of nurses required for 30 bedded unit

- The total working hours per day .... 8 hours/day
- Total number of nurses required as per nursing hours
- For patient calculated as per table 11.3 .... 103/8 = 13 (13 nurses approximately)
- To make up days off, casual leave, privileged leave, holidays (116 days)
- And other leave vacancies extra nurses require .... 116/365 = 4.09 nurses
- Therefore, a grand total of nurses required in that unit = 13 + 4 = 17 nurses

From the above it is very clear that;

- How to categorize the patients
- The nursing hours required by the patient in 24 hours
- The nursing hours required shift wise each category of patients
- Calculation of total nurses allocated in that unit including provision of additional nurses to meet reserve
- We have seen for 30 bedded unit we require 17 nurses and we need to allocate them in each shift.

Table 12.4: Shiftwise nursing hours for 30 bedded unit N = 30

Category of patients	Morning shift nursing hours	Evening shift nursing hours	Night shift nursing hours
Completely dependent patients = 5	3.27 x 5 = 16.35	2.5 x 5 = 12.50	1.45 x 5 = 7.25
Partially dependent patients = 15	1.62 x 15 = 24.30	0.91 x 15 = 13.65	0.56 x 15 = 8.40
Ambulatory patients =10	1.2 x 10 = 12.00	0.7 x 10 = 7	0.17 x 10 = 1.70
Total nursing hours per shift	52.65	33.15	17.35

Total hours = 103.15

Calculation of Nursing Personnel for Each Shift According to Workload

- Staff required in morning shift = 52.65 × 13/103.15 = 7
- Staff required in evening shift = 33.15 × 13/103.15 = 4
- Staff required in night shift = 13 – (7 + 4) = 2

Thus by activity analysis, the study shows in the morning shift 7 nurses, evening shift 4 nurses and in night shift 2 nurses to be allotted.

Box 12.2: Research highlights

Various literature review shows that nursing workforce issues such as recruitment, retention, turn over and work place issues influence staff morale. Both intrinsic and extrinsic factors have an impact on staff morale. Intrinsic factors like professional dignity, respect, opportunities for career development, work group relationship and the type of patient care influence the morale of nurses. Extrinsic factors like organization structure, functioning of ward, leadership of administrator, management styles, communication staffing, and scheduling have an impact on staff morale. Low morale of nursing work force leads to poor patient care outcome (GE Day, 2006)

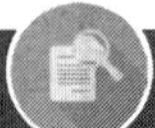

SUMMARY POINTS

- ✓ Staffing is one of the major functions of nursing service administration along with planning, organizing, directing and controlling. It is a process include, series of step in recruiting, selecting, employing, training and delegating activities for effective nursing care, the execution of administrative function depends upon the manpower which is available through staffing function.
- ✓ For organizational effectiveness, nursing manpower is required in quantity and quality.
- ✓ Scheduling is an administrative function that the administrator should keep in mind the following include 24/7 coverage needed for effective care, workload varies by shift by skill level by unit, rotation to off-shifts, multiple skill levels (RN, aide, etc.), covering weekends, meeting shortage of personnel, dealing with daily fluctuations in supply and demand of nursing personnel.
- ✓ Indian nursing council, Staff Inspection units, Bajaj committee and High power committee on nursing and nursing profession has recommended norms for nursing personnel working in hospital and community. Many hospital follow the guideline given by the committee without violating INC recommendations.
- ✓ There are various approaches used to calculate staffing. Patient classification system, nursing hours required by each category of patient. Nursing personnel in each shift for 24 hours, based on number of patients in each category are some of the ways to calculate norms.Activity analysis is one of the best ways to calculate staffing pattern for a nursing unit/hospital.

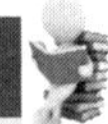

REVIEW QUESTIONS

1. Define staffing. Outline the philosophy of staffing in nursing service administration.
2. Discuss the functions of nursing administrator in scheduling nurses. Outline a duty roaster plan for nurses working in 30 bedded ward for a week.
3. Discuss the staffing norms recommended by Indian nursing council for a hospital.
4. Calculate nursing staff required for a 300 bedded hospital.
5. Define allocation. What are the criteria and objectives of allocation of nursing personnel?
6. **Write short notes on:**
   a. Concepts of staffing and scheduling
   b. High power committee recommendation for staffing norms in nursing
   c. Bajaj committee recommendation for nurse staffing norms
   d. Staff Inspection Unit recommendation for staffing norms for nursing
   e. Objectives of staffing.

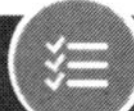

SELECTED READINGS

1. Berkow S, Jaggi J and Fogelson R. Fourteen unit attributes to guide staffing. JONA. Vol 37, no.3 mar 2007.
2. Beyers Marjorie. Nurse executives' perspectives on succession planning. JONA. Vol 36. June 2006.
3. Estimating of nursing staff requirement-
   http://www.slideshare.net/98567/estimating-of-nursing-staff-requirement 10 Jul 2012 ...
4. Gary E Day. Nursing Morale: what does literature reveal?
   Aus Health Rev. 2006:30 (4) 516–524
5. High Power Committee on Nursing and Nursing Profession...
   http://www.communityhealth.in/~commun26/wiki/index.php%3Ftitle%3DHig_Power_Committee_on_Nursing_and_Nursing_Profession 22 Nov 2012.
6. High Power Committee on Nursing and Nursing Profession
   http://www.communityhealth.in/~commun26/wiki/index Last access Nov 22, 2012
7. Koontz H, Weihrich H Management a global perspective 1st edition, New Delhi: Tata McGrawhill Publishers, 2001.
8. Koontz H, Weihrich H. Essentials of management—an international perspective New Delhi: Tata Mcgrawhill Publishers, 2007.
9. Sabitha Jain, Health committees' http://www.slideshare.net/sabithajain/health committees last access Oct 6, 2013
10. Staff Inspection Unit: Ministry of Finance, Government of India
    http://finmin.nic.in/the_ministry/dept_expenditure/staff_inspection_unit/index.asp.
11. Staffing - Management – http://www.slideshare.net/sanchitgangar/staffing-management 24 Jun 2013
12. Staffing Function of Management–Management Study Guide
    http://www.managementstudyguide.com/staffing-function.htm.
13. Staffing: It's Meaning, Nature and Importance | Business Management *http://www.yourarticlelibrary.com/business-management/staffing-its-meaning-nature-and-importance-business-management/27912/*
    http://www.currentnursing.com/nursing_management/staffing_nursing_units.htm

13

Staffing Process

LEARNING OBJECTIVES

This chapter imparts learning about:

- Recruitment, Selection, Placement, Promotion
- Retention
- Personnel Policies
- Termination
- Staff Development Programme
- Supervision
- Duties and Responsibilities of Nursing Personnel
- Research Highlights

RECRUITMENT, SELECTION, PLACEMENT, PROMOTION

Introduction

The first step in staffing is to plan the manpower requirement for the establishment/hospital which means finding out number and type of nurses needed by the hospital in near future.

Manpower requirement is calculated by workload analysis and work force analysis. Workload analysis means finding out number and type of nurses required to perform various jobs in a hospital set-up where as workforce analysis means reviewing existing workforce or nurses already present on the job positions and to study how many of them are overloaded or under loaded. After doing workload analysis and workforce analysis, the administrator compares both an excess of workload over workforce that indicates under staffing and she needs to appoint more nurses whereas excess of workforce over workload indicates over staffing. When there is excess nurses she needs to remove or transfer some nurses to other departments where less nurses are available because understaffing and overstaffing are not desirable in an organization. (Refer Chapter 12) for estimation of manpower requirement.

The concept of staffing includes planning for recruiting, selecting, training and developing employees, as well as compensating them and providing for their health and safety.

RECRUITMENT

It refers to the process of inducing the candidates to apply for the job in the organization. After assessing the number and types of employees required, the manager tries that more and more people should apply for the job so that the organization can get more choice and select better candidates.

Definition

Recruitment is a method of finding suitable candidates to fill various positions in an organization. According to Edwin B Flippo, 'Recruitment is a process of searching for prospective employees and stimulating them to apply for job in an organization.'

Purposes of Recruitment

- To attract and motivate more number of candidates
- To create a pool of candidates and select the suitable candidates as required
- To select the best candidate for the job as specified.

Recruitment is a continuous process. It is a systematic procedure comprising the following steps:

- Identifying vacancies
- Developing criteria for selection of candidate by job specification and candidate specification
- Advertisement for filling vacancies
- Receiving responses from applicants
- Short listing candidates based on criteria developed
- Arrange and inform candidates for interviews
- Conducting interviews.

Identification of Vacancies

The administrator as a first step of recruitment needs to identify the vacancies prevailing in the organization.

Vacancies of posts may arise in the organization due to retirement of employees, death, resignation, disablement or dismissal from the job, transfer to other department or hospitals, and promotion of employees. The administrator may make a list of personnel required in quality and quantity.

Developing Criteria for Selection of Candidate: Job and Candidate Specification

- Job specification denotes the nature of job, work settings, job title and expectation, resource constraints and risk factors involved in job
- Candidate/employee specification include physical specification, such as date of birth, physical fitness. mental and emotional specification include Mental maturity, and emotional stability required for the job.

Advertisement for Filling Vacancies

Advertising for the job could be done through internal and external sources. While advertising the organization's brief profile, title of job vacant, job requirements, number of vacant posts, number of reservation post if any, how to apply, cost of application form and mode of payment, last date for receiving application form and clear details of the addressee of the organization to be given.

Receiving Responses from Applicants

It is expected to have more number of applicants for the post. More the number of applicants, more the chances for getting suitable candidates for the post. After receiving the applications the applications are scrutinized based on the criteria laid.

Short Listing Candidates Based on Criteria Developed

After scrutinizing the applications, the prospective candidates name are short listed based on criteria developed in rank and order.

Arrange and Inform Candidates for Interviews

The administrator arranges for interview for the short-listed candidates. She plans ahead for a suitable date and place for interview so that all the applicants from far and near can appear for the interview. She needs to select a place, time interviewing facilities and prepare interview letters with requirements and to submit to the office prior to interview in detail. Gives landmark for the venue of interview.

Conducting Interviews

The selection committee comprising three to four members conduct interview and make decision on candidates selected and document it in rank and order.

SOURCES OF RECRUITMENT

There are two sources of recruitment:

1. Internal sources
2. External sources

RECRUITMENT FROM INTERNAL SOURCES

In this source the candidates are selected for the job among existing employees working in the same organization. Vacancies are filled-up in the following manner: (a) Transfer and (b) Promotion

Transfer

When a department has surplus staff, they may be transferred to another similar department or other related hospital. The nature of the job, job responsibilities, salary and other benefits for the transferred staff remain the same.

Promotion

In an organization, when a post for higher level position is vacant, the next staff below the vacant position in the hierarchy is promoted to that post and the vacancy is filled. For example when a nursing superintendent post is vacant, the assistant nursing superintendent is promoted to the vacant position. Therefore filling-up of vacancy of a higher position by the next senior staff is called promotion. This position carries higher responsibilities, higher salary and benefits and status in the organization.

Advantages of Recruitment from Internal Source

- Motivates and encourages employees to work with more efficiency
- It boosts up the morale of employee
- The employer is aware of the up-to-date performance of the employee
- Since the newly promoted employee knows well about the organization, it does not require vigorous orientation
- Cost-effective because it does not require advertisement, time spending for scrutiny and employees training.

Disadvantages of Recruitment from Internal Source

- It denies opportunities for talented candidates
- Restricts the best choice of selection
- Innovation and newer outlook in services from the employees is questionable.

RECRUITMENT FROM EXTERNAL SOURCES

The following are the external sources from which the employer can find eligible candidates for vacant posts:

Advertisement

Advertisements in newspaper and professional journals like the Nursing Journal of India brings wide coverage and the employer gets a large amount of applications where as many of the applications may be unsuitable for the post. The employer has to spend a lot of time in scrutinizing the applications.

Employment Exchange

It is a government agency (controlled by Government) where the job seekers register their name with complete profile. When any employer wants to recruit staff can approach this employment exchange, and the agency provides the details of job seekers. Usually employment exchange registers for unskilled job, hence the employers do not approach this agency to recruit nurses for higher position.

Private Employment Agencies

The employers also seek help from these agencies for getting staff for their organization.

On the Campus Recruitment

The employer conducts preliminary interviews to select candidates for the first level position. Usually it is conducted in the campus when the nursing students reached in final year.

Rival Firms

Sometimes employers draw efficient employees from rival organization by offering more salaries specially for the post of Principals, Nursing Director or Professors.

Unsolicited Applications

Sometimes the employer gets applications for job from unemployed candidates who were not called for and are not notified vacancies. These applicants are called unsolicited applicants who apply voluntarily.

Online Recruitment

Vacancies are advertised online and the eligible candidates apply. This includes online interview, online tests and the employer calls for personal interview if the candidate successfully gets through interview on online. This is very common these days.

Telecasting

Television channels play an important role in advertising candidates for certain jobs. In recent times candidates make use of these opportunity.

Advantages of Recruitment from External Sources

- It provides wide choice for the employer to select most eligible candidates for organization
- The candidates are new to the organization. They exhibit their innovative and creative ability in work
- The candidates are more reliable and competitive that enhances the status of the organization
- It is socially advantageous because it promotes employment opportunities for many unemployed in the society.

Disadvantages of Recruitment from External Sources

- It is a long process and consumes lot of time of the employer starting from advertisement to selection interview.
- It is not cost-effective. Lot of money incur in advertisement, scrutiny of application, orientation, employee training, etc. The existing staff may not cooperate or assimilate with the new employees because they feel a sense of insecurity.

FACTORS INFLUENCING RECRUITMENT

A number of factors that influence recruitment are given below:

Size of the Organization

The number of persons to be recruited will depend upon the size of an organization. Larger the organization more number of candidates are recruited at regular intervals while a small organization employs only a few employees as and when needed.

Employment Conditions

The employment conditions, salary and monitory benefits affect recruitment of prospective candidates. At the same time suitable candidates may not be available because of lack of educational and technical facilities in the organization. If the availability of persons are more, then selection from large number becomes easy. On the other hand, if there is a shortage of qualified technical persons, then it will be difficult to locate suitable persons.

Working Conditions

The working conditions of an organization determine job satisfaction of employees. An organization that offering good working conditions like proper sanitation, lighting, ventilation, etc. would give more job satisfaction to employees and they may not leave their present job. On the other hand, if employees leave the jobs due to unsatisfactory working conditions, it will lead to fresh recruitment of new persons.

Growth Rate

The growth rate of an organization also influences recruitment process. An expanding or fast growing establishments require regular appointment of new employees. There will also be promotions of existing employees as an advantage which necessitating the filling up of those vacancies. A stagnant organization can recruit persons only as and when need.

Nature of Vacancy

If the applications are called for temporary posts the number of applicant will be less. Whereas if the vacancy is for permanent post, the employer may get more applications.

Government Reservation Norms

When the applications will be called on the basis of reservation norms there is likelihood of less number of applicants available for the post.

Reputation of the Organization

More the organization is reputed more number of applicants will likely to apply for the post.

SELECTION PROCESS

After recruiting candidates from external or internal source, the selection process is the next step.

Definition

Dale Yoder explains that selection is a process in which the candidates for employment are divided into two classes, those who are to be offered employment and those who are not to be.

The selection process involves the following stages:

- *Receiving application forms*
- ***Scrutinizing committee scrutinizes application:*** The committee ensures by checking age of the candidate, gender, educational qualification and experience, religion and community, references and medical fitness. It helps the employer to eliminate incomplete as well as ineligible application forms.
- ***Conducting preliminary interview:*** When the applications are scrutinized and those applications are complete and found suitable for the job the administrator plans for preliminary interview. This is advantageous because the administrator can see the candidate personally and interact with the candidate. During interaction the administrator can judge his communication, decision-making ability and aptitude for the job. The candidates found unsuitable for the job during scrutiny are not called for preliminary interview.
- ***Tests:*** According to the job different tests are planned and conducted. Aptitude test, attitude tests, personality tests intelligent tests, etc. When a nurse teacher comes for preliminary interview usually a model teaching for actual students are asked to conduct on the candidates specialty area.
- ***Final interview:*** The candidates who clear the tests successfully are called for final interview. The following factors to be kept in mind while planning for final interview:
  1. The date, time and venue for interview to be intimated to the candidates well in advance
  2. Start the interview on correct time
  3. All types of distractions and interruptions to be avoided
  4. Facilitate proper seating arrangement, drinking water facility for the candidate
  5. Ensure adequate light and ventilation in interviewing venue.
  6. The panel of interview to be informed about the interview well in time
  7. Criterion sheet for evaluating the candidate with score to be given to each panel members
  8. After interview all panel needs to sign and justify the cause for the selected and rejected candidates. Rank list is prepared by panel members

9. Candidates are selected provisionally
10. Final selection will be pending to the decision from references and the medical report.

- *Checking references:* The administrator checks with persons who were given in the application form for further verification of the candidates.
- *Medical examination:* A complete medical examination is done by an authorized medical officer to ensure the candidate is medically fit to take up the job.
- *Appointment:* When all the selection procedures are conducted and satisfied the administrator sends an appointment letter showing the title of the post, place of work, date of joining, testimonials to be submitted along with joining report, salary and other benefits, probation and confirmation period, etc.

ORIENTATION AND PLACEMENT

Once the selection process is over, the appointed candidates are made familiar to the job settings and work environment through an orientation programs to make the newly appointed candidates feel a sense of belongingness to that institution/organization. Placement refers to putting right employee on the right job. It is assignment or re-assignment of an employee to a new or different job. Placement includes initial assignment of new employees and promotion, transfer or demotion of present employees. Generally, the candidates undergo a probation period, and when the administrator find the candidates performs satisfactorily will confirm the post and permanent placement is done.

PROMOTION

Promotion is the upward reassignment of an employee in an organization's hierarchy. This is accompanied by increased responsibilities, enhanced status, and usually with increased monetary benefits. Higher the position, the employee is promoted, that increases responsibilities and accountabilities more than the previous position Further it brings changes in the designation, status and work facilities. All promotions are considered for a trial period, to observe whether the promoted employee is capable of handling a job. Normally during this trial period he draws the pay of the higher post, but it should be clearly understood that if he does not make the grade' he will be reverted to his former post and obtains his former pay scale.

Criteria for Promotion Decisions

Promotion policy should optimize the interests of the organizations as well as the needs and aspirations of the individual employee. Some of the criteria for promotion are:

- When the employee demonstrates excellent performance
- Seniority in service or merit and capability of the employee
- Educational/technical qualifications fulfills for the promotional post
- Assessment of potential for growth of the individual and organization
- When vacancy arises in an organization
- When organizational growth is expected.

Promotion Scheme

There should be some promotional scheme established in all organization that promotes uniform opportunities for promotion of employees. The employees may aware that the organization has sound promotional scheme, and they work hard to get next promotion in the hierarchy position.

Advantages of Promotion Scheme in an Organization

- Provides an opportunity to the existing employees to move into higher jobs that provide greater personnel satisfaction.
- Facilitates opportunities to the administrator to ensure recognition and incentives to the better employees.
- Expects hard and better work from the employees that brings desirable outcome in an organization.
- Ensures a systematic, logical and prompt source of recruitment from internal source for management to fill vacancies as they arise.
- Encourages of promotion within the organization, instead of looking outside to fill vacancies in higher posts.

RETENTION OF EMPLOYEES

Employee retention refers to the ability of the organization to retain its employees and it is emerging as a big challenge to health care organization. When an employee leaves the job and in his place another employee is appointed, is called turn over. The top five reasons given by employees who quit their jobs (Kenexa 2011) are:

- Lack of opportunities for professional development (30%)
- Inadequate compensation (28%)
- Boredom/lack of challenge (27%)
- Poor work/Life balance (20%)
- Job stress and unfair treatment (20%).

Reasons for Employees Leaving the Job

Management Causes

- Low salary and benefits
- Poor working conditions
- Lack of avenues for career development, coaching and feedback is lacking
- No promotional avenues
- Overloading work
- Feeling of undervalued, lack of recognition
- Organizational instability.

Employee Causes

- Lack of decision-making ability, lack of skill
- Lack of commitment to quality
- Lack of motivation
- Lack of confidence
- Unhappy with managerial behavior
- Boredom
- Feeling of unfit for job.

Employee Retention Strategies used by Managers

Working Environment Strategies

The first and foremost employee retention a strategy focuses on creating and maintaining a safe workplace consistent with organizational policies that attracts, retains and develops employees. Basically good working environment concentrates on the ethics and values upon which the organization functions, the policies that interpret those values and translate them into day-to-day activities, and the physical environment in which the employee work. An administrator should think the following aspects of work environment strategies:

- Clarify the vision, mission and values of the organization to all employees
- Facilitate upward, downward and lateral communication
- Share information
- Ensure a sense of belongingness to the organization
- Cultivate loyalty toward employees and be fair as well as honest
- Enhance integrity
- Emphasize work place safety.

Employee Relationship Strategies

The employer needs to develop effective employee relationship strategies by providing regular relationship training program to managers and supervisors to develop relationship sensitivity. The employer may find out from employees the reasons for working in that organization and know from them what are the areas needs improvement in the organization. The administrator should think about following employee relationship strategies:

- Help the employee to understand their position in the organization and communicate more effectively
- Help the employee to know the organizational goals and how their goals are matching with organizational goals
- Have informal get together involving family members
- Celebrate organization's achievement
- Build coaching and mentoring relationships with people to increase their emotional bond to the organization. Practice recognition strategy in the organization
- Appreciate the employee who had longer services in the organization by incentives
- Focus on building employee self-esteem
- Give recognition strategically and deliberately

Employee Support Strategies

Employee support strategies involve facilitating resources the employees want to do their job the best. This in turn increases job satisfaction. The basic philosophy behind this strategy is all employees' want to excel in their career, employee is satisfied when adequate equipment and supplies are provided to do the job and facilitating moral and mental support from managers and supervisors enhances the performance outcome. The administrator should think about following employee support strategies:

- Demonstrate a positive attitude towards employees. Keep up the promises that the employer make with employees
- Assign productive, challenging and meaningful assignment to employees
- Facilitate effective communication system
- Assign the right job to right person
- Facilitate job description to know their job responsibilities
- Provide job flexibility in terms of shift and schedule if needed.

Employee Growth Strategies

Employee growth strategies refers to the personal and professional growth of employees. Good employees want to develop new knowledge and skills in order to improve their status and enhance their own self-esteem. In-service education program include seminar, conferences, workshop, skill training, guest lectures from expert in the field, etc. The organization needs to bear the cost of in-service education of employees. This strategies strengthen the employee's knowledge and skill which in turn enhance organizational performance and outcome. The administrator should think about following employee growth strategies:

- Cultivate a learning culture in the organization
- Encourage and motivate the employees to create individual learning plans
- Encourage employees to join professional associations
- Have regular training and mentoring program
- Provide incentives for updating knowledge
- Provide for advantage of internet learning.

Employee Compensation Strategies

Effective employee compensation strategies include both hard and soft employee compensation: Hard compensation means salary and benefits purely on monetary basis. Soft compensation means it include non monitory compensation like rewards, incentives, recognition of the employee.

Pay-for-performance plans involve two basic activities: like defining the job and checking performance against expectations. When employee performs beyond expectations, the management gives bonus to such employees, that brings a positive organizational effectiveness. The administrator should think about following employee compensation strategies:

- The administrator needs to discuss total employee compensation (salary, benefits, bonuses, training, etc.)
- Develop reward systems to motivate employee involvement
- Develop policies for a flexible employee benefits to respond to a changing workforce
- Offer time off, sabbaticals and other forms of non-financial employee compensation
- Provide crèche for women employees having very small children
- Provide employee assistance programs
- Arrange for discounts on purchases and food coupon
- Arrange for professional services specially medical facilities, children education

Role of Nurse Administrator in Retaining Nurses Working in Hospitals

Cultivate a Positive Work Environment

- Makes nurses aware of quality and patient safety is the benchmark of nursing care
- Ensures that nurses are aware of the philosophy, vision, mission and values of the hospital organization
- Creates work setting as a learning environment
- Provides adequate equipment and supplies for nursing care
- Empowers nurses to make clinical decisions
- Facilitates challenging and meaningful work assignment
- Maintains effective communication
- Ensures good interpersonal and collaborative relationship.

Recognition of Skill

- Facilitates skill recognition of nurses on job accomplishment
- Provides adequate supervision and support to novice nurses
- Demonstrates a positive attitude toward nursing personnel.

Benefits and Compensation

- Discusses total nurses compensation (salary, benefits, bonuses, training, etc.).
- Recommends for increment , higher pay and benefits and promotion for eligible nursing personnel
- Develops reward systems to motivate nurse's involvement
- Develops policies for flexible nurse's benefits to respond to a changing workforce
- Offers time off, sabbaticals and other forms of non-financial compensation for nurses
- Provides crèche for female nurses having very small children.

Facilitate Professional Growth

- Cultivates a learning culture in the hospital or unit environment
- Encourages and motivate nurses to create individual learning plans
- Encourages nurses to join professional associations
- Have regular training and mentoring program for nurses
- Provides incentives for updating knowledge
- Foster nurses development through deputation, relieve from duty to attend seminar, conferences and guest lectures
- Use contests and incentives to help nurses keep motivated for learning
- Conducts regular coaching, mentoring and guiding nurses for higher positions

- Provides for advantage of internet learning and make nurses have computer literacy
- Organizes ward library
- Motivate nurses to conduct or participate in research.

Foster a Supportive Culture in Hospital

- Respect nurses as they are an asset to health care services
- Participates in planning and policy-making meeting and speak and support for nurses
- Facilitates for job flexibility by scheduling vacation, leave, shift time, and workload
- Conducts regular staff meeting
- Arrange for informal gathering where family members can participate
- Demonstrates organizational commitment. Highly committed nurses may not leave the hospital
- Proper dealing with low morale.

High turnover, absenteeism, frequent reporting of complaints, negative rumors bring low morale in an organization. The nurse administrator needs to identify them and take proper attention. Stay interviews apart from exit interviews of nurses will be beneficial to know the status of morale of nurses and action should be taken based on the cause.

PERSONNEL POLICIES

Concept and Definition

A policy is a statement developed by the management that guides to decision-making to the employees of the organization in respect of any course of action. Personnel policies are statements developed by the management with respect to manpower management in the organization. Developing personnel policies are one of the staffing functions. According to Edwin B Flippo, 'A policy is a man-made rule or predetermined course of action that is established to guide the performance of work towards the organization. It is a type of standing plan that serves to guide subordinates in the execution of their task.' According to Koontz and O'Donnell, 'Policies are general statements or understanding which guide or channel thinking in decision-making of subordinates.'

- Personnel policy is developed on the basis of objectives of organization.
- A personnel policy is a written document that defines the expectations of management to employees and expectation of employees to management.
- Policy cannot be developed in a day. It includes various steps. It needs lot of decisions taking for the growth organization, management and employees.
- A policy provides guidelines to the employee in organization for choosing a course of action.
- All policies related to personnel decision is compiled and called personnel policy manual.

A personnel policy in nursing is written guidelines that determines a preplanned course of action to work toward desired outcomes and objectives. They are the rules and guidelines that govern how to deal with nursing personnel in specific situation. They are unbiased guidelines to decision-making that help nurses to carry out their functions and for the smooth running of the hospital.

In nursing service administration personnel policy manual is developed by the management and the nursing service administrator with regards to nurse's decision. This manual is given to nurses at the time of induction period.

The nurse administrator ensures to take into account the past policies, management styles and employee challenges when writing or updating nursing personnel policy. To make the policies more effective she ensures that the policies are well-communicated and are available at all times and given to each nurse to preclude complaints of ignorance later.

Purposes of Personnel Policy

- Personnel policies help the management to implement a consistent decision in related situation.
- Policies are managerial tool in reducing perceptions of arbitrary treatment of employees. Everyone from the lowest level employees to top level management should be aware of policies and the management should make sure that everyone knows what is expected of them and how their subordinates or co-workers should be treated in certain situations, including discipline and awards.
- Personnel policies provide a framework for uniform and consistent administration.
- Personal policies help employees understand the reasoning behind decisions and prevent bias and favoritism.
- Policies are revised and amended according to changing trends in health care system.

Contents of Personnel Policy Manuals (Nursing)

- **About the hospital**: History, departments and accreditation if any
- Philosophy of the hospital
- Philosophy of nursing service administration
- Vision, mission and values of nursing
- Channel of communication (organization chart)

- Definition (Governing body/trustees, nursing superintendent, head nurse, staff nurse, etc.)
- Classification of employees (permanent, probationer)
- Bio-data: Record of age, permanent address, present address, personal identification
- Duties and obligation of employees
- Job description of personnel (Annexure)
- Code of conduct
- Confidential reports
- Attendance, absence from work, unauthorized presence
- Penalty for unauthorized absence
- No work- no pay
- Working hours
- Safeguard of hospital property
- **Payment of salary**: Allowances and increments
- Leave rules and procedures
- Station leave permission
- Benefits, incentives, awards
- Redress of grievances
- Service of notice
- Misconduct, penalty for misconduct, disciplinary process
- Cessation of service
- Settlement of accounts and loans if any
- Certificate of service

Personnel policy manual is subject to revision as per the changing trends.

TERMINATION

Meaning of Termination

- It is an act of ending something
- It is the act of making a person leaves a job—the act of dismissing someone.

Terminology Used for Termination

A number of expressions are commonly used to describe situations when employment is terminated. These include 'let go,' 'discharged,' 'dismissed,' 'fired' and 'permanently laid off.'

Employee Termination

Employee termination is very painful function of an administrator. Employee termination is the relieving of an employee against his or her desire. Termination may be, at will, for cause, or for lack of work. The process is sometimes unavoidable for the health of an organization. Terminations, however, are a necessary part of managerial task and must be carried out promptly when the need for such actions becomes obvious in order to preserve the health of the organization.

According to **Employment Standards Act, 2000 (ESA)** a person's employment is terminated if the employer:

- Dismisses or stops employing an employee, including where an employee is no longer employed due to the bankruptcy or insolvency of the employer.
- **'Constructively' dismisses** an employee and the employee resigns, in response, within a reasonable time.
- Lays an employee off for a period that is longer than a 'temporary layoff'.
- In most cases, when an management terminates job of an employee who has been continuously employed for three months, the employer must provide the employee with either written notice of termination, termination pay or a combination.

Reasons for Termination of an Employee in an Organization

- Inadequate job performance
- Unacceptable behavior
- Habitual absenteeism
- Employment at will (Employment at will means that an employee can be terminated at any time without any reason and without notice).
- Damaging company property
- Drug or alcohol possession at work
- Falsifying company records
- Insubordination
- Misconduct
- Poor performance
- Stealing
- Using company property for personal business
- Taking too much time off
- Violating company policy
- Lying on a resume or job application
- Not being able to get along with co-workers or management.

Surveys report shows the following reasons for termination of an employee from job:

- 15% of employers have fired a worker for calling in without a legitimate reason (Career builder)
- 22% of employers have fired someone for using the internet for non-work related activity (Career builder)
- 22% of employees know someone who has been fired for wasting time at the office or disrupting other employees (SHRM)

- 33% of employers have disciplined an employee for violating social media policy (SHRM).

Types of Termination

Voluntary Termination

When an employee in an organization resigns from the job voluntarily due to personal reasons is called voluntary termination. This may be due to getting a better job, spouse's transfer, children's education, parent's sickness, distance from home town and retirement.

Involuntary Termination

- When an employee is dismissed by an employer from his or her job, it is termed as involuntary termination. An involuntary termination is usually the result of an employer's dissatisfaction and many causes are written above paragraph.
- Involuntary termination, such as a layoff, can also occur because an employer lacks the financial resources to continue an employment relationship. Other events that trigger termination can include mergers and acquisitions, a company relocation, and job redundancy.
- With performance problems, the employer most often tries final solutions such as coaching from the employee's supervisor to help the employee to improve.

Role of nurse administrators in termination of nurse for just cause

- Refer personnel policy manual and understand policy for termination.
- Take advice and guidance from human resources administrator, or legal advisor of the hospital.
- Establish an investigation committee and delegate responsibility for investigating when information received about dismissal of nurse that may warrant termination for just cause.
- Meet the employee whose alleged conduct may be just cause for discipline to inform her of the allegation and the initiation of the investigation.
- Decide whether the affected nurse can continue to perform her normal responsibilities without causing any harm to the unit where she works. In the event, this is not deemed advisable, the nurse's duties may be changed, the employee may be reassigned to a different unit of service area, or the employee may be placed on a leave of absence with or without pay as appropriate to the circumstances.
- Any reassignment of duties of the nurse should be commensurate with the individual's qualifications and experience.
- As part of the investigation, give the nurse an opportunity to respond with evidence to address the allegations.
- Meet with the affected nurse upon completion of the investigation to advise her whether the allegations are or are not supported by the evidence.
- Attempt to resolve the issue if the allegations are supported by the evidence and if appropriate.
- Immediately notify the affected nurse of the specific charges, the findings, and the resulting discipline if resolution of the issue does not occur.
- Immediately advise the affected nurse in writing if a determination is made to terminate for just cause.
- Include in the letter the specific charges and findings, the intent to terminate the employment contract, and the effective date of such dismissal.
- Close her personal file attaching the letter duly signed by her.

Employee Rights When a Job is Terminated

- These rights vary according to contract agreement, and personnel policy of the institution. Some of the rights are:
  - Rights to receive the final salary
  - Rights to health coverage
  - Rights to unemployment compensation
  - Rights to service certificate.

STAFF DEVELOPMENT PROGRAM

Developing nurses' knowledge and skills is one of the important functions of nursing service administration. It is the process aiming at enhancing the personal and professional growth of nurses and other personnel while they are on the job.

Today, staff development is emphasized in all health care agencies to improve quality care outcome. The regulatory bodies of nursing at the national and state level recognize the need of staff development to renew the registration of nurses. To bring uniform standard the Indian nursing council has made it mandatory that nurses should obtain 150 nursing credit hours in 5 years or 30 nursing credit hours in a year by attending in-service education program otherwise nurses need to do re-gistration to practice nursing in the country.

Definitions of Staff Development Program

- Staff development program is a process that includes both formal and informal activities which are related to the employee's role expectation within organizations —**Karen J Kelly**

- Staff development program is a term that includes both formal and informal learning, opportunities to assist individuals to perform competently in the fulfillment of role expectations within an agency".
  —American Nurses Association

Need for Staff Development Program

- Societal change and consumerism demands from nurses is the best care for their clients. Today's health consumers are more knowledgeable. Hence, the nurse must have adequate knowledge and competence to deal with patients.
- Staff development program provides opportunity for nurses to continually acquire and implement high quality of nursing care.
- It facilitates nurses for long-term career growth.
- Medical advancement has brought more and more specialization and has an impact of medical specialization in nursing field also. Therefore, nurses must be prepared to function effectively in increasing specialization.
- Fill the gap in the past performance.
- To move ahead and keep up the change due to fast changing technologies.
- To improve productivity and to assist the nurses to improve.

Objectives of Staff Development Program

- Assist each nurse to enhance personal and professional performance.
- To ensure safe and effective patient care by professional knowledge, attitude and professional competency.
- To help nurses to cope with newer trends in health care and nursing system.
- To enhance job satisfaction among nurses.

Types of Staff Development Program

- Orientation
- Skill training
- Continuing education program
- Leadership and management skill training.

ORIENTATION PROGRAM

- It is one of the staffing functions of the nurse administrator. The main aim of this program is to familiarize the new staff nurses with the hospital, departments and the job she or he is going to do. It is a planned activity. Before the arrival of the new staff, it is planned and communicated to all members who are assigned to do the job, areas where the new nurses are oriented and methods to conduct orientation. Usually. It is planned for a week. An evaluation is done by the nurse administrator at the end of the program and recorded.
- A sample of orientation program for new nurses appointed in a hospital is given in Box 13.1.

SKILL TRAINING PROGRAM

Nurses, employers and consumers of health have grown increasingly concern with the level of skills and knowledge of health care providers who perform direct patient care. Many health care institutions conducts nursing skill/competency program for nurses as a part of continuing education program that yield definite credit hours in nursing.

The Benefits of Skill Training Program

- To enhance clinical nursing skills among nurses.
- To update with the functioning and operating of new equipment that is used for patient care as result of technological advancement.
- To meet the statutory body's expectations and accountability.
- To ensure the consumers that the nurses provides care with expert knowledge and skills.
- It brings good nursing standard of the hospital and better patient care outcome.

The nurse administrator can facilitate skill training program for nurses by assessing the needs of nurses. She can plan and coordinate with agencies who provides nursing skill competency program like Cardiopulmonary resuscitation (CPR), BCLS, ACLS, Trauma care, ventilator care, etc. A certificate will be given to nurses after successful completion of the training. The duration ranges from few hours to few days.

The Role of a Nurse Administrator

- Sets the stage using equipment similar to that of the procedure guidelines
- Gives reasons or rationale in each step of the procedure
- Creates in nurse a learner attitude in work situation
- Makes sure that the person has learned by observation
- Demonstrates step by step the procedure
- Provides written outlines for a return demonstration
- Documents program. How to plan an in-service education program in

Box 13.1: Sample orientation program for new nurses

Orientation Program for Staff Nurses

From ....to........2015

Objective: To familiarize the newly appointed staff nurses with hospital, department and job

Date and day	Time	Area of orientation	Assigned personnel
1. Monday AM	9.00	Reporting the Nurse administrator, joining report, submission of documents	Nurse administrator
	9.30	Introduction to hospital, philosophy and objectives, services rendered, various departments, organization chart	Nurse administrator
	10.30	Tea break. Meeting with medical director, Head of the departments and senior nursing personnel	Coordinator of CNE of the hospital
	11.00	Hospital policies	Assistant nursing superintendent
	12.00	Personnel policies	-do-
PM	1–2	Lunch	
	2–4	Observation, visit to hospital	Co-coordinator CNE of the hospital
2. Tuesday AM	9.00	Orientation to special departments, policies and procedures	-do-
	10.30	Tea break	
	11.00	Observation visit to ICU, CCU, OT, NICU	Assistent nursing superintendent
PM	1.00	Lunch	
	2–4	Observation visit to hostel, rules regulation	Warden
3. Wednesday AM	9–1	Visit to school of nursing/college of nursing Integration of service and education	Coordinator CNE, Principal
PM	1–2	Lunch	
	2–4	Methods of assignments, ward policies, procedures and protocol in selected department of posting	Head nurse of the unit
4. Thursday AM	9.00	Discussion on job description, nursing standards	Nursing administrator
	10:30	Tea break	
	11–1	Introduction to hospital CNE program and participation of nursing personnel–Nursing credit hours	Co-ordinator CNE program
PM-	1–2	Lunch	
	2–4	Visit to hospital library-membership	Hospital librarian
Friday AM	9 AM	Ward posting-AM duty	Head nurse of the unit
PM	1–2	Lunch	
	2–3 3–5	Introduction to hospital TNAI unit, membership visit to bank, market, religious institution, other areas of interest	
Saturday	9–1	Performance appraisal Evaluation of orientation program Any other areas of interest shown by the new staff nurse Documentation	Nurse administrator
	1–2	Lunch with all hospital nursing personnel–informal get together	Coordinator CNE

Signature of nurse administrator

Date..................

Continuing Education Program

- Continuing education is all the learning activities that occurs after an individual has completed his or her basic education —**Cooper**
- Continuing education is that education which builds on previous education —**Shannon**

Need for Continuing Education Program

- To ensure safe and effective nursing
- To update nurses knowledge and prepare them for rendering quality patient care
- To prepare for new professional roles
- For career advancements and specialization
- To cope up with new technology emerged
- To acquire specialized skills and leadership capabilities
- To develop competent nurses to provide high quality patient care
- Continuing education is a part of in-service education program
- In-service education is defined as learning experiences provided in the work of setting for the purpose of assisting nurses in performing their assigned functions in that particular health setting
- It is the education given to a nurse while in-service for her professional growth is called in-service education.

Objectives of In-service Education

- To provide better nursing care to patients by improving the knowledge and skills of nurses.
- To improve performance and professional growth of nurses.

A guideline for planning in-service education program for nurses in a hospital: Role of nurse administrator.

Any program with sound planning brings fruitful outcome. The nurse administrator should keep the following in her mind while planning in-service education program.

Decide at What Level, the In-service Education to be Planned?

- Institution level
- District level
- State level.

Assess the Needs of Nursing Personnel Through a Survey

- Felt need identified by the nurses
- Ascribed need felt by the head nurses and supervisors
- Real need felt by the patients and family members
- Need identified by the experts.

Identification of Specific Needs, Establishing Priorities and Objectives

From the data collected from above, the nurse administrator can select the priority needs and establish goals—immediate goals, intermediary goals, long-term goals and instructional goals. (Example: The nurse administrator identifies family planning as topic for in-service education).

Identify Resources

A good planning identifies effective utilization of resources available to conduct the program such as man power, money and materials.

Man Power Resources

Who can help in program planning?

- Assistant Nursing Superintendent
- Nursing supervisors
- Principal and tutors of school of nursing.

Who can help in implementation of program?

- Resource personnel and speakers
  - Professor community health department
  - Principal/tutors of school of nursing
  - Experts from district family planning bureau
  - Extension educator
  - Coordinator CNE program of the hospital
  - Social workers.
- Technical assistants like artists and projectionist
- Guest speakers from Ministry of Health and Family Welfare, Director of Health Services, State Nursing Superintendent.
- Clerical assistance from hospital
- Other agencies who can help in implementation plan like local TNAI unit, NRSI Unit, SOMI unit, regional family planning centre, Health education bureau (District/state level).

Money Resources

Any good program cannot be implemented without financial support. We need money to meet various expenses, e.g. the participants may expect some handout materials/CD, paper, pencil, file, certificates, refreshments, transport, invitation and a copy of the program. Besides this, the program may need to pay for speakers, computerist projectionist, posters, charts, etc. The nurse administrator needs to explore funds from registration fees, advertisements, donation from department of family planning, etc.

Material Resources

The nurse administrator needs to identify availability of sound system, computer system, projected and non-projected teaching aids and other materials required from inauguration to valediction.

Establishment of Program Planning Committee after Identification of Resources

- Select a program coordinator from nursing personnel to assist the nursing superintendent to conduct the program.
- Select a program secretary to keep records of all meetings, sending circulars and other procedures.
- Select a program convener who will convene the whole program. The nursing superintendent shall be the convener of the program.

The functions and responsibilities of program planning committee

- Clarifies the objectives for conducting in-service education for nurses on family planning
- Identify the problems and solutions for them during implementation program.
- Determine the overall content of the program
- Decide duration of program, time period, number and grouping of participants, and venue and dates of the program
- Suggest for resource persons, speakers moderators and chief guest and minute secretaries
- Develop inaugural and valedictory program
- Develop invitation cards, certificates to participants
- Get nursing credit hours from nursing council
- Develop pretesting question paper
- Develop evaluation and feedback strategies from participants
- Throughout the program the committee serves as a continuing resource for the convener informing day to day activities and progress of the program
- Final function of the committee is evaluation of individual sessions, topics, methods of teaching, speakers, participants interaction and media.

Chalking out the Program Schedule

The committee under the guidance of convener decides

- Which group to be educated first—ward sister/staff nurses/supervisors
- Number of participants to be admitted at a time
- When should the participants be relieved from wards and other means to cover total patient care
- Decide how many hours per session/day/week
- Develop program, course contents, units and topics as per objectives
- Decide methods of presenting the program as lecture, seminar, workshop, discussion debate field trip as per the topic
- Speakers to be finalized like teachers from the organization, guest speakers, consultants
- Decide and finalize areas of learning experiences like hospital wards/OPD (family planning clinic)/lecture hall/Health center/laboratory
- Select and facilitate instructional aids
- Finalize method of evaluation of objectives, content, learning experiences, teachers and teaching methods
- Finalize for feedback, follow-up and supervision
- Finalize the venue like classroom, conference hall of hospital and if it is outside of the hospital obtain permission.

Inform the Program with invitation and Schedule to the Departments, Speakers, Participants and Other Areas Concerned with the Program

Implementation of Plan

Evaluation of the Program

Post In-service Education Activities

- Conduct post in-service program meetings
- Settle the finance and prepare balance sheet
- Finalize finance by auditing
- Send thanks letters to all who helped in the program
- Send the report to participants, management, and nursing council
- Ensure complete documentation of the event.

Follow-up Study

It can be done either by sending questionnaire or interviewing the participants or by day to day observation/ report from the authorities for the satisfaction of nurses and patients in relation to the in-service program attended.

LEADERSHIP AND MANAGEMENT TRAINING

To days health care delivery system is more challenging for nurses than ever before. To cope with the changing trends in health care, social change, technological advancements, specialization, demographic transition and consumerism demands on developing nurses as leaders. Nursing leaders today acknowledge that unprecedented level of responsibility is being devolved to frontline workforce in nursing and emphasize leadership knowledge, skills and behaviors needed to improve quality patient care outcome. Effective and successful leadership from nursing workforce is crucial to the delivery of high quality health care to counter the challenge they face today. Studies had shown that there is an important concern regarding the First-line nurse manager's leadership because of the recognition that effectiveness of leadership in this position results in benefits for the whole health care organization. So knowledge and practice of effective leadership behavior are now more essential to nursing than ever before. First-line nurse managers must be effective leaders to meet today's challenge because staff nurses and patients are affected by them.

The nurse administrator must do a need analysis regarding leadership activity among senior nurses, supervisors, and head nurses and plan leadership training program for nursing personnel. Soft skills like interviewing skills, communication skills, decision-making skills, conflict management skills, negotiation skill and team building skills also to be included in the training program. The professional organization of the country (TNAI) imparts leadership and management training program for nurses at national level.

Staff development program is an important component of successful health care systems. The systematic and ongoing provision of opportunities to maintain, update, develop, and enhance professional skills, knowledge, and attitudes can lead to improved health care experiences and health outcomes for the community.

SUPERVISION

Supervision is a managerial tool envisages working together to achieve organizational goals.

Definition of Supervision

- Supervision is an art or a process by which subordinates are helped to make the best use of their knowledge and skill.
- It is a process of guiding, directing, critically evaluating, and correcting the performance of nursing personnel which in turn brings quality patient care outcome.
- Supervision enhances, stimulates, promotes and fosters personal and professional growth.

Definition of Clinical Supervision

Clinical supervision aims to support, motivate and encourage personal and professional growth.

Objectives of Supervision

- To understand the needs and problems of nurses. Good supervision motivates nurses and helps to share their needs and problems to nurse supervisor.
- To understand the working style of nurses. There are various factors that influence the style of working of nurses. Family background, personality traits, educational preparation, professional attitude and professional competency, years of experience, interest to work in the particular unit, and the working environment have an impact on working style of nurses. Through effective supervision, the nurse administrator can help to improve the working style of nurses in a positive way.
- The nurse administrator constantly evaluates the performance of nurses through planned supervision.
- The nurse administrator can provide a feedback of performance of nurses and plans for counseling if needed.
- Good supervision enhances professional growth.
- Supervision is complete when the supervisors reward/recognize or appreciate the nursing personnel for their good performance.

Principles of Supervision

- Good supervision is need-based. The supervision of student nurse is different from staff nurse because their need for growth is different.
- The nurse administrator considers mission and values of the organization while supervising nurses.
- Good supervision is based upon the job description of nursing personnel as job and functions vary. For example the functions of head nurse is different from staff nurse.
- The nurse administrator has a responsibility to conduct well-planned supervision based on objectives, methods and criteria for evaluation.
- Good supervision is always democratic and unbiased.
- It is nurses centered rather administrator centered.
- It is continuous and on-going.
- Good supervision respects and maintain individuality.
- Helps supervisee to set personal goals in line with the organizational goals.
- Establishes good interpersonal relationship.
- Provides freedom for experimentation, self-direction and self-evaluation.

Styles of Supervision

- Autocratic style
  - In this style, the administrator intends at task accomplishment and ignore nurses' priority and needs.

- Benevolent style
  - In this style, the administrator holds a protective attitude always towards nurses. Nurses are provided with constant guidance irrespective of needs.
- Democratic style
  - This style involves nurses in faith and confidence. They are included in decision-making. This style creates work motivation and improves morale of nurses.

Techniques and Tools of Supervision

The nurse administrator uses the following techniques/tools for effective supervision:

- Ward rounds
- Interview and questioning
- Individual/group conference
- Supervisory diary/Journals
- Performance evaluation
- Verbal and written reports
- Orientation and guided experience
- Manuals and protocols
- In-service/continuing education.

Supervisory Skills

The nurse administrator/supervisor possesses the following skills for supervision:

- Subject expertize and competence in supervising nurses
- Possesses leadership qualities
- Demonstrates effective communication skills
- Shows problem-solving ability and decision-making skills
- Demonstrates mental maturity and emotional stability
- Possesses good physical and mental health
- Always shows a good listening capacity
- Demonstrates socially accepted manners.

Barriers to Effective Supervision

- Inadequately prepared supervisor
- Inappropriate nurse-patient ratio
- Lack of dignity and respect for one's own profession
- Poor work environment
- Too rigid/ too flexible personalities
- No evaluative measures
- Less importance to documentation
- Nursing is not placed well in organizational structure.

How to Overcome Barriers of Supervision

- Be in touch with 'recent advances' in nursing practice and administration
- Establish conducive working environment for nurses
- Inclusion of supervisors to various committees
- Promote staff welfare measures to retain nurses
- Develop expertize in supervisory skills
- Be a role model for nurses in the hospital.

Role of Nurse Administrator in Effective Supervision (Fig. 13.1)

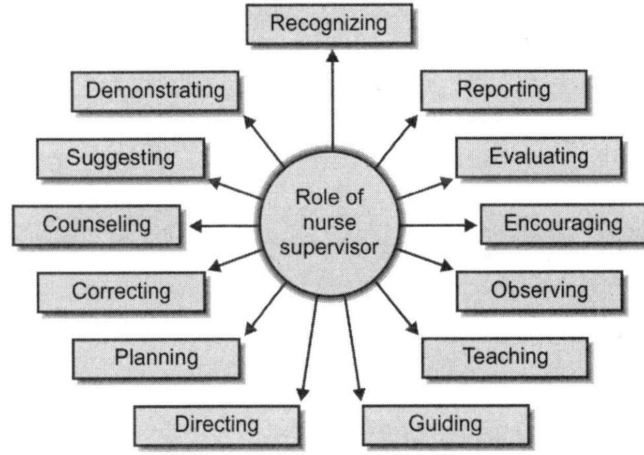

Fig. 13.1: Different roles played by nurse administrator in supervision

JOB DESCRIPTION OF NURSING PERSONNEL

Job Description

Duties and Responsibilities of Nursing Personnel

The success of hospital depends on the performance of its employees. All jobs in an organization must inter-relate to accomplish the organizations, mission, goals and objectives.

Terms Used

- *Task:* A unit of work activity performed by a worker within a limited time period.
- *Duty:* Several related tasks that are performed by a worker.
- *Position:* The set of all tasks and duties performed by a worker.
- *Job:* A group of identical positions.
- *Job analysis:* The process of collecting and analyzing information about jobs to write. Thus, it is a process of documenting the job.
- *Job description:* It is a document that identifies the tasks and duties performed by a job. It is a

written description of a job and its requirements. Job description include job title and location, organizational relationship, primary duties, working conditions and level of financial accountability.

- *Job specification:* A written document that identifies the qualifications required by a job such as education, professional experience, training, mental abilities.
- Physical fitness and skills, judgment and decision-making abilities.

Purposes of Job Analysis

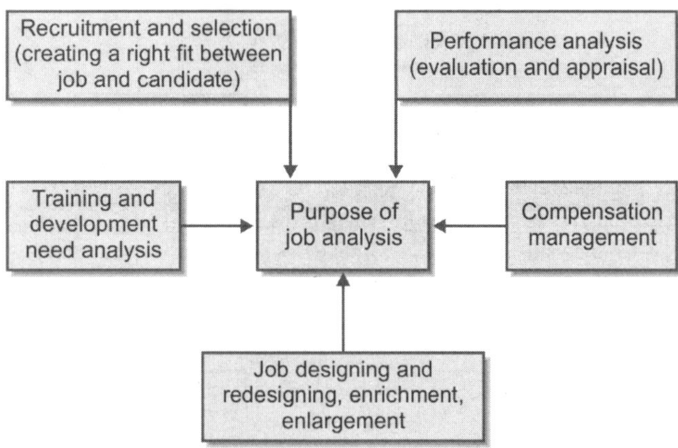

Fig. 13.2: Purposes of job analysis

- *Recruitment and selection:* Job analysis helps the nurse administrator in deciding what kind of nurse is required to perform a particular job. It focuses on the educational qualifications, level of experience and technical, physical, emotional and personal attributes required to carry out a job in desired manner. The objective is to fit a right person at a right place with right job.
- *Performance analysis:* It is done to assess whether the goals and objectives are meeting the particular job or not. It helps in deciding the performance standards, evaluation criteria and individual's output. On this basis, the overall performance of an employee/nurse is measured and he or she is appraised accordingly.
- *Training and development:* Job Analysis can be used to assess the training and development needs of nurses. The difference between the expected and actual output determines the level of training that need to be imparted to nurses. It also helps in deciding the training content, tools and equipments to be used to conduct training and methods of training.
- *Compensation management:* Job analysis plays a vital role in deciding the salary and benefits and incentives to nurses. This depends on the position, job title and duties and responsibilities involved in a job. The process guides the administrator in deciding the worth of an employee for a particular job.
- *Job designing and redesigning:* The main purpose of job analysis is to streamline the human efforts and get the best possible output. It helps in designing, redesigning, enriching and, evaluating responsibilities in a particular job. This is done to enhance the nurses' satisfaction.

Therefore, job analysis is one of the most important functions of staffing management. This helps in fitting the right kind of talent at the right place and at the right time.

Application of Job Analysis

- HR management
- HR staffing
- Job description
- Performance appraisal
- Job design and redesign.

Factors to be considered while doing Job analysis

- *Job context:* It includes the purpose of the job, work environment and its place in the organization.
- *Job content:* It means the duties and responsibilities of the persons who hold the job.
- *Job specifications:* It describes knowledge, skills and competencies required of a person to have a reasonable chance of being able to successfully perform the job.

Process of Job Analysis

The process of job analysis include four phases:

- *Phase I:* The administrator needs to study the scope of the project, decides the purposes of the project and identifies which jobs to include.
- *Phase II:* This phase concerned with method of job analysis. The administrator decides which type of data is needed, identifies sources of data and selects specific procedures for job analysis.
- *Phase III:* This phase focuses on data collection and analysis. The administrator arranges to collect the job data, analyses the data, reports the findings to the organization and recheck the job analysis data collected previously.
- *Phase IV:* This phase concentrates assessment of job analysis methods. The administrator evaluates the results against criteria of benefits, costs and legal aspects.

Functions of Job Description

- It defines the job for performance planning, transfer, promotion, staff planning, career development and disability accommodations.
- It is as standard format, i.e. used for consistent application.
- It gives nurses a written description of their job.
- It is used for comparing salary survey data.

Elements of Job Description

- *Position Summary:* Position overview that identifies purpose and objective of the job.
- *Essential functions:* The task, duties and responsibilities of the job useful for evaluation.
- *Non essential job functions:* Desirable but not necessary aspects of the job.
- *Knowledge, skills and abilities:* Required competencies of the job.
- *Working conditions:* Environment in which the job is performed.
- *Minimum qualification:* Minimum KSA's required to enter the job
- *Success factors:* Personal characteristics that contribute to a person's ability to perform the job.

Guidelines to write Job Description Do's and Don's

- Job descriptions must be based on the specific duties and responsibilities actually performed within the organization.
- Do give a realistic and descriptive job titles
- Do keep the summary brief
- Do list primary duties, tasks and responsibilities
- Do identify essential job functions
- Do review the KSA's (Knowledge, Skill and Attitude) and make sure they are job- related
- Do secure approval and dates
- Do include appropriate disclaimers
- Do not include demeaning titles
- Do not include gender-specific titles
- Do not include percentages.

Box 13.2: A sample job description of nursing superintendent of a district hospital

Job Title.......... Nursing superintendent

Department....... District hospital

Qualification and Experience

Essential: 10 years' experience after BSc (N) out of which 5 years should be administration experience with minimum of 5 years in clinical nursing program.

Desirable: MSc Nursing.

Registration: Registered under State Nursing Council for Nursing, Midwifery and Higher Qualification.

Mode of recruitment: Direct selection/UPSC selection/ State Public Service Commission.

Professional promotional avenue: Assistant director of nursing

Reporting authority: Reports directly to the authority as per the norms of the organizational policy

Job summary: The nursing superintendent acts as an administrator, who controls the overall program of financial, clinical, and research of the hospital in relation to nurses and nursing.

JOB DESCRIPTIONS

Administrative Functions

- Plans and formulates vision and mission statement, philosophy and objectives of nursing service department.
- Plans and develops various policies and objectives for educational program for nurses.
- Maintains recognition of nursing service department of the hospital by accrediting bodies such as INC, State council and other accrediting bodies.
- Determines the staffing requirement as per statutory norms.
- Responsible for recruitment, selection, Appointment, placement and development of nursing and non-nursing personnel.
- Prepares the job descriptions, indicates line of authority, accountability and channel of communication by means of organizational chart.
- Delegates functions and guide subordinates.
- Identifies the professional needs related to educational program and facilitates staff development program in coordination with HODs/coordinators.
- Maintains performance appraisal reports of her subordinate staff and recommend for promotion/other incentives.

Contd...

Contd...

- Attends regularly scheduled meeting with the authorities to share information and concerns of nursing services.
- Chairs nursing committees of the hospital.
- Plans and propose the short-term and long-term budget for nursing service department.
- Acts as drawing and disbursing officer.
- Monitors all expenditures related to nursing service department.
- Ensures internal and external auditing of account.
- Maintains effective public relations
- Acts as member in Institutions Board and Ethical Committee for the approval of research of medical and nursing and faculty students.
- Maintains discipline of all nursing personnel
- Collaborates with disciplinary committee regarding all complaints about nursing staff and take suitable disciplinary actions by disciplinary committee/joint consultative committee.
- Identifies conflict among staff members and identifies resolution
- Allocates workload to the entire nurses as per norms.
- Promotes the morale of staff by facilitating welfare activity.
- Facilitates communication interpersonal relationship both inter and intradepartmental and with other institutions at State, National and International levels.
- Maintains integration of academic and clinical activities
- Establishes a compassionate environment by providing emotional, psychological and spiritual support to nursing personnel.
- Takes responsibility for counseling and guidance of staff.
- Monitors the effective office administration for smooth functioning of the nursing service department of the hospital.
- Maintains all administrative records including personnel policy manual.

Academic Functions

- Coordinates the planning, implementation and evaluation of program with school of nursing
- Facilitates for good clinical experiences for student nurses
- Participates in academic committee meetings in terms of students education
- Maintains supplies and inventory by identifying the needs, anticipated needs supplies, and approving requisitions
- Encourages and facilitate various educational program like workshops, conferences, and seminars
- Ensures clinical experience facilities for students nurses in various clinical areas of the hospital
- Participates in teaching and supervising educational program
- Facilitates in conduct practical examination for student nurses
- Facilitates inspection by various statutory bodies.

Supervisory functions and research

- Supervises and guides all nursing and non-nursing personnel
- Provides the infrastructure facilities and learning environment for students
- Procures and maintains instructional materials for teaching and learning
- Ensures the safety and security of nursing students in the hospital
- Supervises patient care in all units wherever nurses are posted
- Initiates and coordinate research program in nursing practices. Acts as member in Institution Review Board (IRB) and Ethical Committee for the approval of research of faculty, students and nurses
- Promotes evidence-based practices in clinical area

Signature..................
Date............................
Prepared by............
Seal

Box 13.3: Research highlights

A Survey of Needs in Continuing Education for Staff Nurses

Since, the initial training of nurses may not equip them adequately in the discharge of their duties throughout their working life, need for continuing education has become more important

A survey of continuing education for staff nurses was conducted by the author at Agra among 200 nurses. The study investigated the continuing education needs of nurses and the factors that influence their participation in such activities. The study observed that the needs of the nurses vary according to their area of work, interest, age, experience, promotional scope and availability of financial support. Eighty percent of nurses participated in continuing education program in order to improve upon their skills and competence and to keep their professional standards. Ten percent were interested in nursing administration and research. Ten percent nurses wanted to attend but could not attend due to financial constraints and not relieved from ward duties.

The study concluded that continuing professional education for nurses is determined by the circumstances they find themselves and interest to continue to keep up with new developments in the field of and nursing (Raman AV 1973).

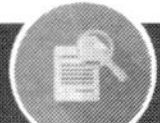

SUMMARY POINTS

- ✓ The concept of staffing includes planning for, recruiting, selecting, and training and developing employees, as well as compensating them and providing for their health and safety. Recruitment is a process of searching for prospective employees and stimulating them to apply for job in an organization. Selection of employees is the next step in which the applications are received and scrutinized for its eligibility based on the selection criteria, various tests are conducted final interview is established, references are checked, medical examination is conducted and appointment is given if the candidates successfully completes all the above.
- ✓ Orientation is a process of making the employee a sense of belongingness to the institution. Placement is given after orientation. Promotion is the upward reassignment of an employee in an organization's hierarchy after successful performance of the employee.
- ✓ Employee retention refers to the ability of the organization to retain its employees and prevent frequent turnover of the employees.
- ✓ Developing personnel policies is one of the staffing functions. Personnel policies are written statements developed by the management with respect to manpower management in the organization. Personnel policies guides employees to choose the course of action as and when needed.
- ✓ Employee termination is very painful staffing function of an administrator. Employee termination is the relieving of an employee against his or her desire for cause, or for lack of work. The process is sometimes unavoidable for the health of an organization. Terminations, must be carried out promptly when the need for such actions becomes obvious in order to preserve the health of the organization.
- ✓ Staff development program is a term that includes both formal and informal learning, opportunities to assist the employees to perform competently in the fulfillment of role expectations within an agency. Various methods include in staff development program are orientation, skill training, continuing nursing education and leadership and management skill development.
- ✓ It is a process of guiding, directing, critically evaluating, and correcting the performance of nursing personnel which in turn brings quality patient care outcome. It enhances stimulates, promotes and fosters personal and professional growth of nurses.
- ✓ Job analysis is the process of collecting and analyzing information about jobs. Thus, it is a process of documenting the job whereas job description is a document that identifies the tasks and duties performed by a job. It is a written description of a job and its requirements. Job description include job title and location, organizational relationship/primary duties, working conditions and level of accountability. However, job specification is a written document that identifies the qualifications required by a job such as education, professional experience, training, mental abilities, physical fitness and skills, judgment and decision-making abilities.

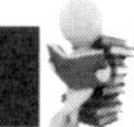

REVIEW QUESTIONS

1. Define recruitment. Discuss the factors influencing recruitment of nursing personnel.
2. Enumerate the causes of turnover of nurses working in a hospital. Discuss the role of nurse administrator in retaining nurses.
3. Define personnel policy. Describe its purposes and contents.
4. What is staff development program? Outline an orientation program for newly appointed ICU nurses.
5. Effective supervision enhances nursing care outcome. Describe the role of nurse administrator in supporting the statement.
6. Differentiate job description and job specification. Outline a job description format for a nursing superintendent working in a district hospital.
7. **Write short notes on:**
   a. Merits and demerits of recruitment of nurses from external and internal sources
   b. Selection process
   c. Promotion and placement
   d. Purposes of job analysis
   e. Termination of job
   f. In-service education.

SELECTED READINGS

1. Abassi, SM and Hollman, KW 2000. Turnover: the real bottom line Public Personnel Management, 2(3): 303-342.
2. Adams, Orvilland Hicks,V. (2000) : Pay and non-pay incentives, performance and motivation, prepared for WHO, December 2000, Global Health Workforce Strategy Group.
3. Booth, S, Hamer, K. 2007. Labor turnover in the retail industry, International Journal of Retail and Distribution Management, 35(4): 289-307.
4. Boxall, P, Macky, K Rasmussen, E. 2003. Labor turnover and retention in New Zealand: The causes and consequences of leaving and staying with employers, Asia Pacific Journal of Human Resources, 41(2): 196-214.
5. Bryant, Rosemary. 2005. Regulation, roles and competency development. Issue Paper. Geneva, Switzerland: International Council of Nurses. http://www.icn.ch/images/stories/documents/publications/GNRI/Issue1_Regulation pdf (accessed July 30, 2012).
6. Campbell, B, G Mackay. 2001. "Continuing competence: An Ontario nursing regulatory programme that supports nurses and employers." Nursing Administration Quarterly 25, no. 2, 22-30.
7. Huffcut, AI (2010). From science to practice: Seven principles for conducting employment interviews. Applied HRM. Research, 12, 121-136.
8. McDaniel, MA, Whetzel, DL, Schmidt, FL, and Maurer, SD (1994). The validity of employment interview: A comprehensive review and meta-analysis. Journal of Applied Psychology, 79(4), 599-61
9. Personnel Policies - Free Management Library management help.org/personnelpolicies/policies.htm.
10. Personnel Selection: Methods: Interviews'. www.hr-guide.com. Retrieved 2015-12-01.
11. Podsakoff, NP, Whiting, SW, Podsakoff, PM, and Mishra, P (2011). Effects of organizational citizenship behaviors on selection decisions in employment interviews. Journal of Applied Psychology, 96(2), 310-326.
12. US Department of Labor Employment and Training Administration. (1999) 'Chapter 1: Personnel Assessment.' pp. 1-7.

UNIT VI DIRECTING

14 Leadership

LEARNING OBJECTIVES

This chapter imparts learning about:
- Concept and Definition of Leadership
- Leadership Theories and Styles, Qualities of Leader and Assertiveness
- Creating a Motivational Climate: Motivation, Concept and Theories
- Organizational Communication Strategies
- Communication Skills
- Research Highlights

INTRODUCTION

Nursing profession depends upon capable leadership to guide nursing professionals and consumers through unprecedented changes. Yet, there is ample evidence in the news and in research reports that even some of the best and most venerable professions are failing to adapt to change or prepare their professionals for more uncertain future.

CONCEPT AND DEFINITION OF LEADERSHIP

Meaning of Leadership

Leadership is a noun. According to World English Dictionary leadership means:
- Position or function of a leader
- The period during which a person occupies the position of a leader
- The ability to lead.

Concept of Leadership

- Leadership is a process. The leader influences the followers to achieve the organizational aims and goals. He or she directs the establishment to make it more cohesive and coherent
- Leadership is not only a process but also is a force that develops a capability among his group members to perform tasks in a better and different manner to achieve the organizational goals.

Concept of Nursing Leadership

- It is the process of influencing nurses to accomplish goals of the hospital or nursing school or community
- Leadership as force for change, and nurse leaders innovate nursing practice
- Nurse leaders focus on nurses empowerment
- Nurse leaders do; influence fellow nurses to achieve goals–long-term and short-term
- Nurse leadership inspire nurses through personal trustworthiness and self-confidence and involvement
- Nurse leaders communicate a vision that turns self–interest to commitment to the profession.

Definition of Leadership

- Leadership is defined as the activity of leading a group of people or an organization or the ability to do this which involves establishing clear vision, sharing that vision with others so that they will follow willingly.

- Providing the information knowledge and methods to realize the vision and coordinating and balancing the conflicting interest of all members and stake holders.
- Leadership is commonly defined as a process of influence whereby the leader influences others toward goal achievement. Leadership – what leaders do; the process of influencing a group to achieve goals something that is different or better
- Leadership is a force that creates a capacity among a group of people to do something that is a different from others.

Formal and Informal Type of Leadership

When an individual, by the virtue of holding highest position in the organization and has assigned the responsibility of the organization to him is described as formal leadership or assigned leadership, e.g. the nursing superintendent, of a hospital is a formal leader.

Whereas, informal leadership is referred as when an individual demonstrates leadership capability and functions as a member of the group. He is not the head of the establishment. He is an emerging leader identified and accepted by members of the group because he can influence others.

LEADERSHIP THEORIES AND STYLES, QUALITIES OF LEADER AND ASSERTIVENESS

The Great Man and Trait Theory

Great Man Theory was an earliest theoretical approach to leadership. Certain traits in individuals were considered responsible for the success/effectiveness of the organization. According to Aristotelian theory, great men are identified as leaders by his followers and some are born as leaders to lead the masses.

Trait Theory

Trait theory believes that individuals with peculiar characteristics or traits makes them good leaders than others. However, the current theories emphasizes that leadership skills are developed not comes as inborn.

Behavioral Theory

This theory describes, leadership capabilities are decided by certain types of action practiced by individuals. However, McGregor et al stressed the change of traits of leadership to situational leadership. Lewin, White and Lippit described three common leadership styles are:

1. Autocratic
2. Democratic
3. Laissez-faire

CHARACTERISTICS OF AUTOCRACTIC LEADER

Autocratic leaders do things by themselves. They possess the power in the organization, and takes all decision alone without involving other members. The leader expects whatever he wants the subordinates to do they have to do it without any clarification or questioning. The nature of autocratic leadership in organization are:

- The leader has strong control over the group members
- Members are motivated to work by force or coercion
- All the activities by members are done by command from the leader.
- There is no provision for upward communication, only one way communication that flows from upward to downward.
- The decision-making authority is only the leader, and members are not involved in autocratic leadership.
- This type of leadership gives weightage to status of the member.
- Punishment is given on criticism by members.

The Impact of Autocratic Leadership on Organization

- Results in well defined group of actions
- Results are predictable and reduce frustration among work group
- Productivity is very high
- Useful in crisis situation
- This type of leadership is common in large organization system.

CHARACTERISTICS OF A DEMOCRATIC LEADER

- A democratic leader exercises and maintains minimum control over his employees
- The leader ensures incentives to motivate the employees
- Others are directed and motivated through suggestions and guidance
- Communication flows from up and down
- Decision-making involves others (employees)
- Appreciation is given on the task done by everybody not the leader alone
- Criticism is constructive.

The Impact of Democratic Leadership on Organization

- Appropriate for groups that works together for extended periods
- Provides autonomy for growth of individuals
- There is organizational effectiveness
- Effective when cooperation and coordination are necessary
- Takes time to make decision because of consultative process
- Less efficient quantitatively.

CHARACTERISTICS OF LAISSEZ-FAIRE LEADER

- Permissiveness—with little or no control over the employees
- Provision of little or no direction to employees
- Communication upward, down ward and flow among members
- Emphasis on work among group members
- Criticism is withheld.

Situational and Contingency Theories

In this approach, leader trait and leader behavior are important aspects but the situation is given more important in this theory.

CHARACTERISTICS OF SITUATIONAL LEADER

This type of leaders believe that there is no single best way to lead. It focuses on maturity and readiness of the followers (ability and willingness). More emphasis is given on task and relationship behavior of leader and followers and integration is stressed in all leadership activities.

SITUATIONAL LEADERSHIP STYLE

- **Telling:** This type of leadership style is exercised when employee demonstrates low readiness, untrained, and inexperienced in their tasks.
- **Selling:** This type of leadership style is exercised when employee demonstrates low/moderate readiness, trained but unexperienced in carrying out tasks.
- **Participating:** When employee demonstrates moderate, high readiness, to participate in tasks.
- **Delegating:** When employee demonstrates high readiness and ready and willing to take responsibility.

Effectiveness of the situational leader is based on the level of maturity of the followers. Hence, less task focuses on leader (Hersey and Blanchard). Leadership skill is exercised by diagnosing, adapting and communicating.

FIEDLER'S LEADERSHIP CONTINGENCY THEORY

This theory focuses on the group and the group effectiveness depend upon appropriate match between leadership style and the demand of the situation. In this theory the success depends upon:

- Leader
- Member relations
- Task structure
- Position
- Power.

BLAKE–MOUTON MANAGEMENT GRID THEORY

The foundation of this theory is that the management should have concern for both the human relations and completion of work and tasks

According to this theory the leaders demonstrate five management styles:

- ***Impoverished management:*** Low concern for people and task
- ***Country club management:*** High concern for people and low concern for tasks
- ***Organizational management:*** This theory assumes that the performance is improved by ensuring the balance between the employees morale and tasks to be done
- ***Authority obedience:*** This philosophy is consistent with autocrat leaders who show concern for tasks not for the employees psycho-social needs
- ***Team management:*** In this style the leader demonstrates interest in the tasks as well as the employees.

PATH-GOAL THEORY

According to this theory, leader's behavior is supportive, directive, more achievement oriented and participative.

SUPPORTIVE LEADERSHIP

Figure 14.1 shows the effectiveness of supportive leadership. It reduces boredom and makes the job more tolerable. This type of leadership increases the intricate valence of work that in turn increases the effort of the employee. It increases confidence among employees and lower anxiety and increases effort to performance expectation.

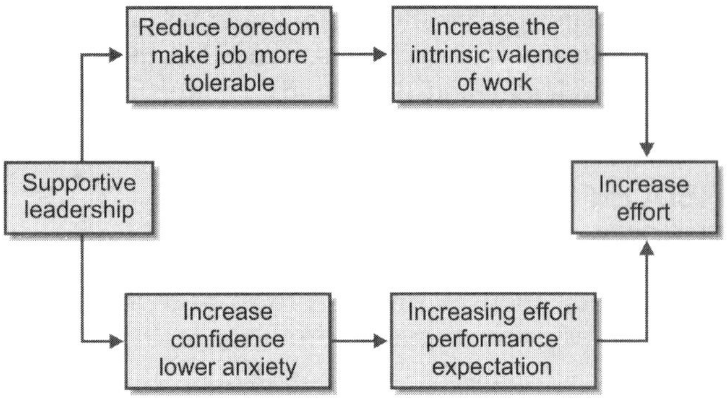

Fig. 14.1: Supportive leadership

DIRECTIVE LEADERSHIP

In directive leadership the Fig. 14.2 shows that it decreases role ambiguity, increases performance, size of incentive, outcome valence of work among employees that in turn increases employees effort to achieve organizational goals and objectives.

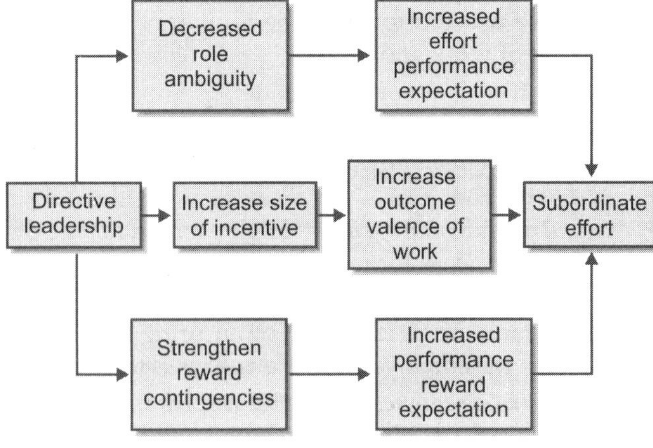

Fig. 14.2: Directive leadership

NEWER APPROACHES IN LEADERSHIP THEORIES (CONTEMPORARY THEORIES)

Transformational and Transactional Theories

Burns (1978) states newer theories focuses on both leaders and followers have the ability to enhance the highest level of motivation and that in turn will raise morale of the organization

- Transactional leaders are of traditional type of leaders who are mostly focus their attention on day today activities
- Whereas, transformational leaders are visionaries, committed to work and the people and empower subordinates to achieve the vision of the organization

Interactional Theory

- Schein (1970) in this theory describes human as a complex being, whose working environment is an open system to which they respond, system consists of objectives, humans and their attributes
- Peter Drucker explains that leadership is more than rank and status in the organization. According to him leadership is a responsibility towards the people and the organization
- Kanter (1989) describes that in leadership title and position authority are not enough to develop the workforce. The employees need to be empowered and encouraged to self-thinking and the leaders must work with the employees enthusiastically as a team
- Brandt 1994 says leaders must ensure to provide a work setting for employees that fosters autonomy and creativity through valuing and empowering others.

In interaction theory, the leadership roles are:

- Guiding
- Directing
- Teaching
- Motivating for goal setting
- Motivating for achievement.

TYPES OF LEADERSHIP

- Leader by the position achieved
- Leader by personality, (charismatic leaders)
- Leader by moral and ideal
- Leader by power held
- Intellectual leader
- Leader because of ability to accomplish things
- Autocratic leadership
- Bureaucratic leadership.

Bureaucratic Leadership Style can be Effective When:

- Employees are performing routine tasks over and over.
- Employees need to understand certain standards or procedures.
- Employees are working with dangerous or delicate equipment that requires a definite set of procedures to operate.
- Safety or security training is being conducted.
- Employees are performing tasks that require handling cash.

Charismatic Leadership

Charismatic leadership is leadership based on the leader's capability to converse and behave in ways that reach followers on a basic, moving way, to motivate and inspire. A charismatic leader should have the gift to speak on a very commanding emotional level, and maybe include some personality traits. Some of the famous charismatic leaders include JF Kennedy, Nelson Mandela and Winston Churchill.

Democratic/Participative Leadership Style

A democratic leader gives importance to the people in organization. He believes that they are an asset and without them organization cannot function. He gives importance to the responsibilities taken by each employee and not with status or title. This leader involves them in making decisions and respects their values and opinion, while making final decisions though he knows the ultimate responsibility for decision-making as his own, and he has to face the consequences of his decisions alone.

Laissez-Faire Leadership Style

The Laissez-Faire leadership style is where all the rights and power to make decisions is fully given to the worker. This was first described by Levin, Lippitt, and White in 1938, along with the autocratic leadership and the democratic leadership styles.

Servant Leadership Style

This type of leaders gives importance to values diverse opinions of employees and develops a culture of trust among employees. They develops future leaders and empower the followers for their development and thinks for others. They are visionaries and humble and humane

People/Relations-oriented Leadership Style

The leader gives importance to the relationships amongst the group and is more concerned with the overall welfare and satisfaction of group members. Relationship-oriented leaders focus on effective communication within the group, trustworthiness, and confidence in group members, and recognizes the good work done with rewards and incentives.

Task-oriented Leadership Style

Task-oriented leadership is a style in which the leader concentrates on the tasks done by the employees to achieve organizational goals. Whatever the problems comes in the organizations, the leader solves them systematically so that the goals are achieved.

TRANSACTIONAL LEADERSHIP STYLE

In this type of leadership the employees are responsive and leaders work within the organizational culture. Employees achieve objectives through rewards and punishments set by leader. The leader motivates followers by appealing to their own self-interest and management-by-exception maintains the status quo; stresses correct actions to improve performance. Some of the characteristics are:

- Leadership exchanges rewards for services.
- Management watches for deviation.
- Keep system operating smoothly.
- Uses rewards and coercive power bases.
- Recognizes what workers wants and tries to deliver it.
- Rewards according to workers effort.
- Responsive to workers self-interest.

TRANSFORMATIONAL LEADERSHIP STYLE

In this type leadership is proactive and leaders work to change the organizational culture by implementing new ideas. The employees achieve objectives through higher ideals and moral values. The leaders motivate followers by encouraging them to present group interests first. Some of the characteristics of the leaders are:

- Inspirational, idea oriented
- Dramatic, arouses intense feelings
- Communicates high expectations and need for change
- Raises level of awareness among values, vision and mission of the organization
- Empower others to develop personally and professionally
- Intellectual stimulation always observed
- Has long-term vision for the organization
- Team approach and group morale
- Maintains organizational climate.

QUALITIES OF A LEADER

One of the qualities observed in all types of leaders is they use good interpersonal skills to influence the members to accomplish organizational goal. They are capable, trustworthy, authentic in their work, accountable and demonstrate enthusiasm, energy, and Commitment

- A leader is always a visionary. A visionary leader shares the power and recognition and she/he must be charismatic, inspirational, respectful, and stimulating, invigorative and creative when leading. A good leader has an exemplary character and integrity.
- A good leader is energetic, vibrant and hardworking about his/her job and also their role as leader. Being a leader with dedication and determination, the members always respond to such committed leader.

- A good leader is confident and always inspired by others Seeing the confidence and skills to lead, the members imbibe such leadership role and the task are easily completed.
- A leader always functions in a systematic and purposeful manner in situations of uncertainty
- Good leaders are tolerant of ambiguity and remain calm, composed and steadfast to the main purpose. They are emotionally stable and mentally matured individuals
- A good leader thinks analytically keeping the main goal in focus. He analyses the whole problem or problem in parts to know the situation and finds alternative solution.
- A good leader is committed to excellence towards his profession
- The good leader maintains high standards is proactive in raising the bar in order to achieve excellence in all areas. (www.GROCO.com)

ASSERTIVENESS

Assertiveness is the quality of being self-assured and confident without being aggressive, it is a learnable skill and mode of communication (Wikipedia).

According to Dorland's medical dictionary, assertiveness is a form of behavior characterized by a confident declaration or affirmation of a statement without need of proof; this affirms the person's rights or point of view without either aggressively threatening the rights of another (assuming a position of dominance) or submissively permitting another to ignore or deny one's rights or point of view.

Assertiveness is a behavior that is demonstrated by self-confidence, and a positive attitude towards self and others. A person being assertive concentrates on his or her goal-being self-aware, true to self, building of self-esteem and nurturing and showing respects to one self and others rights. Psychologists explain that being unassertive demonstrates behavior like weak, passive, compliant of self and others, self-sacrificing self-centered, inconsiderate, hostile, arrogantly demanding behavior.

Some of the behaviors demonstrated by assertive person as from the literature are:

- The assertive persons make requests, ask for favors and respect the dignity of individuals as human being these behaviors reduce the fear and self-depreciation of an assertive person.
- These persons show positive emotions like joy, pride, liking someone, attraction and to give compliments.
- Assertive persons assume responsibility to share and control of the adverse situation and tries to make things better.
- They initiate, continue, change and terminate conversations comfortably and understands one's feelings, opinions and experiences.

Steps to Building Assertiveness

There are four basic steps that can help to become more assertive in every day interactions with others.

1. Realize where changes are needed and believe in one's rights.
2. Chalk out appropriate ways of asserting oneself in each specific situation that concerns to him or her.
3. Give assertive responses
4. Try being assertive in real life situations.

Assertiveness and Nursing

Since, nurses deal with daily staff meetings and interactions with doctors and patients, they must know how important it is to speak assertively and get listened by people. But what exactly does 'assertively' mean and how do they speak without hurting them.

Communicating effectively is pivotal to professional success as a nurse. Some of the tips are given below:

Shows confidence in front of patients who's obviously concerned about their health. Make eye contact to ensure that the nurse is listening to the patient.

Exhibit Leadership Qualities

When a nurse is assertive in communication she is leading the conversation.

Be Specific and Clear

To avoid miscommunication, the nurse should speak clearly and stay on topic. If she is curious or need clarification about something, she should not hesitate to ask, the members of the health team. The nurse should be kind, professional and courteous.

Say Exactly What is Meant

No one likes to listen to someone drone on. Often, the more is said, the less is heard. Keep things specific, use facts, and be conversational—not confrontational.

Listen Carefully

Most times, people just want to be heard. Put the patients at ease and make them more open to listening and understanding with the possible solution. This works wonders on patients!

Do not Feel Guilty for Being Assertive

It is more than good to stand up for self, ideas, and opinions. Being assertive is, very important when communicating with fellow staff members, patients and doctors. Practice, assess the situation and use confidence to emphasize rather than provoke.

CREATING A MOTIVATIONAL CLIMATE: MOTIVATION, CONCEPT AND THEORIES MOTIVATION

Motivation is the characteristic that helps the individual to achieve goal. It is the drive that pushes the individual to work hard. It is the energy that gives the strength to keep going even when things are not going well. It is the internal energizing force which makes the individual to work.

DEFINITIONS OF MOTIVATION

According to Young, motivation is the process of arousing the action, sustaining the activity in process and regulating the pattern of activity.

Morgan and King describe motivation is a state within a person or animal that drives behavior toward some goals. Underwood explains motivation as the classes of operations used to produce and measure changes in performance and changes in energy output.

Motivation refers to all the internal conditions that stir up activity and sustain activity of an individual.

MEANING OF MOTIVATION

Motivation is derived from the Latin word 'movere' which means 'to move' or 'to energize' or 'to activate'.

THEORIES OF MOTIVATION (CONTENT THEORY AND PROCESS THEORY)

Various approaches has been described through theories to study motivation (Fig. 14.3).

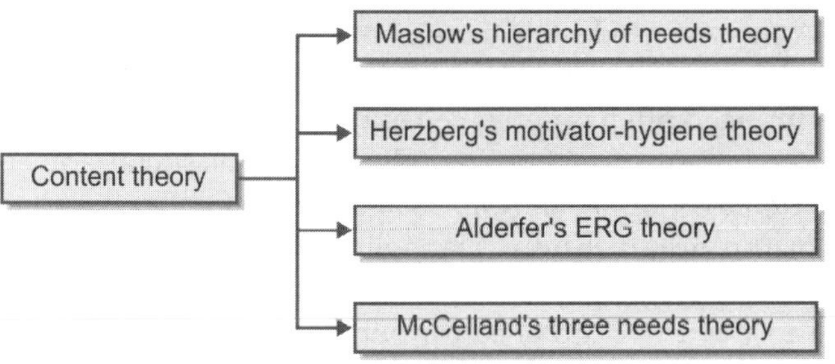

Fig. 14.3: Content theory approach to motivation

CONTENT THEORY OF MOTIVATION

1. Maslow's Theory of Motivation

Human beings have a hierarchy of needs that ranges from lower to higher. As lower needs are fulfilled there is a tendency for other, higher needs to emerge Maslow's theory maintains that a person does not feel a higher need until the needs of the current level have been satisfied. See Maslow's hierarchy pyramid (Fig. 14.4).

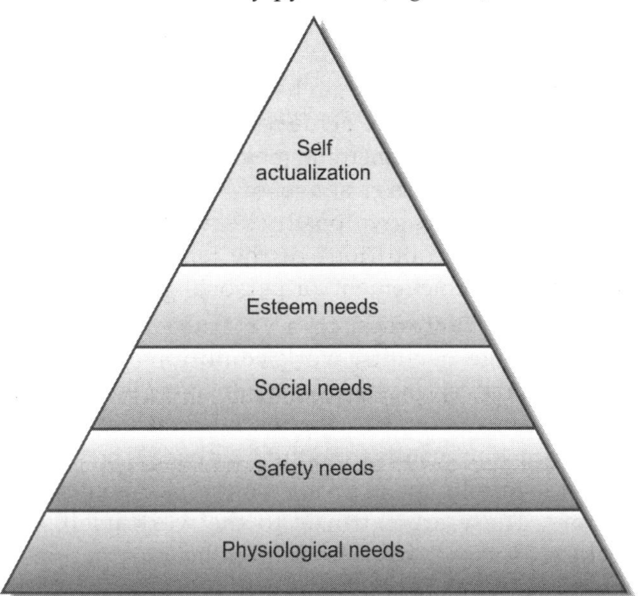

Fig. 14.4: Maslow's hierarchy of needs pyramid

Needs at the lower levels of the hierarchy dominate an individual's motivation as they are unsatisfied once, these are adequately satisfied, the higher needs occupy the individual's attention and efforts.

Application of Maslow's Theory in Nursing Administration

- *Physiological motivation:* Facilitate midmorning/lunch break, pay salaries fair price canteen in the hospital campus that allow nurses to buy life's essentials.
- *Safety needs:* Provide a safe working environment, sufficient job security, and freedom from threats to nurses.
- *Social needs:* Generate a feeling of acceptance, belonging by reinforcing team dynamics and organize informal gathering of nursing personnel.
- *Self-esteem:* Recognize achievements and recognize the exemplary nursing services, assign important and innovative projects, and provide status to make nursing personnel feel valued and appreciated.
- *Self-actualization:* Offer challenging and meaningful work assignments which enable innovation, creativity, and progress according to long-term goals.

2. Two-factor Theory of Motivation

It was initiated by psychologist Frederick Herzberg, who explained that job satisfaction and job dissatisfaction act independently of each other.

The two-factor theory (also known as Herzberg's motivation-hygiene theory and dual-factor theory) describes that there are certain factors in the workplace that cause job satisfaction, while a separate set of factors cause dissatisfaction.

Motivating factors such as challenging work, recognition for one's achievement, responsibility, opportunity to do something meaningful, involvement in decision making, sense of importance to an organization that give positive satisfaction, arising from intrinsic conditions of the job itself, such as recognition, achievement, or personal growth.

Hygiene factors such as status, job security, salary, fringe benefits, work conditions, good pay, paid insurance, vacations that do not give positive satisfaction or lead to higher motivation, though dissatisfaction results from their absence. The theorist used the term hygiene because these are maintenance factors. These are extrinsic to the work itself, and include aspects such as hospital policies, supervisory practices, or salary.

This theory is also known as two factor theory Herzberg's Motivation-Hygiene Theory.

Application of Two-factors Theory in Nursing Administration

The job should have sufficient challenge to utilize the full ability of the nursing personnel. Nurses who show extra ordinary ability should be given increasing levels of responsibility. If a job cannot be designed to use an employee's full abilities, then the person will not be motivated to work.

3. Alderfer's Erg Theory of Motivation

It is the theory of Existence, Relatedness and Growth (ERG). The theory is evolved from Maslow's Hierarchy of needs through efforts to further understand and expand its implications.

ERG is mostly applied to the study of human motivation in the workplace as a device for increasing morale and productivity. It has helped researchers to understand what constitutes job satisfaction and to identify incentives.

Application of ERG Theory in Nursing Administration

ERG is used as managerial tool for enhancing. Job satisfaction, Self-esteem, coworker relationship, and team work. Nursing administration and leadership style influence and contribute to wards the motivation of nursing personnel

4. McClelland's Three Needs Theory of Motivation

David McClelland proposed this theory explains that an individual's specific needs are acquired over time and are shaped by one's life experiences. This is also explained as acquired-needs theory. Most of these needs can be classified as **achievement, affiliation,** or **power**. A person's motivation and effectiveness in certain job functions are influenced by these three needs. McClelland's theory sometimes is referred to as the **three need theory or as the learned needs theory.**

Achievement

People with a high need for achievement seek to excel in their work and thus tend to avoid both low-risk and high-risk situations. Achievers avoid low-risk situations because the easily attained success is not a genuine achievement. In high-risk projects, achievers see the outcome as one of chance rather than one's own effort. High achiever individuals prefer work that has a moderate probability of success, ideally a 50% chance. Achievers need regular feedback in order to monitor the progress of their achievements. They prefer either to work alone or with other high achievers.

Affiliation

The people with high need of affiliation maintain harmonious relationships with others and need to feel accepted by other people. They abide with regulations a policies and norms of their work group. A unique feature of high need of affiliation persons likes a job that provides effective personal interaction and shines well in customer service and client interaction situations.

Power

A person's need could be personal and institutional. Those who need personal power want to direct others, and this need often is perceived as undesirable. Persons who need institutional power (also known as social power) want to organize the efforts of others to further the goals of the organization. Managers with a high need for institutional power tend to be more effective than those with a high need for personal power. A thematic apperception test is used to identify the achievement, affiliation and power need of a person whether it is personal or institutional.

Application of McClelland's Three Needs Theory of Motivation in Nursing Administration

The nurse administrator should understand that people with different needs are motivated differently. Nurses who are high achievers should be given challenging projects with achievable. They should be provided frequent feedback.

Nurses with a high affiliation need perform best in a cooperative environment.

An opportunity to be given to nurses with higher need of power to manage nursing units (Fig. 14.5).

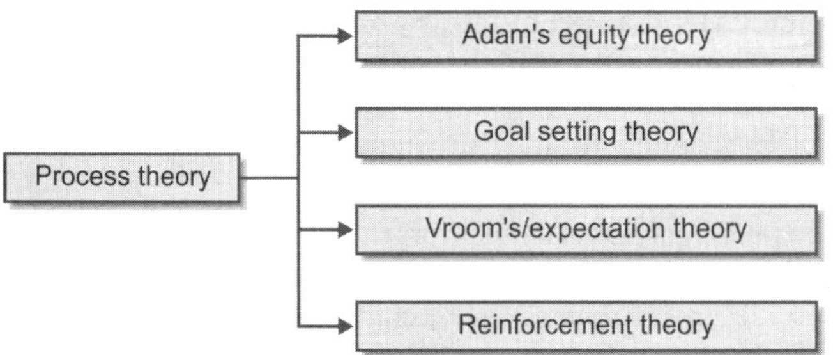

Fig. 14.5: Process theory approach to motivation

PROCESS THEORY OF MOTIVATION

1. Adams' Equity Theory of Motivation

Adams' Equity Theory is named after John Stacey Adams, a workplace and behavioral psychologist, who developed his job motivation theory in 1963. Adams' Equity Theory describes that employees become demotivated, both in relation to their job and their employer, when they feel their inputs are greater than the outputs. Employees feel a disparity between the input and output (Fig. 14.6).

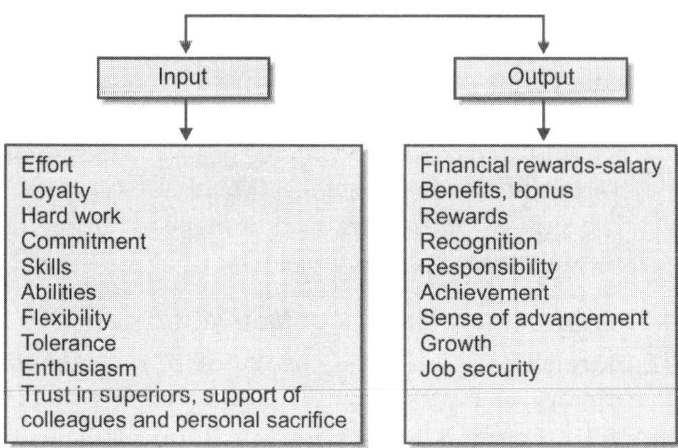

Fig. 14.6: Adams' equity theory of motivation–input and output factors

Motivation is enhanced by facilitating a balance between the input and output. That means, finding this fair balance serves to ensure a strong and productive relationship is achieved with the employee, with the overall result being contented, motivated employees.

Application of Adams' Equitable Theory of Motivation in Administration

The nurse administrator has to keep in mind that when nursing personnel are assessed whether the inputs they demonstrate are fair. The employee will often compare their colleague's work inputs and outputs with their own. The comparison will often be made with an employee at a similar level in the organization.

To motivate nurses the administrator should ensure that they are facilitated with fair number of working hours, work responsibilities, their input and loyalty, and the support and feedback given by the administration.

The administration should facilitate a decent salary benefits, rewards and recognition for outstanding performances, objective performance appraisal, leave benefits and flexibility in dealing with nursing personnel.

When nursing personnel believe that their work outputs are not equal or Lesser than their inputs then the employee will become demotivated.

2. Goal Setting Theory of Motivation

Definition

Goal setting theory is refers to the outcome of established goals on organizational performance. Edwin Locke is the authority of this theory and describes his research findings. He observed in his research that individuals who formulate specific and difficult goals performed better than those who set general and easy goals.

Locke proposed five basic principles of goal setting: clarity, challenge, commitment, feedback, and task complexity.

- ***Clarity:*** A goal that is clear, measurable and well defined is more achievable than one that is poorly defined. One of the criteria for the most effective goals is defining a time frame for completion of the goal.
- ***Challenge:*** The goal must have a reasonable difficulty level in order to motivate a person to work hard towards achieving the goal.
- ***Commitment:*** When a goal is set, the individual put hard work to achieve the goal. He may identify resources to increase the input to strengthen the outcome to meet that goal.
- ***Feedback:*** In order to monitor the progress made in in the performance in achieving the goal, a method of feed back mechanism is important.
- ***Task complexity:*** Give enough time to overcome the complexity. If a goal is especially complex in completing the task. Or, if a goal is really tough, make sure to give some time in addition to complete the goal.

Application of Goal Setting Theory of Motivation in Nursing Administration

Set or Review Organizational Objectives

The nurse administrator needs to define and clarify organizational objectives to nursing personnel.

Ensure the Goals are Attainable and Relevant to the Work Unit

Once the objectives are set the administrator ensures that they are clear to nursing personnel. She makes sure that the goals are attainable and the employees feel accountable.

Encourage Participation in Goal Setting

The administrator encourages nurses in sharing and discussing the goals formulated to understand the reason for formulating such goals. This allows every nurse to set goals to align with the organizational goals and also allows for **an increase for personal responsibility** of their objectives. This enhances motivation among nursing personnel to do better performance as self-direction, decision-making, and responsibility is felt by individual nurses.

Monitor Progress

The goals and objectives are developed based on criteria that are Specific, Measurable, Attainable, Relevant, Time-based, (SMART) can be monitored. She makes sure every goal has mini goals, and adequately monitors goal performance and accountability.

Evaluate and Reward According to Performance

Nurses are evaluated on their performance related to the goal, and retrospectively include rewards, such as compensation and provide appropriate feedback.

3. Vroom Expectancy Theory of Motivation

Victor Vroom proposed Expectancy Theory. This theory believes that all human behavior results from conscious choices among alternatives. The purpose of this conscious choice is to maximize satisfaction and minimize pain.

The key elements to this theory are referred to as following:

- Valence (V)
- Instrumentality (I)
- Expectancy (E).

Valence refers to the perception of individuals psychologically to hold with respect to outcomes or rewards. It may range from the score from –1 to +1. When the individual prefers not attaining an outcome compared with attaining it is termed as negative valence. A zero valence is referred if the individual is indifferent to the outcome.When the individual has the strong preference to the outcome ,it is referred as positive valence. All motivated individuals demonstrate a positive valence.

Instrumentality refers to the first level outcome will lead to the second level outcome. The score value of Instrumentality varies from 0 to 1. If an employee perceives that promotions are based on performance, instrumentality will be rated high. A low estimate of instrumentality will be made if the employee fails to perceive a relationship between performance and reward.

Expectancy refers to an effort that will lead to completion of a task. The score value of expectancy varies between 0 to 1. If an employee sees no chance that effort will lead to the desired performance, the expectancy is zero. On the other hand if the employee is confident that the task will be completed, then as a the expectancy has a value of 1.

Application of Vroom's Expectancy Theory of Motivation in Nursing Administration

- The administrator should know that motivation = Valence × Instrumentality × Expectancy
- Reward system is a motivating factor and makes nurses productive and help in achieving organizational goals
- The nurse's goal is determined by her age, educational qualification, previous clinical experience, economic status, culture, values and belief.
- Assignment to nurses must match the determinants, priorities of the organization and job.
- Facilitate a work environment that must be satisfying nursing personnel.
- The administrator should remember that the activities and the organizational goals depends upon the performance and satisfaction of nurses.
- The success of the organization depends upon the administrator's leadership style.

4. Reinforcement Theory of Motivation

BF Skinner proposed the theory of reinforcement as a theory of motivation. According to this theory the individual's behavior is a function arising from consequences and is based on law of effect. That means individual repeats the behavior again and again because he has experienced a positive consequences, but he never repeats the behavior when the consequences are negative and not satisfying. Thus, according to Skinner, the external environment of the organization must be designed effectively and positively so as to motivate the employee.

There are four approaches of reinforcement to motivate employees

Positive Reinforcement

This denotes giving a positive response when an individual shows positive and desired behavior. For example, when an employee shows punctuality on his job. Immediately praising him for maintaining punctuality will increase probability of repetition of the same behavior again and again. It must be remembered that more spontaneous is the giving of reward, the greater reinforcement value it has.

Negative Reinforcement

This means rewarding an employee by removing negative/undesirable consequences. Both positive and negative reinforcement can be used for increasing desirable behavior.

Punishment

It is an approach of removing positive consequences so as to lower the probability of repeating undesirable behavior in future. In other words, punishment means applying undesirable consequence for showing undesirable behavior. For example, cutting of the weekly off of a nurse for breaking the ward policy.

Extinction

It means avoiding the reinforcements. In other words, extinction implies lowering the probability of undesired behavior by removing reward for that kind of behavior. For instance if a nurse is no longer receives recognition for her good work, she may feel that her behavior is producing no fruitful outcome. Thus, extinction may unintentionally lower desirable behavior.

The Application of Reinforcement Theory in Nursing Administration

Positive and negative reinforcement are common, and often complementary tools used by administrators to motivate nurses. A positive reinforcement is a reward or incentive offered to a nurse for meeting certain performance standards. A negative reinforcement is the use of a consequence, such as loss of pay or a demotion, to discourage an employee from underperforming or behaving offensively or unethically. The nurse administrator uses rewards to reinforce the behavior she expects from nurses in the hospital work environment and uses punishments to prevent the undesirable behavior in work setting. The administrator uses extinction approach to stop nurses from performing a learned behavior.

ROLE OF NURSE ADMINISTRATOR IN CREATING MOTIVATING CLIMATE

- The nurse administrator should apply techniques, skills and knowledge of motivational theory to help nurses to achieve the goals of nursing service department.
- The administrator's role is to influence each nurse's behavior and action towards achievement of organizational objectives.
- Creates a conducive working environment that enhances job satisfaction.
- Facilitates a motivational climate where nurses work with autonomy and able to meet basic needs.
- Provision of counseling and guidance, coaching and training to increase individual nurse's performance and creates a productive climate.
- Applies positive and negative reinforcements, punishment and extinction approaches of motivation to enhance organizational behavior among nurses.
- Monitors performance and provides feedback to nurses for improvement if any.
- She knows clear expectation for nurses, and communicate these expectations effectively to nurses.
- Be fair and consistent when dealing with all nursing personnel.
- Demonstrates effective leadership style.
- Identifies the strengths of nurses and provide experiences that challenge or stretch the employee, and allow opportunity for growth.
- Involves nurses in goal setting and decision-making.
- Creates a trustful and helping relationship with employees.
- Uses her authority to provide formal reward systems.
- Uses positive feedback to reward the individual employee.
- Develops unit goals that integrate organizational and subordinate needs.
- Maintains a unit environment that eliminates or reduces job dissatisfies.
- Promotes a unit environment that focuses on employee motivation.
- Assign work duties commensurate with nurses' abilities and postperformance to foster a sense of accomplishment in them.
- Identifies achievement, affiliation or power needs of subordinates and develops appropriate motivational activities for subordinates. (**Please also read application of motivational theories in nursing administration presented above explained under each theory**)

ORGANIZATIONAL COMMUNICATION STRATEGIES

Introduction to Communication

- Communication is defined as the imparting or interchange of thoughts, opinions, or information by speech, writing, or signs
- Communication is defined as interchange of information between two or more people
- Communication skill is defined as ability to use language and express information
- Communication may be defined as a process concerning exchange of facts or ideas between persons holding different positions in an organization to achieve mutual harmony
- Communication is the process of exchange of ideas, views, facts, feelings, etc. among people. As per literature, 75% of time spent by members in an organization is on interpersonal interactions. One of the causes for organizational problem is poor communication.

Purposes

- To share ideas and opinions.
- To provide feedback to others.
- To get information from others.
- To gain power and influence.
- To develop social relationships.
- To maintain self-expression and our culture.

Communication Process

The communication process is dynamic in nature rather than a static phenomenon. Communication process is considered a continuous and dynamic inter-action, both affecting and being affected by many variables.

They are source, message, encoding,communication channel, decoding, receiver and feed back (Fig.14.7) as follows:

- **Source:** The person who intends to convey the message with the intention of passing information and ideas to others is known as source or communicator.
- **Message:** This is the subject matter or idea of the communication. This may be an opinion, attitude, feelings, views, orders, or suggestions.
- **Encoding:** Since, the message of communication is theoretical and intangible, its further passing requires use of certain symbols such as words, actions or pictures, etc. Conversion of message into these symbols is the process of encoding.
- **Communication Channel:** The person who is interested in communicating has to choose the channel for sending the required information, ideas message, etc. This information is transmitted to the receiver through certain channels which may be either formal or informal.
- **Receiver:** Receiver is the person who receives the message or for whom the message is meant for. It is the receiver who tries to understand the message in the best possible manner in achieving the desired objectives.
- **Decoding:** The person who receives the message or symbol from the communicator tries to convert the same in such a way so that he may extract its meaning to his complete understanding.
- **Feedback:** Feedback is the process of ensuring that the receiver has received the message and understood in the same sense as sender means it.

Barriers to Effective Communication

A barrier means obstruction that exists between two persons and keeps them separate. It can interfere communication process.

- **Badly Expressed Message:** Inadequate vocabulary, usage of wrong words and faulty translations. The translator has to be proficient with both the languages symbols with different meanings
- **Semantic Barriers:** Use of technical jargon, symbols or words with different meanings, unqualified assumptions, body language and gesture decoding
- **Physical barriers:** These are obstacles that prevents the flow of message due to physical factors such as distance, power failure noise in the environment, etc. For example, Power off while working. Unwanted

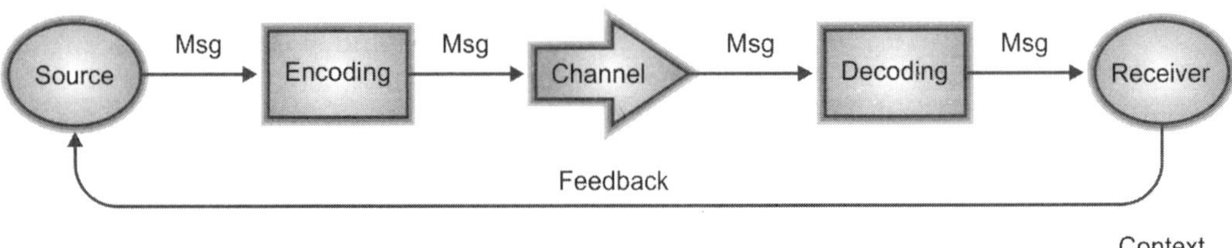

Fig. 14.7: Communication process

sound while meeting. Noise, network down while mailing, etc.

- **An inattentive receiver:** Self-centered attitude of receiver.
- **Psychological barriers:** People who are preoccupied may not pay attention to the message and may react emotionally This is a distraction and become hindrance in effective communication.
- **Faulty transmission:** When we are not paying attention, the message is not registered in our mind. That causes poor retention and partly we retain message.
- **Cultural barriers:** Age, religion, education gender, social status, standards, economic position, cultural background health, priority political belief ethics, values, motives, rules/regulations are some of the cultural barriers influence communication.
- **Organizational barriers:** Organizational policies rules and regulations status complexity, organizational facilities are some of the organizational factors can influence communication in an organization. Organizational structure plays an important role on effective communication among employees.
- **Gender barriers:** There are distinct differences between the speech patterns of man and those in women.
- **Other barriers:** Getting distracted daydreaming, interrupting, listening only to contents, not the feelings, not attending to nonverbal clues prejudging the speaker, jumping to conclusions, talking, not listening failing to express opinion, tone of voice talking too fast, being judgmental, body language. etc.,

Ways to Overcome Barriers

- Use proper of channel of communication
- Hit the right audience
- Listen
- Speak louder than words
- Give explicit message
- Follow-up action.

COMMUNICATION STRATEGIES IN AN ORGANIZATION

Communication is one of the important functions of an organization whether it is a small or very large organization. Even one-to-one communications can be a challenge and sometimes bring misunderstandings. If the management wants positive outcome and good interpersonal relationship it needs to think about effective communication strategies in an organization. Some of the strategies for effective communication is described below.

Open Communication

For the success of the organization, leaders opt for open communication strategy in which the members of the organization irrespective to their level, interact freely, discuss care and share their ideas communicate feedback of their job done including criticism to the management. Committed leaders practice open communication build an environment of a trust culture.

Inclusive Communication

An inclusive communication strategy refers that the management to ensure all employees feel they are involved in decisions that affect their job. Secretive communication in an organization tends to bring poor participation of members in involving major decision that in turn will affect managerial outcome. Employee involvement is basic factor that affects employee satisfaction and success of the organization.

Two-way Communication

Effective communication strategies involve two-way communication, between members of the organization. Establishments whose managers successfully engage employees in communicating about their work, bring out their ideas and their perspectives on issues related to, services, customers and the work environment enhances a communication culture of inclusiveness that brings better results of the organization.

Results-driven Communication

If we want the organizational communication to be effective, it should be goal oriented, to achieve measurable results. Organizations need to respect employees needs related to work environment, job characteristics, effective interaction with members and clients, and to serve as change agent outside of the organization.

Multi-channeled Communication

There is an individual difference among employees. The employer must know these differences and use multi methods of communication system that can be benefitted by all employees. Effective organizational communicators aware of that messages need to be delivered multiple times, in multiple ways to have the most impact. Employee communication needs and preferences differ. Different messages require different methods channeled communication and that brings effectiveness in an organization.

ENHANCING COMMUNICATION SKILLS

Become an Engaged Listener

- **While communication pay attention fully on the speaker,** his or her body language, tone of voice, and other nonverbal cues.
- **Listen the information with patience** and register what is being said
- **Try to avoid any interruption of talk from your interest or redirecting conversation from the track**
- **Show your interest in what's being said by nodding your head on a,** smile at the person, and make sure your posture is shows your concern about him.
- Encourage the speaker to continue with small verbal comments like saying go ahead, that seems fine
- **Be nonjudgmental in communicating with others**
- **If there is a pause or disconnect of sentences from the speaker, reinforce what he had said so far to continue further.**

Pay Attention to Nonverbal Signals

- **Understand individual differences in nonverbal communications from person to person.** People from different cultures tend to use different nonverbal communication gestures, like age, culture, religion, gender, and emotional state take into account when understanding body language clues.
- **Use nonverbal signals that** should reinforce what is being said.
- **Adjust your nonverbal signals according to the situation. It vary from age to age or person to person.**
- **Use body language to convey positive image.**

Keep Stress in Check

- Control of emotion is important to effective communication, you need to control of your emotions in situations such as a job interview, seminar presentation, board meeting, etc.
- **While communicating make a pause to collect your thoughts**—pausing can make you more in control than rushing your response.
- **Make one point** at a time and provide an example or supporting piece of information.
- **Be explicit in your words while communicating,** and make eye contact. Keep your body language relaxed and open.
- Summarize your response and then stop talking.

Assert Yourself

- **Value yourself and your opinions.** They are as important as anyone else's.
- **Know your needs and wants.** Learn to express them without infringing on the rights of others.
- **Express negative thoughts** in a positive way. Its OK to be angry, but you must be respectful as well.
- **Receive feedback positively.** Accept compliments graciously, learn from your mistakes, ask for help when needed.
- **Learn to say no know your** limits and do not let others take advantage of you. Look for alternatives so everyone feels good about the outcome.

Other Communication Skills

- Use conflict resolution skills
- Managing conflicts with humor
- Overcoming loneliness and shyness
- Meeting people and building friendships

EFFECTIVE COMMUNICATION SKILL AND ROLE OF NURSING SERVICE ADMINISTRATOR

- Effective communication is the key factor to a nurse administrator's success. So to grow as a leader and manager, she/he must learn how to be an effective, and skillful communicator. Leadership is a challenge.
- Acts as a communication champion rather than just as an information processor.
- Uses key elements of effective listening and understand why listening is important to leadership communication.
- Recognizes and applies the difference between dialogue and discussion.
- Selects an appropriate communication channel for leadership message and effectively uses nonverbal communication
- Communicates in a way that persuades and influences others.
- Effectively communicates during times of stress or crisis.

Box 14.1: Research highlights

Effectiveness of a leadership development program on leadership competencies of undergraduate nursing students and head nurses

(Dr Usha Marath)

A mixed method study was conducted to find the impact of leadership development package (LDP) on leadership competencies among 30 undergraduate nursing students, and 30 head nurses working in 2 leading private hospitals and 2 leading private colleges of nursing Ernakulum, Kerala state. Second purpose was to assess the organizational climate prevalent in the selected institutions and the readiness and commitment of key management personnel towards the implementation of the leadership development package in their institution. Finally, it was also to find the satisfaction of participants with the leadership development package. The Systems Research Organizing Model (SROM) was selected as the conceptual framework for the study.

The study observed that the leadership development package was instrumental in bringing significant changes in all the Five Exemplary Leadership Practices that served as the basis for learning to lead included: (1) Model the Way; (2) Inspire a Shared Vision; (3) Enables Others to Act; (4) Challenge the Process; and (5) Encourage the Heart among participants. From the feedback of the participants it was clear that the LDP was effective in improving the knowledge and understanding of leadership and highly appreciated the program. The key management personnel expressed the need for such program and were ready to implement such program in their institution.

Nurses often take on leadership positions with enthusiasm when they are provided with tools, training and the active support and encouragement of their superiors. More specifically, increasing general leadership opportunities for all levels and positions, including frontline nurses, would encourage more nurses to consider leadership positions. Nurses cannot improve the culture of their work environment on their own, regardless of the amount and quality of training and support they receive or the depth of their commitment. Lasting cultural and behavioral change requires consistent commitment, leadership and guidance from senior management. It is also recommended that leadership education should be consistently provided. It is preferable to integrate the concept of leadership throughout the nursing education curricula of the program. It is also suggested to integrate it in the extracurricular, in the training of clinical instructors, lecturers, and to provide leadership continuing education courses for nurses.

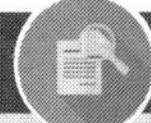

SUMMARY POINTS

- ✓ Leadership denotes to accomplish an objective and directs the organization in a way that makes it more cohesive and coherent.
- ✓ Formal leadership is based on occupying a position in an organization, called assigned leadership. Informal leadership occurs when an individual demonstrates leadership outside the scope of a formal leadership role or as a member of a group.
- ✓ Various leadership styles brings an impact on the organizational effectiveness. Transformational, transactional and servant leadership styles, are used by nursing leaders to days administration. Assertiveness in leadership activities is a great challenge for nurse administrators.
- ✓ Motivation refers to all the internal conditions that stir up activity and sustain activity of an individual.
- ✓ Various theoretical approaches used in motivating employees to create motivational climate in an organization to enhance organizational effectiveness.
- ✓ Communication may be defined as a process concerning exchange of facts or ideas between persons holding different positions in an organization to achieve mutual harmony.
- ✓ Communication is the process of exchange of ideas, views, facts, feelings, etc. People in organizations spend over 75% of their time in an interpersonal interaction. The major cause for organizational problems arising from poor communication.
- ✓ The communication process involves the source, encoding, message, receiver, decoding and feedback.
- ✓ There are barriers observed in communication such as badly expressed message: semantic barriers, physical barriers, psychological barriers : faulty transmission: cultural barriers organizational barriers gender barriers and other barriers
- ✓ The various ways to overcome barriers are use proper of channel of communication hit the right audience listen, speak louder than words, give explicit message and follow-up action.

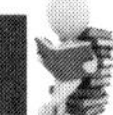

REVIEW QUESTIONS

1. Define leadership. Discuss modern approach to leadership theories.
2. Describe the type of leadership required to meet the challenges in nursing today.
3. What is motivation? Describe the role of nurse administrator in creating a motivational climate in hospital.
4. What are the communication barriers? As a nurse administrator, how will you enhance communication skill among nurses?
5. Define assertiveness. How will you develop assertive leadership among head nurses to promote organizational effectiveness?
6. **Write short notes on:**
   a. Transformational and transactional leadership
   b. Qualities of a nursing leader
   c. Creating motivational strategies in an organization
   d. Maslow's hierarchy of motivational needs
   e. Effective communication
   f. Communication process.

SELECTED READINGS

1. Alimo-Metcalfe, B., Alban-Metcalfe, J 2005. Leadership: Time for a New Direction? *Leadership*, 1 (1), 51-71.
2. Avery, GC (2005). *Understanding Leadership.* London: Sage Publications
3. Beck, RC (2004). *Motivation: Theories and principles* (5th ed.). Englewood Cliffs, NJ: Prentice Hall.
4. Borod, JC (2000). *The neuropsychology of emotion.* Oxford University Press, Oxford.
5. Deckers, L. (2014). *Motivation: Biological, psychological, and environmental* (4th ed.). Boston, MA: Allyn and Bacon.
6. Encyclopedia of Management (2009). Leadership Theories and Studies. In Encyclopedia of Management. http://www.enotes.com/management-encyclopedia/leadership-theories-studies
7. Fisk, P The making of a digital leader. Business Strategy Review, (2002). 13 (1), 43-50.
8. Goleman, D, Boyatzis, R., and McKee, A. The emotional reality of teams. *Journal of Organizational Excellence*, (2002). 21(2), 55-65.
9. Marath Usha and Ramachandra.2015. Impact of Leadership Development Package on Leadership Competencies of Head Nurses. International Journal of Nursing Education. 7(1), 87-93
10. Mumford, MD, Zaccaro, SJ, Connelly, MS, Marks, MA. Leadership skills: conclusions and future directions. *Leadership Quarterly*, (2000). 11 (1), 155-70.
11. Northouse, PG (2007). *Leadership: theory and practice.* 4th ed. Thousand Oaks, CA: Sage Publications. Jutta Heckhausen(Ed.) Motivation and action London: Cambridge University Press,2008
12. Raman, Meenakshi and Sangeeta Sharma. Technical Communication: Principles and Practice. Second Edition. New Delhi: Oxford University Press, 2011.
13. Ref:www.mindtools.com/pages/article/newLDR_84.htm#sthash.cpxDkMwG.dpuf.
14. Rutherford, Andrea J. Basic Communication Skills for Technology: Second Edition. Delhi: Pearson Education, 2007.
15. Seely, John. Writing Reports. New York: Oxford University Press, 2002.
16. Sharma, RC, Krishna Mohan. Business Correspondence and Report Writing: Third Edition. New Delhi: Tata McGraw Hill Publishing company Limited, 2007.
17. Thill, John V, Courtland L. Bovée, Excellence in Business Communication, 10th edition. Boston : Pearson, 2013.

15

Organizational Behavior and Human Relations

LEARNING OBJECTIVES

This chapter imparts learning about:

- Group Dynamics
- Human Relations
- Public Relation in Context of Nursing
- Decision-making
- Delegation
- Conflict Management
- Negotiation
- Collective Bargaining
- Research Highlights

GROUP DYNAMICS

Introduction

Group dynamics is one of the organizational behaviors. Constructive interactions among members of nursing services influence organizational effectiveness and enhances patient care outcome

Definition of Group

- A group is defined as when two or more people interacting and come together to achieve particular goals (Harold Koontz, 2004).
- An aggregate of individuals who interact and mutually influence each other (Shaw, 1981).
- A group—refers to a collection of people who are attached to one another and held together by forces.

Definition of Group Dynamics

The group dynamics is defined as a change that occurs within groups in a social setting due to interactions that influence the attitudes and behavior of members of the group or in other words, it is concerned with the forces working within a group to achieve certain goals.

Group dynamics is two way communication implies a situation where not only two parties talk to each other as well as it helps in clarification of confusion misconception and understanding with each other by receiving and giving of feedback.

Group dynamics is viewed from the perspective of internal nature of group: how they are formed, why groups are formed, what are their structure and process, and how they affect individual members, other groups and the organization (Mamori, 1996).

Group dynamics describes how a group should be organized and conducted. Democratic leadership member participation and overall cooperation are stressed in group dynamics.

Group dynamics, is a field of study that explains how people interact and build unity.

Classification of Groups

The groups are mainly classified as:

- ***Psychological group:*** This group is the one in which two or more individuals who are interdependent to each other influences every other individuals. For example, family as a group that interact with each other to make a decision

- ***Social group:*** A group is formed with individuals who work together as an integrated system to achieve an established goals. For example, a political party.
- ***Formal group:*** A group that is formed under the legal or formal authority with the view to achieve a particular end result. For example military force in which individuals works for nation's safety.
- ***Informal group:*** A group of individuals works in an aggregate manner. In other words, Informal groups are social structures which connect people naturally over a period of time. For example, clique or groups among hospital employees.
- ***Primary group:*** It is a small group of individuals who communicate and interact among members. Example family is a primary group.
- ***Secondary group:*** It is a large sized group and the members possess certain values and beliefs prevailing among them rather actual interaction. For example, trained nurses association, society of midwives, nursing research society of India.
- ***Command group:*** It is a group formed by members of an establishment who directly report to a particular manager/officer. For example. Assistant Superintendents of Police and Superintendent police forms a command group.
- ***Task group:*** The task group are members of a group who work together to perform a task but involve a cross command relationship. It is a temporary task force group. For example, trained nurses association of India (TNAI) organized a task force committee to develop job description for nursing personnel.
- ***Interest group:*** The interest group involves individuals who come together to accomplish a particular goal with which they are concerned. For example office staff of college of nursing.
- ***Friendship group:*** In friendship group individuals are formed a group having one or more common concern. For example, friendship group supported flood calamity at Chennai.

Purposes of Group Formation

Individuals prefer to join such group that are stable and help the members in achieving their objectives.

- When the individual belongs to a particular group, he perceives a sense of security.
- When the group has a positive vision, the members are recognized as a member of that particular group. It gives a status to the individuals.
- It enhances self-esteem, worthiness and a sense of belongingness to the group members.
- Becoming a member of a group, it satisfies the social needs of the individual and members enjoy group interaction.
- When the individual is a member of a group, he achieves power and strength as he closely interact with members of the group.
- When there is a group effort, it is easier to achieve goals of individual members.

CHARACTERISTICS OF GROUPS

- Common motives conducive to group interaction.
- A group structure with a hierarchical status system.
- Standardization of norms and values.
- It has one or more common goals.
- Interactions and communication occur among members.
- Members with in a group assume roles.

STAGES OF DEVELOPMENT OF GROUP

Groups develops through six stages:

- ***1st stage Orientation:*** In this stage, the group members are oriented with an outline of their purpose, goals, rules, responsibilities and each members schedule.
- ***2nd stage Forming:*** In this stage, the group members acquaint with each other through verbal and nonverbal communication. According to the problem identified, a plan is developed with group concentrating on the problem. The leader facilitates trust, and openness, participation and creativity among members and their views, ideas, opinions and thoughts are encouraged to bring outThe leader is more directive in this stage.
- ***3rd stage Storming:*** In this stage, group members begin to trust and become cohesive. Leader gives fewer directives but refocuses the group and starts to assign tasks to each member. There is concern, criticism, confrontation and conflict in this phase.
- ***4th stage Norming:*** Here, there is cohesion, commitment and cooperation, and trusting relationship among leader and members.
- ***5th stage Performing:*** The leader delegates the task and the members start performing the tasks. The leader also concentrates on developing group members.
- ***6th stage Termination:*** In this stage, the groups discontinue or terminate their tasks as soon as the

assignment or project is completed. If the project is not fixed for a short period, the members continue to work till it is completed. This stage poses difficult for some members because the members of the group worked very closely, interacted and developed working relationship throughout the five stages.

Group Process

Group process means to how an organization's members work together to get the work done. Organizations spend a lot of time and energy in establishing and achieving its goals. Though in the organization members are a great resource and asset but seldom the organization shows concern over its members. No doubt the achievement of goals is a difficult task, it is essential that the members' needs are taken care of. When an individual becomes member of a group, he gets an opportunity to develop self-confidence, refines skills and makes friends which cannot happen on their own. Effective organizations take a close observation as how members work together, and the roles and function they play to achieve the organizational goals. These observations and regular meetings helps the administrator to identify and analyze their needs and problems early to prevent adverse occurrence and allow smooth running of the organization. Communication, participation, decision-making and role fulfilment are some of the elements of an organization. The administrator needs to be a good observant that will give clues of communication like who is leading, who is influencing, who is interrupting and who is assertive in the group, etc. It will also help to understand the amount of involvement and participation among members. In the same way, decisions are made in groups without considering the effects will have on other members. Some individuals impose their own decisions on the group, while others want all members to participate or share in the decision-making process. Organizational roles and related tasks are performed by group members for the success of the organization. The administrator applies process observation sometimes that requires patience and the ability to pay attention or focus on each member in the group.

Principles of Group Dynamics

- There must be a sense of belongingness among members to the group.
- The more attraction a group member is to its members, the greater influence it would exercise on its members.
- The successful efforts to change individuals sub parts of the group would result in making them confirm to the norms of the group.
- Information relating to the need for change, plans for change and the consequences of the changes must be shared by the members of the group.
- The changes in one part of the groups may produce stress in the other parts, which can be reduced only by eliminating the change or by bringing about readjustments in the related parts.
- The groups arise and function owing to common motives.
- The intergroup relations, group organization, member participation are essential for effectiveness of a group.
- There are three essential dynamics of the group process: Group membership, social reality and group development.

Functions/Roles of Group Leader in Group Dynamics

- The leader leads and directs team members, establishes vision, mission statement and goals for the group and group members.
- Develops structure and process to achieve the goals and to realize the vision.
- The leader establishes confidence and positive relationship among group members.
- The leader identifies the problems and conflicts within the group and helps and supports the members to resolve conflicts.
- Counseling, guidance and coaching is facilitated to members as and when needed. Training is given to members on assertive skills and conflict management skills.
- Delegates tasks and individual responsibility to achieve goals.
- Appreciates and rewards for the successful achievement of goals to each members.

Role of Nurse Manager in Group Dynamics

- Communicates, the vision and mission statement of nursing service department to all nursing personnel.
- Ensures that each nurse knows the goals of the department.
- Delegates roles and tasks according to the level of preparation and experience to nursing personnel.
- Supervises and manages the overall performance of staff in department. Develops future strategies based on analysis and reporting of data from nurses.
- Achieves organization goals, visions and objectives by involving employee selection, career development, succession planning and periodic training.

- Works out compensations and rewards for nursing personnel.
- Identifies problems, creating choices and providing alternatives courses of actions.
- Shows concerns for the growth and increase in the organizations' finances and earnings.
- Knowledge of group dynamics is needed by nurse managers to improve leadership competencies and facilitates group discussions and communication.
- Groups are a common platform of a majority of experiences of all nurses.
- Identifying problems, creating choices and providing alternatives courses of actions are important functions of the nurse administrator.

HUMAN RELATIONS

Introduction

Successful nursing service administration depends upon the competency of the administrator. One of the basic skills required by the nurse administrator is Human Relation (HR) skills that is the ability of the administrator to work effectively as a member of the nursing team and develop cooperative efforts within the nursing team she leads.

Definition

Human relations is an area of management practice which is concerned with the integration of people into a work situation in a way that motivates them to work productively, cooperatively and with economic, psychological and social satisfaction. — **Keith Davis**

Characteristics

- It is a combined approach through which the goals of the organization and the employees' interest working in the organization are synchronized. The main aim of HR in an organization is to enhance employee satisfaction and to increase the productivity of the organization.
- Human relation is a study of human behavior. It utilizes the philosophy and knowledge from various interdisciplinary sciences like sociology, psychology, anthropology and other sciences. Human relations are an action oriented process to build human cooperation towards achieving organizational goals.
- It ensures employees happy and productive workers.
- Scope of HR is wide. It is widely integrated in health care institutions, industries, defense and other organization where large number of people are worked.

Purposes of HR

- To remove conflicts between management and employees
- To remove individual differences among employees
- To achieve organizational goals
- To facilitate effective work environment
- To establish cooperation and coordination with different departments in an organization
- To enhance quality of services.

Advantage of HR

- It ensures higher performance
- It promotes optimum use of resources
- Maintains individuality and moral justification
- It is a basis for understanding of human behavior
- It gives importance to persons
- It recognizes individual differences
- Respects common interest
- Facilitates favorable conditions in work settings
- Encourages collective efforts
- Recognizes inter-relationships
- Recognizes human needs and work
- Employees participate in decision-making
- Employees develop leadership and communication skills.

Approaches of HR

Human relation approaches are classified as:

- ***Negative Approach:*** According to this approach, the individuals by nature are lazy and self-interested. They need close supervision as they are not trustworthy in their day to day work. Therefore, this approach recommends that such individuals need to be monitored closely.
- ***Natural Approach:*** According to this approach, the individual's behavior and adaptation to work setting is developed through his experiences. The characteristics of the behavior of the individual are based on the type of situation he is exposed to. Therefore, it is very important for the administrator to create and maintain a conducive work environment for employees for smooth running of the administration.
- ***Positive Approach:*** In positive approach, employees intend for personal and social well being. They are trustworthy to put in a good work. They work sincerely and loyally without supervision provided with that they get internal satisfaction with their job. Therefore it is the task of administration to facilitate challenging task to every employee. This approach requires democratic leadership and participative decision-making.

Problems in HR

- Conflict between individual and organization
- Individual differences
- Interpersonal conflicts
- Incongruence between roles.

Techniques of HR

- Integration employee participation is one of the important technique of human relation
- Congenial work environment increases job satisfaction
- Open communication promotes sense of belongingness
- Adaptive leadership influence employee to do work better
- Resolving conflicts prevents negative events in an organization
- Personnel counseling encourages and supports employee

Theories of HR

There are two important theories of human relations:

1. Mary Parker Follett (1868–1933) who is also known as a visionary genius, proposed a human relation theory that emphasizes when people are working together in an organization, mutual influence and trust are developed.
2. George Elton Mayo (1880–1949) was an academic and psychologist found out the basic concept of human relation. He stressed that working place should be like a social environment and good working relationship should be maintained between the employer and employees. In such work environment, people are motivated to work (For details refer Chapter 3 Management theories).

Role of a nurse administrator in creating human relation climate in hospital

A nurse administrator's success in leading her department depends on her ability to create a healthy human relation climate. Nursing leaders need to understand that nurses are human beings with social and emotional needs

- Demonstrates transformational leadership, optimistic and positive outlook towards nursing personnel
- Ensures trust in nurses
- Smiles and shows sense of humor
- Maintains individuality and call nurses by their name
- Communicates effectively
- Shows concern about nurses' satisfaction
- involves nurses in planning, implementing and participatory decision-making
- Establishes work environment that focuses on the needs of nursing personnel
- Always demonstrates a positive social skill in administration.

PUBLIC RELATION IN THE CONTEXT OF NURSING

Introduction

Public relation is a part of nursing service administration. It is focused with the promotion of a positive image of nursing service administration and nursing professional.

Definitions of Public Relation

- It is defined as the management of communication between an organization and its publics'.
  —Grunig and Hunt
- 'Public relation is using communication to adapt relationships between organizations and their publics'. **—Carl H Botan**
- 'Public relations is the deliberate, planned and sustained effort to establish and maintain mutual understanding between an organization and its publics.' **—Institute of Public Relations, USA**
- 'Public relations is the attempt by information persuasion and adjustment to engineer public support for an activity, cause, movement or institution.'
  —Edward L Bernays
- 'Public relations is a combination of philosophy, sociology, economics, language, psychology, journalism, communication and other knowledge into a system of human understanding.'
  —Herbert M Baus
- Public relation is a planned deliberate and sustained effort to establish and maintain mutual understanding between the organization and the public
  —British Council of Institution of Public Relations
- Public relation is a philosophy and function of management expressed in policies and practices which serve the public and secure its understanding and goodwill.—**Public Relation Society of America**

Purposes of Public Relations

- To help the organization to achieve its goals and objectives
- To attract, encourage and motivate the public to utilize the services of the organization
- To create and develop the image of individual employee as well as the organization to the public
- To remove the conflict or misunderstandings between the employees and organization.

Functions of Public Relations

- Public relations is establishing the relationship among organization and members.
- It is an art and science of establishing reciprocal of understanding and goodwill
- It focuses on analyzing the public perception about the individuals and organization
- Public relations is assessing the attitude of the public
- Public relations identifies the interests and needs of the public
- It execute the program for communicating with people.

Elements of Public Relations

According to Raymond Simon, the elements of public relations are:

- It is a managerial function
- It requires good planning
- It involves the relationship between the public and organization
- The main focus of evaluation is the attitude and opinion of public
- The policies, procedures and actions related to the public of the said organization
- Execution of policies and procedures are at the interest of public and socially responsible
- Utilizes effective communication to execute the plan
- The public activities seeks development of rapport, goodwill, understanding and acceptance as an end result.

Tools and Techniques of Public Relation

Various tools and methods both traditional and advanced are used to maintain public relations with organization today. Some of the methods are described as below:

- ***Attendance at public events:*** In order to attract public attention and opinion, public relation specialist from the organization speaks about the organization. By this method, the organization can directly reach to the public.
- ***Press releases:*** These are the oldest methods of public relation tools TV or/and radio program, film, newspapers, magazines and other types of media regularly communicates with the information that catches attention and achieves a bigger impact than advertisements among public because the public believe that these tools reliable, meaningful and trustworthy.
- ***Newsletters:*** To the target audience, the organization sends periodical newsletters, news bulletins, and other pamphlets which contains relevant information about the organization. For example TNAI sends periodical newsletters to nurses to communicate on important events of TNAI.
- ***Blogging:*** We are living in the era of information and technology. To reach the online audience, public relation specialists use the digital forms of press releases and newsletters. It can be a two-way communication also.
- ***Social media marketing:*** It is used in industry to promote sale of product. In this method, the public relation specialist communicates directly to the public/consumers.
- ***Traditional methods:*** If audience is illitrate, method such as folk dance, music, drama street play, exhibition etc. are used to pass the information.
- ***Parent-teacher meet, annual day celebration of the organization, reading reports and activities:*** During institutional program are some of the methods that maintain public relations.

Hospital is a new and unknown place for many individuals. The public should know regarding the profile of hospital, services rendered, qualified medical and medical personnel, visiting hours, emergency department, ambulance services, contact numbers, domiciliary services for follow-up care, the financial aspect of care, etc. This publicity should be done through public education.

In many hospital, at the entrance hall itself is communicated in boards fixed on walls. There are pamphlets available describing the profile of the hospital including vision, mission and objectives.

The functions of nurses in promoting public relation are listed below.

The administrator and nursing personnel should be aware of the vision, mission and philosophy of the hospital. The other public relation activities are:

- Identification of needs and problems of individual patients, family and affiliated community
- Develop trust with individual patient and their families
- Systematic and meticulous planning of publicity program based on the needs of the community relevant to the age group because they are the audience
- Coordinate the program with intra and inter departments

1. Collaborate the program with other agencies
2. Plan and conduct a detail orientation program to all patients/family members regarding hospital services
3. Facilitate high quality of nursing care and ensure patient safety
4. Attend problems/complaints of patient promptly and ensure relevant solution
5. Ensure clean and healthy ward and hospital environment
6. Ensure the best care from admission to discharge
7. Provide suggestion box in each unit for patients/ relatives
8. Organize exit interviews for patients
9. Invite patients who were discharged from hospital for any hospital developmental program
10. Be in touch with the patients after discharge through community health department of the hospital

DECISION-MAKING

Introduction

Decision-making within an organization is a complex process which is influenced by several factors. Decision-making is the heart of all administrative and managerial functions. Taking right decision at the right time is unique caliber of a good administrator.

Definition

Decision-making is the intellectual process leading to the selection of a course of action among alternatives. Every decision-making process produces a final choice called a ***decision***. It can be an action or an opinion.

'A decision in its simplest form, is defines as a selection of alternatives'. —**RA Killian**

'Decision making is a course of action which is consciously chosen for achieving a desired result'.

—**Haynes and Massie**

Types of Decisions

- *Mechanical decision:* It usually occurs in a situation involving a limited number of decision variables where the outcome of each alternative is known. Tools used for this type of decision include charts, lists, decision tree. etc. This is useful for daily routine and scheduled activity.
- *Analytical decision:* It involves a problem with a large number of decision variables, where the outcomes of each decision's alternative can be computed. Such as network analysis, statistical analysis and so forth. This decision helps to solve complex problems.
- *Judgmental decision:* It involves a problem with a limited number of variables, but the outcomes of decision alternatives are known. These kinds of decisions are useful in marketing, investment and to solve personal problem.
- *Adaptive decision:* It involves a problem with a large number of decision variables where outcomes are not predictable because of uncertainty and complexity. In such situation, strategies have to be frequently modified to accommodate new development in technology and environment, e.g. application of research findings.

Managerial Decisions

The administrator takes various methods to take decision when she/he encounters problems.

- *Strategic decision:* Made by top executives that commit valuable agency resources to achieve major long term goals.
- *Administrative decision* are those made by mid-level managers to resolve unusual problems and develop innovative methods for improving agency function.
- *Operational decision* are routine decisions governing day to day events that have been delegated to first level managers.
- *Experimental decision:* These types of decisions are not final until the first results appear and prove them to be satisfactory.
- *Decision by trial and error:* A certain course of action is selected and is tried out, if the results are positive, the action is carried further.
- *Decision made in stages:* Here, the decisions are made in steps until the whole action is completed.
- *Cautious decision:* It allows time for contingencies and problems that may crop up later at the time of implementation.
- *Conditional decision:* Such types of decisions can be altered if certain foreseen circumstances arise. It is an 'either/ or' kind of decision with all options kept open.
- *Delayed decision:* Such decisions are put on hold till the decision maker feel that the time is right.

Decision-making Approaches

- *Optimizing approach:* It is an approach in which an individual analyses a problem, determines desired outcomes, identifies possible solutions, predicts the consequences of each action, and selects the course of action that yields the greatest amount of preferred outcomes.
- *Satisfying approach:* It is an approach, whereby an individual chooses a problem solution, that is

non-ideal, but that is good enough to meet a set of minimum requirements.

- *Mix scanning:* Making a decision that satisfies to remove least promising solutions, and then select best of remaining options. Opportunistic making a decision for the solution is chosen by problem identifier.
- *Eliminate critical limiting factor:* Making a decision that satisfies to remove least promising solutions, and then select best of remaining options.
- *Do nothing:* Taking decision after waiting for the storm to pass.
- *Maxima:* An optimistic approach in which, while assuming the highest possible payoff from use of any action.
- *Mini regret:* An approach designed to minimize the surprise resulting from any action decision by selecting the action alternatives that will yield a result midway between the most desired and the least desired outcome.
- *Precautionary:* Making a decision by choosing action that will maximize gain or minimize loss regarding of opponents actions.
- *Chameleon:* Taking decision by making vague plan, adjusted to changing circumstances.

Decision-making Process

The following steps are used in decision-making process:

- *Step 1 Identify and analyze the problem:* The first step in the decision-making process is defining the problem. What is wrong? Where is improvement needed? As long as the supervisor concentrates on the symptom instead of the problem, the difficulties will arise. It is only when the real problem has been identified that effective decision-making can be initiated.
- *Step 2 Explore suitable alternatives for the problem analyzed:* When solving a problem, the administrator should determine first whether the situation is covered by policy or not and then he should determine alternatives. He can consider some other alternatives such as conducting professional meeting correspondence and brainstorming with staff, etc. inductive and deductive reasoning is both appropriate.
- *Step 3 Choose the most desirable alternative:* The following questions may be asked: Will this decision accomplish the stated objectives? If it does not, it should not be enforced and another option should be used. Does it maximize effectiveness and efficiency? One should use available resources before seeking outside assistance. Finally, can the decision be implemented? If not it obviously will not solve the problem. Leadership quality of supervisor prevents immediate acceptance of an apparently obvious solution and facilitates group exploration of decision making opportunities usually increases the number of alternatives and the quality of problem-solving.
- *Step 4 Implement decision:* The administrator will need to communicate the decision to appropriate staff in a manner that does not arouse antagonism. The administrator will need to select the associate to implement the decision and provide the direction to initiate action. Once the decision has been implemented, it should be evaluated.
- *Step 5 Evaluate the results:* Audits, checklists, ratings and ranking can be used to review and analyze the results. Because solutions to old problems sometimes create new problems, additional decisions may need to be made and evaluated.

The Role of Nurse Administrator in Decision-making

A nurse administrator's role usually requires a prompt decision making.. Decision making process is a cognitive activity by which the nurse administrators respond to opportunities, threats, analyze all the available options and make a practical decision which is consistent with the goals of the organization.

Mintzberg (1973), described managerial roles are as follows:

- *Decisional roles:* It involves decision-making. This role is again subdivided into the following:
  - Entrepreneur role: In this role, the administrator makes decisions and initiating new ideas to improve organizational performance.
  - Disturbance handler's role: In this role, the nurse administrator taking corrective action to cope with adverse situation in the organization.
  - Resource allocators role: This is very important role of the nurse administrator to decides and allocate human, physical, and monetary resources.
  - Negotiator role: Negotiating with trade unions, or any other stakeholders and makes sound and practical decision for nurses and nursing.
- Ensuring Patients' Welfare is another function of nurse administrator. The primary responsibility of a nurse administrator is to ensure that patients and their families are receiving the highest level of care possible from the nursing staff. Many nurse administrators play an important role in determining what services the health care facility will offer to patients.

- Supervising nursing personnel is important function of nurse administrator. She needs to make correct decisions regarding recruiting new nurses, scheduling employees, training personnel, performing employee evaluations, conducting employee counseling and making hiring and terminating decisions with regard to the nursing staff, all of which usually involve working a great deal with the human resources department.
- A nurse administrator is also responsible for making sure that each staff member's registration, credentials and certifications are up-to-date. She acts as a role model and mentor for other nurses.
- Representing nursing personnel is a challenge for nurse administrator.
- The nurse administrator facilitates communication between the nursing staff and other areas of the organization, such as the medical and administrative staff. She typically acts as a liaison between the nursing staff and senior management of the hospital or care facility. To effectively achieve these tasks, the nurse administrator must have exceptional communication, decision-making and negotiation abilities, in addition to strong leadership skills.
- The nurse administrator is not only expected to manage and represent the nursing staff, but also be involved in creating and implementing a budget for his/her department. She must ensure that patient needs are met first and foremost, and she is also responsible for making sound budgeting decisions from determining what patient services are to be offered to deciding which medical equipment to purchase. The nurse administrator is generally responsible for making sure that her department is running as efficiently as possible.
- A nurse administrator is often involved in developing and implementing policies, ensuring that her staff members understand and follow the guidelines and policies of the organization. She is expected to periodically assess the effectiveness of policies and recommend appropriate decision for revisions whenever necessary.

DELEGATION

Introduction

Delegation is the managerial process of giving decision-making authority to lower-level employees. For the process to be successful, a worker must be able to obtain the required capability and cooperation needed for successful completion of the delegated task. An enabled employee has both the authority and the responsibility to accomplish the work. Although authority can be delegated, the delegator is ultimately responsible for its success. The delegator is therefore accountable for meeting the goals and objectives of the task.

Definition

Transferring to a competent individual the authority to perform a selected nursing task in a selected situation. (National Council of State Boards of Nursing (1995).

Transfer of responsibility for the performance of a task from one individual to another [American Nurses Association (1996)].

Concept of Delegation

Achieving performance of **care outcomes** for which you **are accountable** and **responsible** by sharing activities with other individuals who have the **appropriate authority** to accomplish the work (Yoder-Wise, 2008).

Thus the components of delegation are:

- Care outcomes—patient care is safely provided
- Accountable and responsible—both delegator and delegatee have an obligation to care for that patient and ensure the task is completed
- Sharing activities—both the delegator and delegatee work together to accomplish care
- Appropriate authority—the delegator selects the appropriate person to delegate the task.

Elements of Delegation

Authority

In context of a business organization, authority can be defined as the power and right of a person to use and allocate the resources efficiently, to take decisions and to give orders so as to achieve the organizational objectives. Authority must be well-defined. All people who have the authority should know what is the scope of their authority is and they should not misutilize it.

Authority is the right to give commands, orders and get the things done. The top level management has greatest authority. It always flows from top to bottom. It explains how a superior gets the work done from his subordinate by clearly explaining what is expected of him and how he should go about it. Authority should be accompanied with an equal amount of responsibility. Delegating the authority to someone else does not imply escaping from accountability. Accountability still rest with the person having the utmost authority.

Responsibility

It is the duty of the person to complete the task assigned to him. A person who is given the responsibility should ensure that he accomplishes the tasks assigned to him. If the tasks for which he was held responsible are not completed, then he should not give explanations or excuses. Responsibility without adequate authority leads to discontent and dissatisfaction among the person.

Responsibility flows from bottom to top. The middle level and lower level management holds more responsibility. The person held responsible for a job is answerable for it. If he performs the tasks assigned as expected, he is bound for praises. While if he does not accomplish tasks assigned as expected, then also he is answerable for that.

Accountability

Accountability means giving explanations for any variance in the actual performance from the expectations set. Accountability cannot be delegated. For example, if 'A' is given a task with sufficient authority, and 'A' delegates this task to B and asks him to ensure that task is done well, responsibility rest with 'B', but accountability still rest with 'A'. The top level management is most accountable. Being accountable means being innovative as the person will think beyond his scope of job. Accountability, in short, means being answerable for the end result. Accountability can not be escaped. It arises from responsibility.

RELATIONSHIP BETWEEN AUTHORITY AND RESPONSIBILITY

Authority is the legal right of person or superior to command his subordinates while accountability is the obligation of individual to carry out his duties as per standards of performance. Authority flows from the superiors to subordinates, in which orders and instructions are given to subordinates to complete the task. It is only through authority, a manager exercises control. In a way through exercising, the control of the superior is demanding accountability from subordinates. The marketing manager directs the sales supervisor for 50 units of sale to be undertaken in a month. If the above standards are not accomplished, it is the marketing manager who will be accountable to the chief executive officer. Therefore, we can say that authority flows from top to bottom and responsibility flows from bottom to top. Accountability is a result of responsibility and responsibility is a result of authority. Therefore for every authority, an equal accountability is attached.

Difference Between Authority and Responsibility

Authority

- It is the legal right of a person or a superior to command his subordinates.
- Authority is attached to the position of a superior in concern.
- Authority can be delegated by a superior to a subordinate.
- It flows from top to bottom.

Responsibility

- It is the obligation of subordinate to perform the work assigned to him.
- Responsibility arises out of superior-subordinate relationship in which subordinate agrees to carry out duty given to him.
- Responsibility cannot be shifted and is absolute
- It flows from bottom to top.

Needs for Delegation

- Increased acuity of patients
- Increased registered nurses (RN) responsibilities in the management of the nursing unit/organization
- Accelerated pace and changing health care environment.

ADVANTAGES AND DISADVANTAGES OF DELEGATION

Advantages

Effective delegation can benefit the employer, the employee, and the organization. It improves the quality of work. Delegation enhances the quality of work by allowing the employees who have knowledge of services to make decisions promptly and complete tasks. This in turn increases motivation among employees. Employees may do a better job because they feel a personal accountability for the outcome. Motivation is enhanced as delegation enriches the worker's job by expanding the types of tasks that are involved in it.

Employers who delegate effectively have more time to do their own jobs when they assign tasks to others Effective delegation frees the manager to focus on managerial tasks such as planning and control. It helps to develop employees skills. When there is a highly skilled workforce in the organization, they have more flexibility in making assignments and are more efficient decision makers.

Disadvantages

Many employers lack knowledge to delegate effectively, and thus delegation (or lack of delegation) may be detrimental to the organization. Other reasons for a lack of motivation to delegate are lack of trust in subordinates, fear of being seen as lazy, reluctance to take risks, and fear of competition from subordinates lack of competency in delegating, and sometimes they select wrong tasks to delegate. This will result in poor outcome of the organization. This will affect the career of employer and employees. Both the employer and employee blame each other and causes poor organizational outcome.

Five Rights of Delegation

Right Tasks

Questions to ask when determining the right task

- Is there potential for harm?: If there is a great potential for harm, if the task is done incorrectly, be careful with delegation.
- How complex is the task?: If the task is very complex, be careful with delegation.
- What problem-solving is required to carry out the task?: If significant problem-solving measure is required while performing the task, be careful with delegation.
- What is the predictability of the outcome?: If in completing the task there is potential for many different outcomes, be careful with delegation.
- Patient interaction/ability: If the patient has limited ability to assist or respond to the task, be careful with delegation.

Right Person

Nurse Practice Act—each state has a nurse practice act that will define and determine what task can be delegated to what level of personnel.

- Determines the scope of practice for each position
- Issues standards of care that guide practice
- Renders official opinions which guide practice.

Organization guidelines—each organization has statements that guide practice.

- Mission statement
- Policies and procedures (determine what can be done and what level of personnel can carry out the task)
- Job descriptions—identifies job responsibilities.

Right Circumstances

Delegating a task under the right circumstances includes:

- Considering the condition and acuity of the patient
- An awareness of the staff mix—distribution of professional and non professional nurses
- Organization documents—the job descriptions, policies, and procedures within the organization will guide to whom and what can be delegated.

Right Communication

- Clear and concise communication is imperative from the delegator to the delegatee. This communication should include the following:
  - Task with clear expectations of what is to be done, why it is being done, and when the task should be completed
  - Correct patient
  - Information that should be reported back to the nurse and when that information should be given to the nurse
  - Expected outcome of the task.

Right Supervision

The delegator must provide sufficient follow-up including:

- Checking on the progress of the task
- Checking on the outcomes once the task is performed
- Obtaining feedback about the completed task from the delegatee
- Evaluate the effectiveness of the delegation with the delegatee
- Effective supervision.

Role of Delegator and Delegatee in Caring Patients

Role of delegator

As the delegator, the head nurse must:

- Have a view of the big picture in the care of the assigned patients
- Select the appropriate activities to delegate
- Select the appropriate staff to carry out the activities
- Clearly communicate the expectations and required follow-up
- Follow-up periodically while the task is being completed
- Evaluate and provide feedback on the effectiveness of the delegation to staff.

Role of Delegate

The delegate also has responsibilities including:

- Accepting the delegated activities as directed by the head nurse
- Give report to head nurse as requested on the delegated task

- Give feedback to delegator on the effectiveness of the delegation process.

Legal Authority to Delegation

Legal responsibility for the nurse to delegate a task is determined by:

- Nurse Practice Act
- Employer's statements including job descriptions, policies, and procedures
- National standards of care
  - Indian Nursing Council Act—if any
  - Trained Nurses Association of India—if any.

Why Delegation Fails? Problems of Delegation

- Delegatee refuses to accept the delegated task.
  - Fear of inability to complete the task correctly and safely
  - Told not to do by others—other nurses have told the delegatee never to carry out this task
  - Lack of confidence—the delegate may be new or lack the confidence to complete the task
  - Overwhelmed—may be concerned about the workload already assigned.
- The delegator's belief system—the nurse feels that because of the responsibility of care, the tasks need to be completed by herself
- Lack of confidence in delegatee and therefore is not comfortable with delegation
- Nonsupportive environment
  - Organization culture that restricts delegation
  - Lack of resources
  - Lack of training.
- Insecure delegator or delegate
  - Lack of trust
  - Lack of liability.
- Unwilling to delegate
  - Inexperience
  - Fear or failure.

Delegation Errors

- Inadequate delegation
- Failure to identify higher purposes served
- Lack of clarity
- Emphasizing outcome to the exclusion of method
- Failing to delegate developmentally
- Failing to anticipate radial impact
- Abdication
- Deliberate redundancy
- Failing to impose accountability
- Delegating to weakness
- Assigning responsibility in excess of responsibility
- Under delegation (false assumption-employee)
- Over delegation
- Improper delegation (wrong time, wrong person to the wrong reason).

Role of Nurse Administrator in Effective Delegation

For achieving effective delegation, a nurse administrator has to work in a system and to function as follows:

- ***Assesses the qualification and experience:*** required to do the task before delegating to nursing personnel when delegating the tasks.
- ***Defines the task*** and duties to the nurses before delegation.
- ***Clarifies the task*** and the result expected is determined as a first step in delegation.
- ***Defines responsibility and accountability.***
- ***Allows nurses to participate in the delegation process.*** When nurses who accept their assignments are more likely to be committed to their success. This acceptance is enhanced when nurses have some say in the process. Thus, nurses should be allowed to participate in determining when and how the delegated task will be accomplished and, when possible, what the assignment will be.
- ***Ensures from nurses that if he or she is available to do a task,*** rather than telling him/her to do it. Participation can also increase when nurse administrator/ nursing staff communicates, which may minimize problems due to misunderstandings.
- ***Specifies standards.*** To avoid problems related to performance standards, the nurse administrator specifies performance standards expected from the nurses. Such as, expected level of performance, dates for feedback, proper reporting timings and problem faced in carry out the tasks. The suggestion from nurses are also invited to know their choice of task and input they can provide regarding modification of assigned tasks.
- ***Balances responsibility and authority:*** To avoid delegation errors, the nurse administrator assigns responsibilities with the freedom to make decisions and the authority to implement them. She communicates to all nurses regarding the task and provides support,
- ***Ask nurses as what resources they require to complete the task*** like coaching, training and other supports that may empower them to complete the task by themselves.

- *Facilitates adequate support and encouragement:* This will enhance the nurses' motivation and authority for future assignments
- *Acknowledges for successful completion of tasks:* by recognition and rewards.
- *Delegates consistently:* The administrator delegates not at the time of crisis, but it is always considered for the development of nursing personnel.
- *Balances the assignments:* It avoids overloading to one nurse and less work to the other. All types of task whether it is challenging or not is delegated to nurses as per their level of knowledge and experience
- *Focuses on results:* The nurse administrator is accountable for nursing service department. She supervises and closely monitors nursing personnel whether the job is completed and the outcome is achieved.

CONFLICT MANAGEMENT

Introduction

Conflict management plays a very important role in preventing conflicts among individuals in any organization. A conflict arises when individuals strongly oppose each other's opinions and ideas. A conflict starts when individuals think on different lines and find it very difficult to accept each other's ideas. Conflict must be avoided as it lowers the productivity as well as morale of the organization and demotivates the individuals. All the factors leading to a conflict needs to be identified and the administrator must make efforts to prevent a conflict. The administrator requires conflict management skills as a conflict in an organization is not that easy to control.

Meaning

The word conflict originates from the Latin word '**confligere**' which means clash, contend, fight or struggle.

Definition

- It is a clash or struggle that occurs when a real or perceived threat or difference exists in the desires, thoughts, attitudes, feelings or behaviors of two or more parties.
- It is a situation in which someone believes that his or her own needs have been denied.
- The struggle for scarce organizational resources is organizational conflict.
- A perceived opposition or antagonistic process at the individual—organization level is called job conflict
- A competitive conflict rules based conflict with the goal to win or beat an opponent employee
- A disruptive conflict activity designed to attack, defeat, or eliminate an opponent through disruption
- Conflict often about gap between want and have as well as gap between need and unmet needs.

Types of Conflict

- *Intrapersonal conflict:* It occurs within an individual. The experience takes place in the individual's mind. Hence, it is a type of conflict that is psychological in nature involving the individual's thoughts, values, principles and emotions. It can affect the major decisions such as choosing a career path. This type of conflict can be quite difficult to handle. It leads to restlessness and uneasiness, or can even cause depression. In such occasions, it would be best to seek a way to let go of the anxiety through communicating with other people. Eventually, when a person finds himself out of the situation, he becomes more empowered as a person. Thus, the experience evoked a positive change which will help him in his own personal growth.
- *Interpersonal conflict:* It refers to a conflict between two individuals. It is common between people whose positions require interaction with other persons who fill various roles in the same organization or other organizations. This occurs typically due to how people are different from one another. We have varied personalities which usually results to incompatible choices and opinions. Apparently, it is a natural occurrence which can eventually help in personal growth or developing relationships with others. In addition, coming up with adjustments is necessary for managing this type of conflict. However, when interpersonal conflict gets too destructive, the administrator who has a conflict management skill needs to intervene to resolve the situation.
- *Intragroup conflict:* It occurs within a team of individuals. It occurs when the group faces new problem, when new values are imposed on the group from outside, or when an individual's extra group role conflicts with her intragroup. It is a type of conflict that happens among individuals within a team. The incompatibilities and misunderstandings among these individuals lead to an intragroup conflict. It arises from interpersonal disagreements or differences in views and ideas or opinion. Within a team, conflict can be helpful in coming up with decisions which will eventually allow them to reach their objectives as a team. However, if the degree of conflict disrupts harmony among the members, then some serious guidance from an administrator with conflict management skills will be needed for it to be settled.

- *Intergroup conflict:* It occurs when a misunderstanding arises among different teams within an organization. For instance, the dietary department of a hospital can come in conflict with the nursing service department. This is due to the varied sets of goals and interests of these different groups. In addition, competition, rivalry, resources also can contributes for intergroup conflict
- *Inter-organizational conflict:* It is referred as conflicts developed between organizations. Inter-organizational conflict occurs when there is high level of competition between two organizations. The different philosophy, attitudes and values which are opposite to each other can lead to high level of inter-organizational conflict. Besides, it develops when situations in which managers in one organization feel that other organization is not behaving ethically and is threatening the existence of the organization. A majority of inter organizational conflicts result in better outcome of an organization rather than deterioration in performance. Some level of inter-organizational conflict is essential for organizations to compete in the market. It must be handled in a positive way in order to make it beneficial to the organization (Gross and Guerrero, 2000). Organizations must avoid adopting unethical practices to resolve such a conflict. Inter-organizational conflict can be resolved only in few situations. However, due to varied culture, structure and policies existing in different organizations, the conflicts remain unresolved most of the times.

Causes of Organizational Conflict

- Unrealistic expectations from the employer and employees. Many times the expectations are unclear to the employees
- Stressful working conditions
- Poorly defined roles and responsibility or role ambiguity
- Lack of information due to poor or inadequate communication. Many times incorrect facts are communicated to the employees
- Fear, lack of security, and support from the organization
- Management styles such as lack of team work, perception of favoritism, with different priorities
- Lack of respect and trust
- Feeling of being exploited
- Not being appreciated for good work.

Causes of Person to Person Conflict

- Personality clashes between individuals in a group
- Differences in work styles of individuals
- Communication styles differs from person to person
- Individual preferences among individual's desire to get own needs met
- Gap between needs and un met needs cause conflicts in and among individuals
- Stress level varies and is subjective
- Prejudice and bias among individuals can cause conflict
- Conflict causes according to variation in culture gender, age
- Inflexibility, narrow mindedness, competition spirit, goals and priorities can cause person to person conflict

CONFLICT SOURCES FOR NURSES

- *Interpersonal conflict:* Nurses are working in an environment where they interact with nurses, nurse administrators/managers, members of the health team and patients and their families. Nurse to nurse conflict can arise from different personality, attitude, goal and aims of individual nurse with other and different working styles. Role conflict is a cause for conflict between nurses and members of health team. Power divisions, and unpleasant management styles can cause conflict between nurses and administrator. When patient and family's expectations for nursing care from nurses are not satisfactory that may also cause conflict; lack of peer cohesion and poor working relationship among nurses.
- *Lack of communication:* Nurses are the largest working group in an organization. When they are receiving incorrect facts, poor or inadequate communication and avoidance from the nurse administrators, that will affect their work and can cause conflicts.
- *Leadership style:* Lack of supervision, inadequate delegation, lack of team work and lack of negotiation skill, leads to negative emotion, poor work-related attitude, absenteeism, turnover of nurses, decreases organizational commitment and job dissatisfaction among nurses. Subjective criticism not being listened to and threats by the administrator can cause organizational conflict.
- *Increasing workload:* There is a huge cry in all over the world that there is a shortage of nurses in hospitals that causes increasing workload with less benefits, creates conflicts.
- *Scarcity of resources:* Inadequate budget, nursing shortage lack of retention of nurses policy, equipment and supplies for nursing care increasing the demand

of quality care from consumers causes organizational conflict.

- ***Inadequate policy*** for managing organizational conflict and violation of work place norms.
- ***Work place stress*** among nurses
- ***Role conflict:*** When there is no clear-cut role definition for nursing personnel that causes conflict among diploma, degree and postgraduate nurses. There is a generational conflict also occur when novice graduate nurses enter into the wards where senior nurses show different attitude and causes conflicts.
- ***Personal or organizational goals and values*** when differs, conflict may arise.

Impact of Conflicts in an Organization

It can be discussed under constructive and destructive impact.

- ***Constructive impacts:***
  1. Improves decision quality
  2. Stimulates creativity
  3. Encourages interest
  4. Provides a forum to release tension
  5. Fosters change
  6. Enhances job satisfaction
  7. Increases organizational outcome.
- ***Destructive impacts:*** Studies observed that 24% of total management time is spent on listening to complaints countering rumors/giving correcting feedback, searching for solutions, disciplining conflict-related behavior and monitoring compliance of agreements. Some of negative effects of conflict in the organization are:
  1. Constricts communication among employer, employee and among employees
  2. Lowers morale of the organization as well as individual
  3. Decreases cohesiveness among members in the organization
  4. Causes undesirable behavior
  5. Causes more and unpleasant fights
  6. Hinders organizational performance occur.

Symptoms of Conflict

- Tensions occur among employees
- Work is not done properly
- Conduction of disastrous meetings
- Anger occurs quickly and easily
- Failing productivity
- Slipping of organizational morale
- Absenteeism
- Accidents
- The employee (or employees) involved display, no desire to communicate.

Options for Conflict Management

In every situation, we are responsible for our actions. Conflict situations offer among each one of us and we select an opportunity to choose a style for responding to the conflict. Some of the common approaches used by managers are:

- Avoiding
- Withholding or withdrawing
- Smoothing over or reassuring
- Accommodating
- Forcing
- Competing
- Compromising
- Confronting
- Collaborating
- Bargaining and negotiating
- Problem-solving.

The following are the most common styles used by administrators in conflict management:

- ***Cooperative problem solving style:*** Choosing a cooperative problem-solving style, enables people to work together so everyone can win. Using this style, people try to find a solution that will help everyone to meet their interests and help everyone to maintain a good relationship.
- ***Competitive style:*** Choosing a competitive style means that a person who is assertive and uncompetitive is putting his/her interest before anyone else's interests. In fact, sometimes people who use the competitive style try so hard to get what they want that they ruin friendships.
- ***Compromising style:*** People choose a compromising style when it is important for them to satisfy some of their interests, but not all of them. People who compromise are likely to say 'let's split the difference or 'something is better than nothing.'
- ***Avoiding:*** People who chose the avoiding style do not get involved in a conflict. A person choosing the avoiding style might say 'you decide and leave me out of it.'
- ***Accommodating style:*** People who choose an accommodating style put their interests last and let others have what they want. Many times these people believe that keeping a good friendship is more important than anything else.

- *Collaborating style:* The person using this approach is more assertive and, cooperative. This person attempts to work with the other person to find a solution that fully satisfies both parties. Collaborating works on identifying each other's problem and insights, or collaborating to solve an interpersonal problem.

Steps in Conflict Resolution

Conflict in the workplace is inevitable, as employees and employers have different personalities, goals, and opinions. Knowledge on managing conflict is the basis for prevention of conflicts in an organization. The following are the steps in conflict resolution process: which can work to resolve conflict between individuals and between groups.

- *Step 1: Identify the source of the conflict*: In this step, the administrator gathers maximum information regarding the source of conflict. The more information she gathers about the cause of the conflict, the more easily she will be able to resolve it. The administrator uses a series of questions toi identify the cause of conflict such as What is bothering you?, 'When did you feel upset?', 'When and how did the incident take place?, Do you see a relationship between your feeling and incident?' The administrator as a mediator gives time to both persons a chance to share their problem. It gives better information about the situation and an impartial process. Occasionally, nodding head to encourage the disputants to continue to speak so that the administrator gathers very clear information regarding the cause of the conflict.
- *Step 2: Look beyond the incident*: In this step, the administrator observes the visible disruptive evidence of the conflict in between the disputants and the level of stress experienced by them. She calls them in her office and tries to find out the cause of conflict or the factors responsible for conflict, the occurrence time as when they felt there is a problem exists between them and she asks the view points on the conflict.
- *Step 3: Request solutions:* After getting the disputants' viewpoint on the conflict, the next step is to get each to identify how the situation could be changed. As a counselor, the administrator asks the disputants as how they can make the conflict solved. She behaves like an active listener, observes the disputants' body language, emotional status and their verbal language during conversation with them Slowly the disputants stop blaming each other and come to a cooperation level. Till such time the nurse administrator keep silence and listen to the disputants carefully.
- *Step 4: Identify solutions and both disputants can support:* The administrator listens and finds the most suitable courses of resolution at the cost of the benefits to the organization as well as individuals' point of view.
- *Step 5: Agreement:* The nurse administrator allows the disputants to agree to one of the alternatives identified in the previous step. They select one course of action and agrees to resolve the conflict. The disputants ensure that in future how they can help in preventing conflict in the organization. The step concludes agreement between two disputants and shaking hands with each other.

ROLE OF NURSE ADMINISTRATOR IN CONFLICT MANAGEMENT

- Communicates vision, mission and philosophy of the service administration to all nursing personnel.
- Ensures all nursing personnel understand and aware of channel of communication through the organization chart.
- Establishes clear cut expectation from nurses by facilitating well-defined job description.
- Ensures sufficient resources for effective patient care.
- Provides a conducive work environment for all nurses.
- Periodical counseling, coaching and training given to nurses to empower their services.
- Maintains democratic, transformational and servant leadership styles.
- Facilitates adequate supervision to ensure quality care and patient safety.
- Conducts periodical in-service education program on conflict management, workplace stress management and interpersonal relationships in hospitals.
- Establishes a cohesive group of nursing personnel by organizing periodical formal and informal meetings
- Ensures work load balancing to the preparation and qualification of nurses.
- Develops effective policies on conflict management.
- Identifies and resolve Generational work force conflict immediately Her mentoring role here is very important for novice nurses.
- Maintains good public relations in the hospitals.

NEGOTIATION

Introduction

Nursing is a practice profession and today's health care delivery system is becoming more complex than ever before. Nurses are the largest workforce in health care system and they experience frequent conflicts, disputes, and other situations that require negotiation. These conflicts include differences of opinion among nurses, between members of health team, between nurses consumers of health with regards to quality nursing care.

Definition

- Negotiating is the art of reaching an agreement by resolving differences through creativity.
- Negotiation is a dialogue between two or more people or parties intended to reach a mutually beneficial outcome, resolve points of difference, to gain advantage for an individual or collective, or to craft outcomes to satisfy various interests (Ricardo Buettner, 2006).
- Negotiation is a strategic discussion that resolves an issue in a way that both parties find acceptable. In a negotiation, each party tries to persuade the other to agree with his or her point of view (investopedia).
- Negotiation is a managerial tool/strategy or technique useful for avoiding head on competition or a win-lose conflict outcome.
- Negotiating is the process of communicating back and forth, for the purpose of reaching a joint agreement about differing needs or ideas.
- Negotiation is a dialogue intended to resolve disputes, to produce an agreement upon courses of action, to bargain for individual or collective advantage, or to craft outcomes to satisfy various interests. From the above definitions, one can find the following characteristics of negotiation.

Characteretics of Negotiation

Negotiation involves a common interest that connects two or more parties. They need each other's involvement in achieving a desired outcome.

- The parties start with different opinions or an objectives that prevents agreement between both parties.
- The parties are willing to cooperate and communicate to meet their goals.
- The parties can mutually benefit or avoid harm by influencing each other.
- The parties realize that any other procedure will not produce desired outcome other than negotiation and the parties think that negotiation is the best way to resolve their differences.
- Each has some influence over the others actions.
- Negotiation process itself involves interaction between people or group.

Terms Used in Negotiating Process

According to Michelle Maiese (2003), the various terms used in negotiation are:

- *Issues* or problems that needs to be to be negotiated or resolved.
- *Deadlock:* The result of that occurs when no agreement can be reached by the parties.
- *Impasse:* The result that occurs when an issue cannot be resolved to the party's mutual satisfaction.
- *Concession:* An agreement is given to provide satisfaction to the other party to advance towards a settlement.
- *Power:* It is the ability to influence other party's behavior.

Principles of Negotiation

- Negotiation is a process that utilizes human behavior and open about feelings and motives in individuals. This will enhance trust between individuals and group.
- Identifies and prioritizes the very important issue and avoids presenting so many issues.
- Avoids deadlines, lessening the chance for needless concessions.
- Summarizes frequently reinforce, the discussion held.
- Presents arguments calmly and objectively , without personalization, personal opinions, argument, personal judgment, and make sure they are logically supported the individuals.
- The next principle is to avoid ultimatums and other forms of non-negotiable demands.
- If the other party's argument is found valid and appropriate, no harm in admitting them.
- Develop a good relationship and rapport with the other party before you negotiate.
- Discussion should be moved towards organizational objectives.

ELEMENTS OF NEGOTIATION

- Goals that are conflicting and non-conflicting.
- Values that vary as to urgency and priority as information is exchanged.
- Mutual victory when both sides realize satisfaction and feel something has been won.

- Incomplete information since parties never reveals all information and thereby shift the negotiating power.

The Factors Influencing Negotiation

There are many factors that influence the process of negotiation. The goals interest, interdependency, past relations, persuasive ability and temperament which exist between the two negotiating parties are some of the most common factors influence negotiation. According to PD Chaturvedi and Mukesh Chaturvedi in their book, Business Communications: Concepts, Cases and. Applications described some of the factors influencing negotiations are the following:

- ***Place of meeting:*** The place of meeting influences one's level of confidence. When one chooses his own place for negotiation the strength of the person is increased during the course of discussion if any paper or materials required that is available.
- *The choice of time:* For effective negotiations action to be taken timely. The achievement of goal is expected when negotiation is done as early as possible. According to mutual convenience of negotiating parties, if the time for negotiation is fixed that brings fruitful effect. There should be enough time for the negotiating parties to discuss the issue that will facilitate more interactions and exchange between the parties, exploring possible compromise and searching for common ground to reach the agreement. The time to prepare for negotiation and the time for implementing the agreement should also be carefully fixed for action before and after the meeting. So that both negotiating parties can review and reinforce the agreement.
- ***Subjective factors:*** As objective factors are important, the outcome also depends on subjective factors of influence negotiating parties.
    1. ***Personal relationship:*** The conduct of negotiation is influenced by not only by the real situation of the matter but also by the relationship between the two persons or parties involved in the process of discussion.
    2. ***Fear:*** often our bargaining power is conditioned by our fear of the other party's authority, power, higher connections and the capacity to harm.
    3. ***Mutual obligation:*** The memories of good done in the past by the other party also act as an influence on us.
    4. ***Future considerations:*** When personal relationships are at stake, we may not wish to win the argument, especially when good relations between the two parties are likely to be affected.
    5. ***Practical wisdom:*** Fear of losing good opportunities in the future is a strong factor in our bargaining and negotiation positions and power.

NEGOTIATING PROCESS

Smeltzer in 1991 described the following in negotiating process:

- Preparing for negotiation
- Communicating a general overview of what is to be accomplished
- Reviewing why negotiation is required
- Redefining the issue or issues
- Selecting when issues will be addressed
- Encouraging discussion throughout the process
- Addressing the fallback or compromise position for both parties on each issue
- Agreeing in principle during settlement stage
- Recapping and summarizing the agreement
- Monitoring compliance with the agreement after settlement.

NEGOTIATION TECHNIQUES

- Prepare- prepare- prepare
- Pay attention to timing
- Leave behind your ego
- Ramp-up your listening skills
- If you don't ask, you don't get
- Anticipate compromise
- Offer and expect commitment
- Do not absorb the problem of negotiating parties
- Stick to your principles
- Close with confirmation.

EFFECTIVE NEGOTIATION SKILLS

The key to effective negotiation is **clear communication. Communication** involves three important skills: Speaking, listening and understanding.

- **Speaking:** Negotiation begins with a clear, concise explanation of the problem as each person sees it.
- **Listening**: Listening is an active process of concentrating all of one's attention on the other person.
- **Understanding**: Before two sides can look for solutions; a common understanding must be reached. If two people do not understand each other's problems and concerns, then the process of negotiation will either be broken off or will end with

solutions that do not work. The negotiator should be aware of negotiating parties speech, body language while conducting discussion.
- **Objectives** define the objectives that should be specific and flexible to be achieved through negotiation.
- **Explore** the possibilities for a wide range of options.
- **Prepare** well in advance for negotiation including date, time and place.
- **Set priorities as** which problems is more important.
- **Be emotionally stable.**
- **Demonstrate** self-confidence and self-assertiveness, but without unnecessary aggressiveness.

The Role of Nurse Administrator

- Negotiation is an organizational behavior and the nurse administrator miust have negotiation skill.
- Usually nurses are blamed for inadequate quality care by the health care consumers. A nurse administrator needs to mediate between conflicting sides of patients' families, and nurses. She advocates for various care protocols. Negotiating skills can help to deal with these demands of patients and nurses.
- Because nurses are on the front line of the delivery of health care, and because there are major changes in the organization of health care delivery, nurses need to use negotiation skills for the smooth running of the organization. The following skills are required for effective negotiation.
- Communicate clearly, listen and understand the issue presented listen both sides carefully.
- Recognize and clearly define the problem. Prepare questions in advance.
- Seek solutions from a variety of sources.
- Respect the negotiating parties. Be reliable and emotionally stable.
- Collaborate to reach a mutual solution. Preserve the relationship.
- Avoid rush to make the decision.
- Understand the time factor give enough time for mutual discussion.
- Be prepared for compromise.
- Never make your desperation apparent to the other party.
- Negotiate for agreements—not winning or losing.
- Use data/evidence to strengthen your position.
- Focus on patient care interests and organizational goals.
- Always remember that the process is a problem. solving one and the benefit is for the patient and family.
- Clearly identify the priority and arrive at common goals. Avoid using pressure.
- Identify and understand the real reasons underlying the problem.
- Be knowledgeable about organizational policies and procedures.
- Try to understand the other side and ask questions and seek clarification when uncertain.
- Be concrete and flexible.
- Be reasonable and fair.
- Use only factual statements.
- Keep an open mind because negotiation always provides the potential for learning.
- Always discuss the conflict.
- Try to focus on preventing recurrence of further conflict.
- Never tell the other party what you are willing to negotiate totally.
- Take a brake if either party becomes angry or tired during negotiation.

Common Negotiation Errors

- Unclear objectives.
- Inadequate knowledge of other side's goal.
- Incorrectly viewing the other party as an opponent.
- Insufficient attention to the other party's concerns.
- Lack of understanding of other side's decision-making process.
- Nonexistence of a strategy for making concessions
- Too few alternatives and options prepared before negotiation.
- Unskillful use of negotiating power.
- Poor sense of timing for closing the negotiation.

COLLECTIVE BARGAINING

Introduction

Health care delivery system is more complex today. As we enter into the 21st century, more and more challenges are confronted by health care providers especially nurses.Shortage of nursing workforce, increasing nurse patient ratio, scarcity of resources for patient care, consumerism, role conflict, unsafe work environment and oppressive management practices poor nursing practice environments, poor salary benefits, etc are few issues causing concern among nurses for providing quality patient care. To enjoy organizational autonomy and control over nursing practice, a collective bargaining strategies, is emerged as an important solution to the nursing challenges.

In any establishment, the employee has the freedom to bargain for self to safeguard his own interest like better service condition , better term of employment like salary benefits, work place safety and security. To simplify collective bargaining is that arrangement whereby the conditions of employment of the employees are settled through a bargain between the employer and employees collectively.

The concept of collective bargaining was originated from western world when there was an industrial conflict and a trade union movement In India, collective bargaining movement was born in 1920 at Ahmadabad to regulate labor management relation. In 1940, Coir factory workers union and coir mat manufacturers association, in Kerala was instrumental in establishing a joint negotiation body widely known as Industrial relation committee for negotiation with regards to settling terms and conditions of employment in industry.

Meaning and Definition

Collective bargaining consists of two words—'collective' means a group action through its representative and 'bargaining' means negotiation.

It is the process of negotiating the terms of employment between an employer and a group of workers. The terms of employment are likely to include items such as conditions of employment, working conditions and other workplace rules, basic pay, overtime pay, work hours, shift length, work holidays, sick leave, vacation time, retirement benefits and health care benefits **(Investopedia).**

Collective bargaining refers to a process by which employers on the one hand and representatives of the employees on the other attempt to arrive at agreements covering the conditions under which employees will contribute and be compensated for their services'
—Michael J Jucius.

'Collective bargaining is a process of discussion and negotiation between two parties, one or both are a group of persons acting in consent. The resulting bargain is an understanding as to the terms and conditions under which a continuing service is to be performed. More specifically collective bargaining is a procedure by which employees and group of employers agree upon the conditions of work.' **—Encyclopedia of social sciences**

'Negotiation about working conditions and terms of employment between an employer and a group of employees or one or more employees organization with a view to reaching an agreement where in the terms to serve as a code of defining the rights and obligations of each party in their employment relation with one another and for a large number of detailed conditions of employment (ILO).

Collective bargaining is an agreement between single employer or an association of employers on one hand and a labor union on the other which regulate the terms and conditions the employment **(Ludwig Teller).**

From the above definitions, it is clear that collective bargaining is an agreement under which the employees association collectively under take to resolve their existing or future oriented problem with or without the assistance of a third party.

Objectives of Collective Bargaining

- To provide an opportunity to the employees/workers, to voice their problems on issues related to their job.
- To arrive at an agreement on wages and other service conditions of their job.
- To protect the interests of employees through collective actions.
- To negotiate voluntarily, yielding some concessions and sacrifices by both parties.
- To bargain from a position of strength without exploiting the weakness.
- To resolve the differences between employees and management through negotiation.
- To resolve and prevent all conflicts and disputes in a mutually agreeable manner through mutually signed agreements.
- To facilitate reaching a solution that is acceptable to all the parties involved.
- To develop a conductive environment to enhance organizations stable, and peaceful relations.
- To enhance the productivity of the organization by preventing strikes lock–out, etc.
- To have a peaceful co-existence for the mutual benefits and progress.

CHARACTERISTICS OF COLLECTIVE BARGAINING

- It is a group action initiated through the representatives of employees. It is collective work in nature.
- According to the changing needs and problems of employees, it is flexible. It is a dynamic and continuous process.
- In collective bargaining, both parties are strong and equal to negotiate.
- It is the involvement of the two parties to negotiate and reach to the agreement.

- It is constructive in nature, where both the employer and employees are satisfied that in turn bring positive organizational outcome.
- It is a formal process (Fig 15.1). Employee related issue are registered with local, state or national level depending upon the severity of the issue.

Collective Bargaining Process is discussed below:

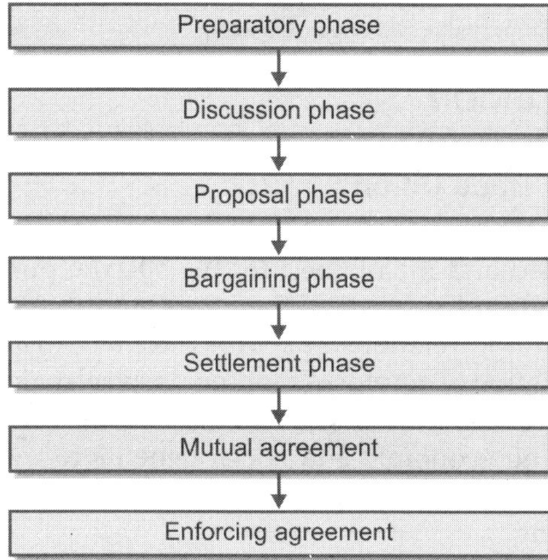

Fig. 15.1: Steps in bargaining process

- ***Preparatory phase:*** This phase is very important in collective bargaining. In this phase, both parties select their representative and members and establish a negotiation team. This team should be knowledgeable regarding the issue and should be able to communicate effectively during discussion. The main function of the team is to identify the relevant issue, and examine the situation to negotiate. The team also collects the relevant data to support the discussion.
- ***Discussion phase:*** After deciding the time and place for negotiation, the both parties discuss the issue in a conducive environment. The parties maintain trust, understanding and cooperation. This phase involves active interaction, listening, clarification and summarizing the discussion.
- ***Proposal phase:*** In proposal phase both parties think about possible alternatives to resolve the issue seriously
- ***Bargaining phase:*** In this phase, the proposals are presented and the problem solving is continued.
- ***Settlement phase:*** It is an important phase in which both the parties come to a common consensus and agreement and negotiates.
- ***Finalizing the mutual agreement:*** When both the parties are satisfied, the agreement is drafted in a clear, concise and simple language. Both the parties read the draft of terms and conditions and sign the agreement.
- ***Enforcing agreement:*** For better effectiveness, the agreement is executed immediately and collective bargaining comes to an end process.

Advantages of Collective Bargaining

- Collective bargaining process in an organization enables a continuous relationship between the employer and the employees.
- It helps to update policies, procedures and standards of the organization that meets the expectations of employer and employees.
- Since, collective bargaining is a dynamic and on-going process, it decreases the risk of disruption to the work environment when one side or the other makes an unexpected move or demand.
- Even when the two parties in disagreement, it is helpful for everyone in the organization to know the context of the conflict and to understand the position of each side.
- Collective bargaining increases ongoing communications between all parties and helps to enhance productivity.

Disadvantages of Collective Bargaining

- Collective bargaining curtails the freedom of the managements. The authority and liberty of the management would be limited and may be curtailed if the trade unions are far too influential and strong.
- The concept of collective bargaining is to bridge the communication gap between the employers and employees, they can easily create further conflicts instead of bridging the gap. Vested interests of elected representatives by competitive organizations and rivals can ruin the foundation of an establishment through collective bargaining.
- Collective bargaining is time consuming.
- It slows down the decision-making process and makes more complicated since there is no authoritarianism. Instead, there is increased bureaucratization.
- Reduces individuality, other union members may outvote one's decisions.
- Disputes are not handled with individual and management only; less room for professional judgment.

PROFESSIONAL ASSOCIATIONS AND UNIONS

What is an Association?

An association is considered as the organization that brings members of the same profession together for the exchange of information and experience for the advancement of their profession. It has its members of the same profession. For example, Trained Nurses Association of India (TNAI) is big association and all registered nurses are members of this association. The members do not violate code of ethics, bye laws and its philosophy, The main objectives of the associations are to uphold the dignity of each nurse, and the profession, to maintain esprit-de-corps among its members. The association meets its general body members once in two years however, the executive committee meets periodically as per by-laws of the association. The members discuss their problems and share experiences. They remain in touch with administrative officials, political leaders, etc. They voice collectively through the executive body to discuss nurse issues with concern agency like government.

The Role TNAI in Collective Bargaining

- TNAI has a grievance committee. The TNAI cannot be legally appointed as a negotiating body either at a local, state or national level. But there are association like government nurses association, Rajakeeya nurses sangh in U.P. Government Nurses Service Associations. These association has a TNAI representation to prevent members from joining other unions. For the improvement of nursing services to the community, the TNAI members may support a strike action.

What are the conditions under which a strike by Nurses may be approved by TNAI?

- Where grievances exist, they should be thoroughly investigated by the Government Nurses Association and reported to the local or State TNAI Executive.
- The State Branch Executive, TNAI, should also know all facts regarding the situation and be satisfied that justice requires some action.
- All possible approaches through legal efforts should be made to the authorities for correction of the situation.
- If no action is taken by the authorities despite all efforts, the situation should be put before the members of the Government Nurses Association for vote regarding strike.
- At least two months notice should be given before the date set for the strike
- Ensure that the patient care in the hospital will not be affected All possible arrangement for 24 × 7 day care must be assured
- It must be clearly understood that the TNAI and its members will not support any strike controlled or supported by any union, or organization which includes employees other than Nurses.
- It must be planned, voted, and carried out with the above stipulations in a dignified manner and with the assurance that the public understands and will support the Nurses demands and that the Nurses will make every effort to prevent harm to patients that might be caused by which might be caused by the strike.

TRADE UNION

What is Trade Union?

Trade union is a permanent association of employees, established and maintained for the specific purpose of advancing and protecting the interests of members in their working relationships with their employers. It is an association of employees for the purpose maintaining and improving the working conditions. It is established for gaining economic and social benefits to members. Its focus is on joint, co-ordinate action and collective bargaining.

Purposes of Unions

- The main purpose of union is to solve economic, social, political and psychological problems of the members of the union.
- To secure the better wages, better working conditions.
- To facilitate self-respect and dignity.
- To meet the social needs.
- To ensure stability of employment.
- To move into the trend of union activities which seems to be necessary to better conditions.

The Role of Nurse Administrator in Collective Bargaining

- As a nurse administrator she knows the law, and ensures the rights of the nurses as well as management.
- Formulate policies in this regards and communicates to all nurses about collective bargaining from induction period.
- Encourages nurses to become member of professional Nurses organization.
- Discourages nurse joining in any union other than nurses.
- Identifies and explores the reasons for collective bargaining.
- Before determining for collective bargaining, negotiates the problem at her level by discussing the problem directly with nurses

- Refers and confirms the action whether it is within the jurisdiction of law.
- If it is not possible to negotiate at her level, a collective bargain is supported by her. The district collector is informed about employees problems.
- While nurses are on collective bargaining, ensures that the patients are not neglected.
- Keep all nurses informed through regular meetings held close to the hospital or institution.
- Speaks for nurses and nursing supports nurses while taking agreement.
- Takes immediate action of the agreement.
- Documents the events.
- Follow-up the action taken.

HEALTH CARE LABOR LAWS IN INDIA

Box 15.1: Laws enacted by the Central Government, where the Central Government has the sole responsibility for enforcement

- The Employees' State Insurance Act, 1948
- The Employees' Provident Fund and Miscellaneous Provisions Act, 1952
- The Dock Workers (Safety, Health and Welfare) Act, 1986
- The Mines Act, 1952
- The Iron Ore Mines, Manganese Ore Mines and Chrome Ore Mines Labour Welfare (Cess) Act, 1976
- The Iron Ore Mines, Manganese Ore Mines and Chrome Ore Mines Labor Welfare Fund Act, 1976
- The Mica Mines Labour Welfar Fund Act, 1946
- The Beedi Workers Welfare Cess Act, 1976
- The Limestone and Dolomite Mines Labour Welfare Fund Act, 1972
- The Cine Workers Welfare (Cess) Act, 1981
- The Beedi Workers Welfare Fund Act, 1976
- The Cine Workers Welfare Fund Act, 1981.

Box 15.2: Labor laws enacted by Central Government and enforced both by Central and State Governments

- The Child Labour (Prohibition and Regulation) Act, 1986.
- The Building and Other Constructions Workers' (Regulation of Employment and Conditions of Service) Act, 1996.
- The Contract Labour (Regulation and Abolition) Act, 1970.
- The Equal Remuneration Act, 1976.
- The Industrial Disputes Act, 1947.
- The Industrial Employment (Standing Orders) Act, 1946.
- The Inter-State Migrant Workmen (Regulation of Employment and Conditions of Service) Act, 1979.
- The Labor Laws (Exemption from Furnishing Returns and Maintaining Registers by Certain Establishments) Act, 1988
- The Maternity Benefit Act, 1961

Contd...

Contd...

- The Minimum Wages Act, 1948
- The Payment of Bonus Act, 1965
- The Payment of Gratuity Act, 1972
- The Payment of Wages Act, 1936
- The Cine Workers and Cinema Theatre Workers (Regulation of Employment) Act, 1981
- The Building and Other Construction Workers Cess Act, 1996
- The Apprentices Act, 1961

Box 15 3: Labor laws enacted by Central Government and enforced by the State Governments

- The Employers' Liability Act, 1938
- The Factories Act, 1948
- The Motor Transport Workers Act, 1961
- The Personal Injuries (Compensation Insurance) Act, 1963
- The Personal Injuries (Emergency Provisions) Act, 19628
- The Plantation Labour Act, 1951
- The Sales Promotion Employees (Conditions of Service) Act, 1976
- The Trade Unions Act, 1926
- The Weekly Holidays Act, 1942
- The Working Journalists and Other Newspapers Employees (Conditions of Service) and Miscellaneous Provisions Act, 1955
- The Workmen's Compensation Act, 1923
- The Employment Exchange (Compulsory Notification of Vacancies) Act, 1959
- The Children (Pledging of Labour) Act, 1938
- The Bonded Labour System (Abolition) Act, 1976
- The Beedi and Cigar Workers (Conditions of Employment) Act, 1966 (d)
- (Source-Report of the working group of labor laws and other regulations, Government of India)

Box 15.4: Research highlights

According to literature review, the antecedents factors like personality, value, and expectation differences and complexities of organization often result in interpersonal conflict between health care professionals. Nurses' individuality can result controversies. Indefinite job descriptions and decision-making disagreements, especially those between nurses and physicians and inter departmental competitions are problematic and conflict inducing. This can result in negative conflict. While functional conflict can help an organization make necessary changes, dysfunctional conflict bears negative results that can lead to medical errors, job dissatisfaction, stress, psychosomatic illnesses, stress, decreased productivity, poor employee retention, and lack of collaboration. In order to mitigate these effects, education about different styles of dealing with conflict and conflict resolution processes is recommended. (CM Patton, 2010)

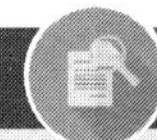

SUMMARY POINTS

- ✓ Organizations spend a lot of time and energy in establishing and achieving its goals. Though in the organization members are a great resource and asset but seldom the organization shows concern over its members. No doubt the achievement of goals is a difficult task, it is essential that the members needs are taken care of. When an individual becomes member of a group, he gets an opportunity to develop self-confidence, refine skills and make friends which cannot happen on their own. Constructive group dynamics enables to achieve organizational goals.
- ✓ Human relation is a study of human behavior. It utilizes the philosophy and knowledge from various interdisciplinary sciences like sociology, psychology, anthropology and other sciences. Human relations are an action oriented process to build human cooperation towards achieving organizational goals.
- ✓ Public relation is a specialization. The nurse administrator handles the internal and external communications in a hospital. She interacts with physicians, nurses, managers, administrators, and patients, and therefore must have excellent communication skills. Some of her responsibilities include writing for internal publications such as newsletters, handling calls from the media, as well as writing and creating various material that promote the services offered at that hospital. She organizes events between the organization and the public, or they might prefer to correspond by publishing press releases.
- ✓ Decisions are made at all levels of hospital nursing services. The nursing administrator makes decisions concerning goals and strategies of nursing service department. The head nurses make tactical decisions concerning ward management goals and strategies to accomplish them in relation to their own nursing service unit (wards). Frontline nurses or first level nurses make decision for day-to-day patient care to bring quality care outcome.
- ✓ Delegation is an organizational behavior consisting three components: authority, responsibility and accountability. The nurse administrator makes careful decision to delegate the right task, right nurse and right situation The accountability remains with the nurse administrator.
- ✓ Conflict management is managerial skill to identify and handle conflicts sensibly, fairly, and efficiently. Since conflicts in a hospital are a natural part of the work environment, it is important that the nurse administrator must understand how to resolve conflict and what style of conflict management she can adopt. When the conflicts are not resolved it may cause disruption in hospital setting.
- ✓ Negotiation is a method by which the employer settle differences with employees. It is a process by which compromise or agreement is reached while avoiding argument and dispute between the nurse administrator and nursing personnel. The principles of fairness, seeking mutual benefit and maintaining a relationship are the keys to a successful outcome of negotiation.
- ✓ Collective bargaining is an agreement under which the employees association collectively under take to resolve their existing or future oriented problem with or without the assistance of a third party. The ideals of collective bargaining in professional association and trade union differs.

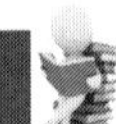

REVIEW QUESTIONS

1. Define group dynamics. Discuss the role of nurse administrator in enhancing group dynamics in nursing service department.
2. Discuss the importance of public relation in the context of nursing.
3. Describe the decision making process in nursing service administration.
4. Discuss the components of delegation. Discuss the functions of nurse administrator in effective delegation.
5. What is collective bargaining? Describe the role of professional organization in supporting nurses.
6. Write short notes on the following:
   a. Purposes of human relations
   b. Delegation errors
   c. Conflict management
   d. Principles of negotiation
   e. Association and trade union
   f. Types of group.

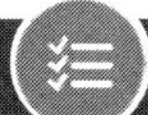

SELECTED READINGS

1. Bruce, K and Nylan, C 2011, 'Elton Mayo and the Deification of Human Relations', Organization Studies, Vol 32, No 3, pp 383-405.
2. Bruce, Kyle. 'Henry S. Dennison, Elton Mayo, and Human Relations historiography.' Management and Organizational History 2006, 1: 177–199.
3. Carl H. Botan "International public relations: Critique and reformulation" in Public Relations Review, Vol. 18, No. 2, 1992: 149-152)
4. C M Patton , Conflict in health care. : a literature review. IJHA, 2010, volume 9: number .1

   http://smallbusiness.chron.com/top-ten-effective-negotiation-skills-31534.html. Government of India, report of the working group of labor laws and other regulation, New Delhii1
5. DuBrin, AJ (2007). Human Relations Interpersonal Job-oriented Skills (9 ed.). New Jersey: Pearson Prentice Hall. p. 2.
6. Gardner, Margo; Steinberg, Laurence (July 2005). "Peer influence on risk taking, risk preference, and risky decision making in adolescence and adulthood: an experimental study" (PDF). Developmental Psychology 41 (4): 625–35.
7. Gross M A and Guerrero L K (2000), "Managing conflict appropriately and effectively: an application of the competence model to organizational conflict styles," International Journal of Conflict Management, London
8. Grunig and Hunt, Managing public relations, (1984)
9. J Taneja, S, Pryor, M G and Toombs, L A 2011, 'Frederick W. Taylor's Scientific Management Principles: Relevance and Validity', Journal of Applied Management and Entrepreneurship, Vol 16, No 3, pp 60-78.
10. J, Weiss S. and Lewin D (1992), "Models of conflict, negotiation and third party intervention," Journal of Organizational Behavior, USA
11. Likert and Likert (1976), New ways of managing conflict, Tata McGraw-Hill, New York
12. MacNamara, C. (n.d.). Group dynamics: Basic nature of groups and how they develop.
13. Neill, JT (2002). Social support helps people grow. Horizons, 17(Spring), 32-34.
14. Neill, JT, and Dias, KL (2001). Adventure education and resilience: The double-edged sword. Journal of Adventure Education and Outdoor Learning, 1(2), 35-42.
15. Raymond Simon, Public relations: concepts and practices, 2nd ed.(Columbus, O.Grid, 1980), pp 9, 11.
16. Ringer, TM (2002). Group action: The dynamics of groups in therapeutic, educational and corporate settings. London: Jessica Kingsley.
17. Roebuck, Chris. Effective Delegation. New York: American Management Association, 1998.
18. Straub, Joseph T. The Agile Manager's Guide to Delegating Work. Bristol, VT: Velocity Business Publishing, 1998.

UNIT VII CONTROLLING

16

Quality Assurance

LEARNING OBJECTIVES

This chapter imparts learning about:

- Introduction to Quality Control
- Concept of Quality Assurance in Nursing Service administration
- Quality Assurance Models
- The Importance of Nursing Audit
- Description of Continuous Quality Improvement
- Description of Quality Improvement Models

INTRODUCTION

Quality health care provides the patient with appropriate and consistent health care in a clear and safe environment in which the patient is treated with respect resulting in desired health outcome. Today, nurses play a key role in providing high quality of patient care and patient safety in health care setting. Activities to assure the adequacy and performance of hospital nursing, improve quality, and achieve effective control of hospital costs requires to be harmonized. That is possible only when the nursing service administrator possesses effective leadership and aware of quality assurance in nursing.

QUALITY CONTROL

Definition

What is Quality?

'A standard of something as measured against other things of similar kind; the degree of excellence of something'.

'A distinctive attribute or characteristics possessed by someone or something (Oxford dictionaries)'.

According to Joint Commission on Accreditation of Health care Organizations (2002) quality is referred as the extent which health services for the individuals and communities improves the possibility of desirable health outcomes and is consistent with current health care professional's knowledge.

International Organization for Standardization (ISO) defines quality of service as the totality of services that satisfies the actual and potential needs of patients under care. Thus, quality refers to the pursuit of excellence with zero defects.

Quality Control (QC)

It is a procedure or set of procedures intended to ensure that a manufactured product or performed service adheres to a defined set of quality criteria or meets the requirements of the client or customer. (Software development glossary)

It is a process through which a business seeks to ensure that product quality is maintained or improved and manufacturing errors are reduced or eliminated. Quality control requires the business to create an environment in which both management and employees strive for perfection. This is done by training personnel, creating benchmarks for product quality, and testing products to check for statistically significant variations. (Investopedia)

Thus, QC is a system of routine technical activities, to measure and control the quality of the inventory as it is being developed.

Purposes

The QC system is designed to:

- Provide routine and consistent checks to ensure data integrity, correctness, and completeness
- Identify and address errors and omissions
- Document and archive inventory material and record all QC activities.

DIFFERENCE BETWEEN QUALITY CONTROL AND QUALITY ASSURANCE

In any health care facility, quality is an important factor with reference to its services. In this competitive health care field, quality has become the benchmark for its services. Therefore, all service providers vigorously working on improving quality of services rendered. Health care administrators utilize QC and quality assurance (QA) as desirable techniques to maintain and enhance the quality of the services.

The administrators use a wide variety of techniques to achieve a desirable standard of health care services such as Total Quality Management (TQM), and internal and external standards. The standards are the processes and procedures for organizational activities that assist to enhance and maintain the quality of organizational functioning at all aspects. For example, ISO is one of the prominent bodies for defining quality standards for different hospitals or health care institutions. Many health care facilities try to adhere to the quality requirements of ISO.

Quality Control (QC) Function

QC and QA are different concept. Many organizations have its own internal quality standards, processes and procedures; that are developed from its inception or periodically and functions accordingly. These standards are monitored and verified periodically against definite criteria, its quality and effectiveness.

Every organization possesses a QC manual that outlines the quality focus and the objectives of the organization and guides practices to achieve QC goals. Each employee in the organization needs to be aware of this manual and his or her responsibilities mentioned in the quality manual.

Quality Assurance (QA)

It is a broad practice used for assuring the quality of services. There are many differences between QC and QA.

It is an administrative effort to enhance the quality practices in the organization. Continuous improvements are expected in quality functions in the hospital set up. For this, there is a dedicated team established. In a multispecialty or complex health care facility, a process team is established for enhancing the processes and procedures in addition to the quality assurance team.

The main responsibility of QA team is to define a process for achieving and improving quality of nursing care. Sometimes the hospitals go for accreditation and adopt standard process like ISO.

There are many tools used by administrators to improve QA in hospital setting from simple tool to sophisticated software system.

The QA teams of organizations constantly work to enhance the existing quality of services by optimizing the existing services and introducing new processes. Thus, QC is the outcome oriented and the QA is the process oriented function. Therefore, QA can be identified as a proactive process, while QC can be noted as a reactive process.

QUALITY ASSURANCE

What is Quality in Health Care?

Lohr KN 1990 explains QA as the extent to which individuals and communities achieve desired health outcomes and are in accordance with knowledge of health care professionals.

It started with Florence Nightingale identifying the role of nursing in health care quality and began to measure patient care outcomes.

Definition

As per Webster's Dictionary, QA is an activity/program for the monitoring and evaluating the various aspects of a project, service, or facility, systematically to ensure the desired standards of quality are being met.

It is the process of verifying or determining whether products or services meet or exceed customer expectations. It is a process-driven approach with specific steps to help define and attain goals. It is managed by a special department in many establishments. The main aim of this unit is to evaluate the product or service developed by the establishment in meeting the specified standards. This a systematic process. The advantages of QA are:

- It increases customer's confidence and a company's status.

- Improves work processes and efficiency
- Enables a company to better compete with others and identify the defects of the products before it reaches to the consumer. (Tech target, 2007)

Kozier refers QA is a dynamic, systematic and comprehensive evaluation of health care services and the impact of those services on health care of consumers.

According to Neetvert (1992), QA is referred to all activities undertaken by an establishment to prevent poor quality.

The key terms used in QA are Quality Improvement (QI), Total Quality Management (TQM), Quality Control (QC), and Quality Circles.

Purposes of Quality Assurance

- To assess the product or services in a systematic and comprehensive manner and find any fault and errors so as to rectify them.
- To Identify the areas which have not met the criteria or standards and to correct them immediately.
- To improve the efficiency and effectiveness of the service or product.
- To motivate for research effort by finding the relationship of services provided with expected outcome.
- To identify and address various problems.

Objectives of Quality Assurance in Nursing

According to Jonas (2000), the objectives are:

- To ensure delivery of quality client care.
- To demonstrate the efforts of the health care providers to provide the best possible outcome.
- To provide good quality of service to public.
- To improve efficiency and effectiveness of nursing service.

Quality Assurance Models

There are many models developed by doctors and nurses and health system researchers. However, the following models are widely used in QA:

Donabedian Quality Assurance Model, 1960

This model represents three dimensions of assessing quality.

Structure

In this model, structure refers to all the factors that influence the delivery of health care services. This includes the infrastructure and physical facilities of the hospital, equipment and supplies for delivering care to patients, staffing structure in quality and quantity and other human resources, It also include hospital and personnel policies, procedures, protocol, training, and use of technology. These factors are measurable based on defined criteria.

Process

In this model, process refers to the sum total of all activities that influence health care. These actions include diagnosis, treatment, preventive care modalities, patient and family education and their response in technological interventions, evidence informed care culture, and interpersonal processes, etc. According to Donabedian, the measurement of process is nearly equivalent to the measurement of quality of care because process contains all acts of health care delivery. These information about process can be obtained from medical records, exit interviews with patients and practitioners, or direct observations of health care.

Outcome

Outcome is the result of structure and process that include changes to health status, behavior, or knowledge as well as patient satisfaction and health-related quality of life. Outcomes are measured by certain indicators (discussed in nursing Audit). However, accurately measuring outcomes that can be attributed exclusively to health care is very difficult although it is widely recognized and applied in many health care related fields; the Donabedian model was developed to assess quality of care in clinical practice.

Wilson's Quality Assurance Model, 1987

This model is a slight modification over Donabedian model and describes the practical aspect of framework that emphasizes QA in health care. It is beneficial for both the health care providers and health consumers. His model is redefined the three dimensions as input, methods or procedures and outcome in place of structure process and outcome as in Donabedian model. In this model, input refers to resources for patient care such as personnel and equipment and supplies. Methods and procedures refers to the professional and technical activities carried out everyday, Outcome is described as the target of services rendered and is measured by productivity, quality and client satisfaction. This model complements TQM.

Quality Health Outcome Model

This model was published in 2000 by the members of the American Academy of Nursing expert panel. This model has the conceptual framework that describes multiple factors affecting quality of the care outcome. It is a model which envisages broad perspective of quality care outcome. This model is used to:

- To guide development of databases for quality improvement and outcomes management.
- To suggest key variables in clinical intervention research.
- To provide a framework for outcomes research and outcomes management that compares not only treatment options, but organizational or system level interventions. The model also has several policy implications.

Quality Management Model

This model is based on the theory of cause and effect in long term care i.e. higher the quality of care received by the client, higher the level of functioning or higher the level of Quality of Life (QoL) experienced by the patient, The model describes three dimension of quality:

1. Assessment
2. Care planning
3. Functional outcome.

Quality assessment leads to meticulous care planning. The outcome of the care is measured and compared with standard. The outcome is symbolized by (+) and (–) sign. (+) sign indicates the outcome exceed the standard quality and (–) sign indicates, there is shortfall in quality.

Marker's Umbrella Model, 1987

It is a model emphasizing a system for providing continuous, and competent clinical nursing care. According to this model, QA is achieved through:

- Nursing standard development for QA.
- Facilitating advanced training to provide competent care.
- Caring person should be technically an authority in nursing care.
- Assess the outcome of care.
- Measure the outcome with standards.
- Risk management.
- Effective use of resources.
- Problem identification and resolving the problems.

PDCA model by WE Deming

The most popular tool used to determine QA is the Shewhart Cycle, developed by Dr W Edwards Deming. This cycle for QA consists of four steps: *Plan, Do, Check,* and *Act* (PDCA) (See Fig. 16.1)

- **Plan:** Establish objectives and processes required to deliver the desired results.
- **Do**: Implement the process developed.
- **Check:** Monitor and evaluate the implemented process by testing the results against the predetermined objectives including customer feedback.
- **Act:** Apply actions necessary for improvement if the results require changes.

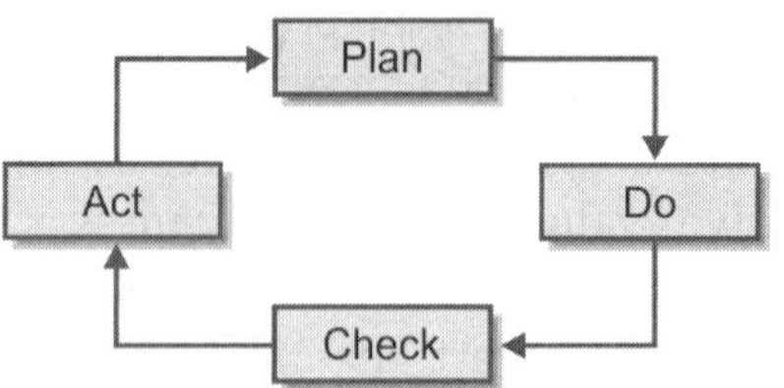

Fig. 16.1: PDCA model

Quality Assurance in Nursing

Pre-requisite for a QA program, the nurse administrator should follow the following steps:

- Set up a system for collecting and reporting data
- Write clear definition of all activities
- Agree methods for establishing current performance
- Identify resources and list them
- Agree data formats, its consolidation
- Identify and list the possible sources of benchmark data
- Develop a calendar for reporting
- Define roles and responsibilities
- Identify the training need requirement
- Plan for training personnel
- Establish a quality assurance committee in hospital.

QUALITY AUDIT

Next step is to prepare for quality audit.

Quality audit is the process of systematic examination of a quality system carried out by an internal or external quality auditor or an audit team. It is an important part of an organization's quality management system.

Purposes

- To identify and monitor the progress achieved against organizational goals.
- To find out chances for improvement.
- To compare the performance of employee with internal and external standards.
- To ensure the program to meet the requirements and needs of the customer. To be able to set sensible objectives and comply with them.
- To establish standards for establishing comparisons.
- To ensure each employee is aware of their level of performance.
- To identify and highlight quality-related-issues and decide the areas for priority action.

- To provide feedback for the successful performance.
- To make auditing as an integral part of regulatory requirements.

Audit Framework

The nurse administrator has to keep in mind the following when establishing audit framework. Audit framework must be based on:

- Focusing on health consumer and measure the correct thing.
- Meaningful, unambiguous and easily understood.
- Managed by the team within the organization.
- Improvement focus.
- Based on organizational goals.

Identify the Tools to Measure Quality Assurance

- Standards set by Indian nursing council, (INC), professional bodies (TNAI), university (Board of Nursing Studies)
- Nursing audit of patients records
- Patients opinion on exit interview on discharge
- Review of infection control records
- Patient's family's opinions
- Critical incident technique by nurses
- Reports on nursing rounds
- Adhering the unit philosophy and objectives
- Effectiveness of team conferences and reports
- Effectiveness of patient teaching program
- Review of staffing pattern for each unit
- Use of nursing care plans
- Observation of nursing activities.

What are the Outcome of Quality Care that can be Measured?

- Hospital acquired infection, surgical site infection, Inpatient mortality, neonatal mortality, perioperative mortality.
- Unplanned re-admission, unplanned admission after outpatient procedures.
- Patients 'falls.
- Incidence of health care associated pressure ulcers
- Incidence of health care associated infections; Catheter Associated Urinary Tract Infection (CAUTI).
- Patients' experience of pain management.
- Patients' experience of the provision of educational information.
- Health-care Associated Infection (HAI) rate: The number of individuals who develop any infection while in an inpatient setting.

NURSING AUDIT

What is Nursing Audit?

- It is a detailed review and evaluation of selected clinical records by qualified professional personnel for evaluating quality of nursing care.
- It is a part of the cycle of QA.
- It incorporates the systematic and critical analysis of care given by nurses.
- Nursing audit critically evaluates the planning, execution and evaluation of nursing services rendered to individual, family or community.
- It appraises the use of available resources and the impact of it on patient care outcome.
- According to the findings of audit, it introduces change or modification, of care (NHS ME, 1991 Framework for Audit for Nursing Services).

To conclude, nursing audit is tool to perform systematic evaluation of nursing services rendered which results in an improvement in the quality of patient care.

Purposes

- To evaluate the nursing care given.
- To achieve the deserved and feasible quality of nursing care.
- To improve the quality of documentation.
- To focus on the care provided and not on the care provider.
- To contribute towards research.

Common Approaches to Nursing Audit

- Organizational audit
- Peer review
- Prospective review
- Concurrent review
- Retrospective review.

Nursing Audit Cycle

According to FBA Clinical Governance and Nursing Audit Workshop (www.quis.org.uk) the nursing audit cycle describes to start with deciding the selected area to measure, review against standard, identify the gap, decide action, implement action and review standards.

- **Defining the standard***:* It is based on Donabedian quality assurance models. The three dimensions measured are structure, process and outcome.
    a. **Structure***:* Environmental elements required to deliver care. For example, all infrastructure facilities, policy, procedures, equipment, record keeping system, etc.

   b. **Process:** Professional and technical elements required to deliver care.
   c. **Outcome**: Measurable elements demonstrating results of care. For example, leg ulcer healing time, immunization levels, pressure ulcer prevalence, falls, infection rate mortality etc.
- Identify the problem regarding quality nursing care by conducting a baseline survey.
- To read widely from available literature.
- Identify gaps in providing care by analyzing.
   a. What are the reasons for not meeting the standard?
   b. How can the service be implemented?
- Implement action:
   a. This is the hardest area to address and involves the input from the whole team.
   b. An action plan needs to be developed.
- Review standards.
   a. To know whether the developed standards met the needs and to assess the status of standard whether they are high or low level standard.

Advantages

- It can be used as a method of measurement in all areas of nursing.
- Scoring system is fairly simple.
- Results easily understood.
- May be a useful tool as part of a QA program in areas where accurate records of care are kept.

Disadvantages

- Appraises the outcomes of the nursing process, so it is not so useful in areas where the nursing process has not been implemented.
- Many of the components overlap, making analysis difficult.
- It is time consuming.
- Requires a team of trained auditors.
- Deals with a large amount of information.
- Only evaluates record keeping; serves to improve documentation and not nursing care.

QUALITY IMPROVEMENT

Quality Improvement (QI) refers to improving a system by gathering data on performance and proposing changes.

Need for Quality Improvement

The following factors are responsible to necessitate quality improvement:

- Rapidly developing and expensive technology.
- Inability to pay the full cost of the treatment.
- Aging population with increased life expectancy.
- Legal environment leading to defensive medicine with high costs.
- Wide variations in efficiencies and quality of care.
- Inequalities and variations in income.
- Variety of providers despite efficiency or quality.
- Demand to deliver quality health care.

Why do we need continuous quality improvement in nursing?

The rising costs of health care, along with knowledgeable consumers and their awareness, interest, knowledge, and access to information about 'the right care, at the right time, at the right place, by the right provider, have now, more than ever' required that health care providers demonstrate the quality of their care.

—***Millenson, 1997***

Principles of QI

It should be customer focused, identifies key process to improve quality, use quality tools and statistics for evaluation and collaboration for problem-solving.

- QA targets on currently existing quality whereas;
- QI target is ongoing and always improving quality. Thus, the two models together emphasize ongoing nature of QI include TQM. (QA+QI=TQM).

QI is Japanese philosophy developed by Edward Deming which focuses on the following:

- Production and service depend on the individual.
- Quest for quality is an ongoing process.
- There is always room for improvement.
- Customer needs and experiences with the product are constantly evaluated.
- Preventive or proactive approach to problems prevents crisis management.
- Empower employees with positive feedback and reinforce attitudes and behaviors.
- Knowledge, on the job training and being valued.
- Encourage employees to improve quality through risk-taking and creativity.
- Trust the employees to be knowledgeable, accountable, and responsible.
- Provide education and training to employees at all levels.
- Quality is important than profit but high-quality attracts customers and more profit.

Principles of Total Quality Management (TQM)

Deming has described 14 principles of TQM. They are:

- This quality management program enumerate the purposes for improvement of product and service of the organization.

- The philosophy of TQM is continuous improvement.
- One of the principles of TQM is to emphasizes improving process rather inspection of product.
- End practice of awarding business on price alone; instead, reduce total cost by working with a single supplier.
- It continuously focuses on improve each process for planning, production and service.
- Ensures on the job training and plans for retraining.
- Develops the leadership capabilities at all levels of employees in the organization.
- Encourages employees to involve actively in the organizational process.
- Promotes interdepartmental cooperation, and remove breakdown barriers between departments.
- Eliminates slogans, exhortations and targets for workforce.
- Focuses on quality, and not just quantity; eliminate quota systems if they are in place.
- Promotes teamwork rather than individual accomplishments. Eliminate ratings systems or merit system and ensure pride of workmanship.
- Educates employees to maximize personal development and empowerment.
- Gives all employees responsibilities to carrying out the total quality management package. [*Deming, WE (1986)*]

QUALITY IMPROVEMENT MODELS

The following are some of the Quality Improvement models (Donna M Daniel,) which can be applied in health care management system they are classified as:

Quality Improvement Models Organizational Frameworks/Quality Management Model

This models include:

- **Baldrige evaluation process**. The main concept in this model is increasing performance excellence (quality of services)
  - **The Baldrige Performance Excellence Criteria is:** Leadership, strategic planning, customer and market focus measurement, analysis, and knowledge management. The Baldrige Criteria does not instruct organizations to use any specific improvement tool, but allows the organization to select the tool appropriate to their improvement efforts in health care.
- **ISO 9001 certification**: The idea behind this model is increasing performance excellence (Internal Process) ISO 9001 Certification is a series of international standards initially published in 1987 by the ISO, Geneva, Switzerland. The standards specify requirements and recommendations for design and assessment of a management system, the purpose is to ensure products and services meet customer requirements. ISO 9000 registration determines whether a company complies with its own quality system.
  - **Criteria for ISO Certification:** The following criteria used for ISO certification are: Customer focus, leadership, involvement of people process approach, system approach, continual improvement factual approach to decision-making, mutually beneficial relationships (Hoyle, David 2000).
  - Key tools used of ISO 9000 certification are flowcharting, process mapping cause and effect diagrams Plan-Do-Check-Act cycles, etc.
- **Balanced scorecard approach**: It is an approach that brings increasing performance excellence (measurement of business processes and external outcomes) balanced scorecard developed in the early 1990's by Drs Robert Kaplan and David Norton.

Quality Improvement Methods

Six Sigma

It is defined as 'a comprehensive and flexible system for achieving, sustaining, and maximizing business success. Six sigma is uniquely driven by close understanding of customer needs, disciplined use of the facts, data, and statistical analysis, and diligent attention to managing, improving and reinventing business processes.'

—Pande P, Neuman R, and Cavanagh R, 2000

Six critical elements of Sigma are:

1. Genuine focus on the customer.
2. Data and fact-driven management
3. Processes and the action is for improvement
4. Proactive management
5. Boundary less collaboration
6. Drive for perfection.

Human Factors

It is the science of designing tools, tasks, information, and work systems to be compatible with the abilities of human users. This includes both physical and cognitive abilities. Human factors include errors like execution errors, planning errors, and intervention errors. This model identifies these errors and designs tools in such a way that improves performance of the employees.

Lean or TPS (Toyota Production System)

Lean thinking is a way to do more and more work with less and less-less human effort, less equipment, less time, and less space-while coming closer and closer to providing customers with exactly what they want. The aim of lean is to eliminate waste.

PDCA Cycles or Model for Improvement: (This model is discussed already in quality assurance model).

FUTURE TRENDS IN QUALITY IMPROVEMENT IN NURSING PRACTICE

Clinical Pathway

A clinical pathway is a blueprint that guides the clinician in the provision of care. Clinical pathways are pre-conceived patient care algorithms, or paths, that are intended to reduce variability and cost, increase efficiency, and ultimately improve patient care. (Ped CCM: Clinical Pathways and Guidelines) Clinical pathways have four main components. They are:

- A timeline,
- Categories of care or activities and their interventions
- Intermediate and long-term outcome criteria
- The variance record. **–Hill 1994, Hill 1998**

What are the characteristics of clinical pathway approach to nursing care?

- It is patient-centered approach
- Systematic and consistent best practice evidence informed
- Tracks variance
- Multidisciplinary approach
- Maps clinical and non-clinical care
- Includes guidelines, protocols.
- Nursing standards and outcomes.

Benefits of Clinical Pathway Approach in QI

- Clinical pathway is a road map of treatment plan.
- Helps efficient and effective inpatient care.
- Disease specific and individualized care given for hospitals patients.
- It details the steps in the care for a specific problem, progress and facilitates practice of clinical guidelines, audit and communication with patients.
- Clinical pathway guidelines describes when, why and how to use the guidelines.
- The potential risks, benefits, and costs of care given.
- Summary of supporting literature with links to the actual studies and alternative approaches.

Demand Management

Demand management is referred to directing patients to the most appropriate level and intensity of medical care using planning and forecasting skills. It helps patients make decisions about self-care, whether to seek medical attention, or treat themselves, thus reducing the demand for professional health care. It helps the patient to choose when he/she wants to go to his/her doctor.

It is also a patient–centered tool that combines patient empowerment through self-care and health promotion information with professional support through a 24-hour hotlines and triage services. It is aimed at to improve the patients' health status and their decision-making in care.

The mission of demand management is that if people are informed about what they can do for themselves and in partnerships with providers, they will get better quality care, be more satisfied with their care, and save money (Mettler).

Benefits of Demand Management Approach in QI

- It reduces unplanned hospital admissions that is good to all patients.
- Predicting type and source of demand are the key to managing it.
- Clinical referral protocols help to increase consistency of referrals.
- Demand management will change the practice of nursing, on a broad base of clinical and communication skills. It will eventually include utilization review, case management responsibilities and health education.

Disease Management

It is a community-based systematic approach that identifies the individuals who are at risk, execute interventions and measures the outcomes, and thus provides continuous quality improvement. A nurse requires a knowledge base to identify patients, intervene, and measure outcomes.

What are the characteristics of Disease Management?

- It is a systematic information-driven approach, clinical encounters are computerized, summarized, and shared.
- Interventions detected from a central data-base.
- Practice guidelines in practice setting available
- Initiatives evaluated in terms of health outcomes.

Prerequisite for a Disease Management Approach

- Training and orientation of nurses on analysis and program development.

- Uniform collection of data and transmission.
- Consent from patients to provide the data.

What a Nurse should know Regarding Disease Management Approach?

- In depth knowledge and understanding of the natural history of disease process in man and to determine the lifecycle of disease and an intervention should be implemented.
- Chronic diseases have a long natural history, the same intervention (for example, lipid lowering to benefit atherosclerosis) could be implemented for patients who have pre-existing disease (secondary prevention) or for those who do not (primary prevention).
- Information on managing a successful disease management program.
- Knowledge on inefficiencies in health care delivery.
- Disincentives for the patient or provider such as access and cost issues.
- Relative cost-effectiveness of alternative treatments.
- Success of different interventions in modifying behavior such as compliance.

Evidence-Based Practices (EBP) or Best Practices Evidence Informed

Evidence-based nursing practice is necessary to build a nursing knowledge base and to meet accountability and credibility among other health disciplines (Rafael, 2000) Using evidence-based practice in the clinical setting is different from nursing research and the important aim of using EBP is to adopt the latest evidence from research and guide patient care to achieve the best possible outcomes for the patient (Saba, VK and McCormick, KA, 2011).

Evidence-Based Practice and Quality Improvement

It has been proven that integration of evidence-based practice has a lot of benefits in health care (Cullen, L and Adams, S 2010). One of the advantages of implementing evidence-based practice by nurses and other health professionals results in higher quality of care that leads to improved patient outcomes, since EBP incorporates the latest research evidence that are made available to health care providers at the point of care (Prior, Wilkinson and Neville, 2010). Also, the current use of evidence in health care would result in increase patient outcome since EBP includes healthcare recommendations that would help nurses in addressing questions related to best client care (Pipe et. al, 2005). EBP in nursing increase the nurses' confidence, adaptability, improve their skills, critical thinking and decision-making since they have to constantly evaluate various research that would support and be beneficial in their practice (Hamberg and Brown, 2006). Evidence-based practice not only enhance the nurse's clinical performance, but also lead to higher job satisfaction and better group cohesion which promote job retention in health care (Saba, VK and McCormick, KA, 2011). Also, another benefit of using evidence-based practice is reducing cost in health care compared with the care that is based in tradition and outdated policies and practices (Saba, VK and McCormick, KA, 2011). Implementation of evidence-based practice would manage available resources, since it would be used efficiently and effectively instead of being wasted in the process of determining ways of providing competent client care (Hamberg and Brown, 2006).

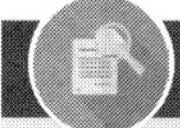

SUMMARY POINTS

- ✓ Quality health care provides the patient with appropriate and consistent health care in a clean and safe environment in which the patient is treated with respect resulting in desired health outcomes. Today nurses play a key role in providing high quality of patient care and patient safety in all health care setting.
- ✓ Quality refers to the pursuit of excellence with zero defects.
- ✓ Quality control is to create an environment in which both nursing service department and nurses strive for perfection in caring. This is done by training personnel, creating standards and criteria for nursing service quality, and evaluating continuously.
- ✓ In orders to maintain and enhance the quality of the services nursing administrators use two techniques, quality control and quality assurance. These two practices make sure that the services provided to the consumers of health meets the quality requirements and standards defined for the service.
- ✓ Quality assurance is any systematic process of checking to see whether a product or service being developed is meeting specified requirements. Many hospitals have a separate department devoted to quality assurance. Quality assurance function of an organization uses a number of tools for enhancing the quality practices. These tools vary from simple techniques to sophisticated software systems.

- ✓ Some of the models used in health care for quality assurance are: Donabedian Quality assurance model, 1960; Wilson's quality assurance 1987; quality health outcome model; Quality management model; Marker's umbrella model (1987) and PDCA model by WE Deming.
- ✓ Quality audit is the process of systematic examination of a system concerned with quality carried out by an internal or external quality auditor or an audit team. It is an important function of any organization.
- ✓ Nursing audit is the systematic evaluation of nursing which results in an improvement in the quality of patient care. Nursing audit is based on Donabedian quality assurance models. The three dimensions measured are structure, process and outcome.
- ✓ We need quality improvement in nursing because of various reasons such as the rising costs of health care, along with knowledgeable consumers and their awareness, interest, knowledge, and access to information about 'the right care, at the right time, at the right place, by the right provider' have now, more than ever, required that health care providers demonstrate the 'quality of their care'.
- ✓ Various models are used to bring quality improvement in health care delivery system.
- ✓ Some of the future trends to bring quality improvement in nursing practices are Clinical pathways; Disease management; Demand management and evidence based practice.

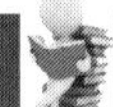

REVIEW QUESTIONS

1. Differentiate quality control and quality assurance. Discuss various quality assurance models that can be used in nursing.
2. What is nursing audit? What is the responsibility of nurse administrator in conducting nursing audit?
3. Define quality improvement. Describe the quality improvement models used in health care.
4. Describe the future trends in quality improvement for nursing practice.
5. Describe the principles of total quality management.
6. Write short notes on the following:
   a. PDCA model
   b. Quality control
   c. Six sigma
   d. Evaluation of nursing standard
   e. Steps in quality assurance in nursing
   f. Principles of continuous quality improvement.

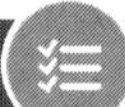

SELECTED READINGS

1. Clinical governance. website http://www.clinicalgovernance.scot.nhs.uk.
2. Cullen L, Adams S (2010). What is evidence-based practice? Journal of Perianethesia Nursing 25(3): 171-173.
3. Donabedian A (1986) Criteria and standards for quality monitoring. Quality Review Bulletin, 12(3):99-100.
4. Hanberg A, Brown S (2006). Bridging the theory–practice gap with evidence-based practice. Journal of Continuing Education in Nursing. 37(6): 248-49. Retrieved from EBSCOHost.
5. Hoyle, David. ISO-9000 Quality Systems Handbook. Butterworth-Heinemann Ltd, Oxford, 1998.
6. Kitson A, Hyndman S, Harvey G, et.al (1990) Quality Patient Care: The Dynamic Standard Setting System London: Scutari Press
7. Lohr KN (ed,) Medicare: A Strategy for Quality Assurance. Vols I and II. Washington, DC: National Academy Press, 1990.
8. Malby R. (1995) Clinical audit for nurses and therapists.London: Scutari Press.
9. Marquis, Bland Huston, CJ Leadership Roles and Management Functions in Nursing, Theory and Application,6th edition, India: Lippincott Williams and Wilkins, 2009.
10. Melnyk BM, Fineout-Overholt, E (2011). Evidence-based practice in nursing and health care: A guide to best practice. 2nd ed. Toronto: LWW.
11. NHS e-library. http://www.elib.scot.nhs.uk/portal/elib/pages/index.aspx

12. Pande, P, Neuman, R, and Cavanagh, R.The Six Sigma Way. McGraw Hill, 2000.
13. Pipe, T, Wellik, K, Buchda, V, et al., (2005). Implementing evidence-based nursing practice. Urologic Nursing. 25(5). Retrieved from ProQuest Nursing and Allied Health Source.
14. Prior P, Wilkinson J and Neville S (2010). Practice nurse use of evidence in clinical practice. A descriptive study. Nursing Praxis in New Zealand, 26(2): 14-25. Retrieved from EBSCOHost.
15. Sherwood, LM, Epstein RS; From Outcomes Research to Disease Management: A Guide for the perplexed. Annals of Internal Medicine; May 1, 1996vol. 124 no. 9 832- 837.
16. Wildman G (1988), Monitoring and Evaluation: The Joint Commission's-9-Step Model. Journal of Quality Assurance, 10: 18-23.

17

Performance Appraisals

LEARNING OBJECTIVES

This chapter imparts learning about:

- Concept of Performance Appraisal
- Description of Performance Appraisal Tools
- Importance of Mentoring and Coaching
- Discipline–Constructive versus Destructive Discipline
- Disciplinary Strategies
- Grievance Procedure

INTRODUCTION

One of the important functions of administration is controlling. Earlier days in personnel administration, controlling functions focused on periodical assessment of employees at work and maintaining organizational discipline. However, the modern management system gives more emphasis on employees performance appraisal that enables the administrator to facilitate the employees regarding job security, promotion, transfer training needs, rewards and punishment, retirement benefits, termination, etc. The feedback mechanism in performance appraisal communicates the employees to know their strengths and weakness constructive or adverse comments by the employer, and their performance level. This motivates the employees to improve their job performance that in turn enhances individual employee's morale.

Definition

Performance appraisal is the process of enhancing the employee's performance of the job in terms of the requirement of the job. It is an objective assessment of the individual's performance against well-defined bench-mark.

—Springel

Performance appraisal is a systematic, periodic and impartial rating of an employee's excellence in the matter pertaining to the present job and his potentials for better job.

—Flippo

Performance appraisal is the systematic description of an employee's job related to strength and weakness.

—C Wayne

Performance appraisal is the systematic evaluation of the individual with regards to his or her performance on the job and his or her potential for development

—Beach DS

From the above definitions, it is clear that performance appraisal is a systematic and planned process to assess the performance capabilities of the individual on his job based on criteria, and serves as an effective control mechanism in organization.

OBJECTIVES

Performance appraisal in an organization is aimed at the following objectives:

- To provide a basis for determining employee's salary, benefits, promotion, training and incentives
- To identify the potentials of employee and give placement where they are found better suitable

- To identify strength and weaknesses of each employee in an organization
- To determine training program to improve performance
- To communicate each employee regarding their strengths and weaknesses.

Advantages of Performance Appraisal

Performance appraisal is beneficial for both the employee and employer.

Advantages for Employee

- Helps the employee to identify his/her potentials and limitations regarding work performance
- Performance reports are necessary to determine individual's promotion, placement, transfer, rewards, compensation, etc.
- Performance appraisal motivates the employee to improve his/her performance and boost up his/her morale
- It provides a basis for coaching, mentoring, training and counseling for the employee.
- Since, it is a continuous process, the employee can evaluate his/her progress made in performance
- Provides for self-evaluation.

Advantages for Employer

Performance appraisal is a tool for motivating employees and brings improved care outcome that in turn brings organizational success.

- It helps the administration in implementing organizational control and enhances employer-employee relationship.
- It provides data for organizational policy decisions like promotion, training, transfer and termination.
- It increases job satisfaction and reduces grievances among employees.
- It serve the purpose of evaluating unit/departmental supervisors contributions in developing their subordinates.
- Well-documented performance appraisal reports serves as a legal document to protect the management against defamation or charges.

Disadvantages

- Performance appraisal may not serve the purpose if the criteria or standard developed are irrelevant to the job.
- There is possibility of subjectivity.
- It consumes time.
- While appraising, if the supervisor is highly charged with emotion, the psychological factor may affect the result.

Principles of Performance Appraisal

- The criteria developed for performance appraisal should be based on job position, and job description of the employee.
- Rating scale should be based on the task that should be observable and measurable.

  For example:

  Job position: Head nurse

  Type of role: Maintaining equipment and supplies

  Major tasks: (These tasks are observable and measurable. We can use a five-point rating scale to appraise the task performance) (Always observed (5 score); Almost always observed (4 scores); task observed when initiated (3 score); seldom observed (2 score) and never observed (1 score). For example, some of the tasks to be carried out in terms of equipment are:

  a. Identifies the need for equipment and supplies
  b. Makes timely requisition to the concerned store in a standard format
  c. Verifies the materials received from store
  d. Makes entry in the stock book in appropriate column provided
  e. Informs the staff nurses about the new arrival of materials
  f. If it is a new equipment, arranges for demonstration
  g. Communicates the cost of valuable or scare item
  h. Plans and conducts periodical inventory
  i. Arranges for condemnation of in serviceable items
  j. Maintains exchange of costly equipment with hospital workshop till the item is repaired
  k. Maintains a standard for materials according to number of patients in her/his unit
  l. Materials are always available and accessible for patient care
  m. Prepare and helps for auditing stock with nursing service administrator.

- The performance standard should be goal oriented.
- The performance appraisal should include criteria for appraisal, who will appraise, when and how it will be assessed, how it will be communicated to the appraisees and follow-up activity after appraisal.

- There should be a provision for counseling, coaching, training or mentoring for the employee if needed after performance appraisal.
- There should be follow-up interview and observation of employee after training.

PERFORMANCE APPRAISAL TOOLS (METHODS)

Performance appraisal is conducted by individual employee's evaluation and multiple persons evaluation methods.

Individual Employee's Evaluation Methods

- **Annual confidential report:** This is one of the traditional methods of performance appraisal used in governmental health care facilities. There is a printed proforma available for that purpose which describes mostly the nurses personal characteristics, leadership role, attitude and the nature of work. This is filled once a year by the nursing superintendent and seldom communicated the report to nurses.This appraisal report gives a basis for confirmation on the job, feasibility for higher education in nursing, promotion increments and transfer of employee.
- **Critical incident method:** This concept was originated from Armed Forces, U.S.A. during Second World War. In this method, the supervisor observes the subordinate's performance throughout the period of review regarding any critical or important incident whether it is positive or negative and this observation is recoded. Though it is an objective method of appraisal, the supervisor may show subjectivity.
- **Essay appraisal method:** It is one of the simple and traditional methods of performance appraisal. The supervisor writes an essay emphasizing the strengths and weaknesses of the employee on seeing the performance of the employee. The main disadvantage of this method is subjectivity of the supervisor may happen:
- **Checklist appraisal:** Checklist consist of detailed list of statements or items related to the job with dichotomous Yes or No answers for observation made. When the observation of the statement or item is present a score of 1 and if the observation of statement is absent a score of 0 (Zero) is given. The supervisor mist have thorough knowledge regarding the job while the checklist is made. At the end of the appraisal, the scores are added and documented for future reference.
- **Graphic rating scale:** This method is widely used in all establishments for performance appraisal that constitutes personal characteristics such as leadership capability, initiation, decision-making ability, etc. and professional contribution such as the quality and quantity of the job performed. The format includes 10–15 factors that to be appraised. Each factor is qualified with outstanding, very good, good, fair and poor. The supervisor appraises the employee and evaluation is made which is based on the scale. The limitations of the methods are subjectivity of the supervisor and sometimes the supervisor may give high ratings to avoid criticism.
- **Appraisal interview:** In health care industry this method is used widely. In this method, the appraiser communicates the employee regarding the job done by him/her, his potentials and limitations. This method is a natural type of conversation and no bossing over or controlling over the employee. The support of the supervisor encourages the employee that in turn helps in his professional growth and development Since the supervisor has given time and content of the interview, the employee is motivated and satisfied. This increases performance level and more objectivity is observed in this method.
- **Self-evaluation:** It is the modern trend of appraisal by the employee self The employee is asked by the supervisor regarding his performance during the period of review. The employee includes in his/her self-evaluation report as follows:
  - The period from-to-the task was completed
  - The nature of job
  - Whether the objectives of the task assignment was achieved, if achieved what were the reasons? If not what were the obstrucles?
  - What were the strong and weakest factor experienced during that appraisal period?
  - Any outstanding work done during the period
  - What are suggestions from employee to improve performance?
  - Signature of the employee.
  - Date of submission to the supervisor.

This method helps the administrator to improve the factors for which the suggestion is made

- **Peer rating:** Peer review is done by peers with similar competencies who are actively present on job. An established standard performance appraisal format is used. This method shows highly professionalism and identifies the strengths and weaknesses of the employee.

MULTIPLE PEOPLE'S EVALUATION METHODS

Forced Distribution Method

This system is designed to force the appraiser to fit the employees being appraised into a pre-determined ranges of scale. It is assumed that employees in an organization can be divided into five point scale, such as outstanding, above average, average, below average and poor. The appraiser distributes the employees into these categories in such a way that outstanding 10%, above average 20%, average 40%, below average 20% and poor 10%. Thus this method reduces bias. The main disadvantage is that it is difficult to categorize employees when they are in small number according to different scale.

Ranking Method

It is a simple method that permits comparison of all employees in any stage rating group irrespective of the type of job they do. All employees are evaluated on the same factors and are rated according to their job performance. The best is placed in first rank and the poor at last rank. The main disadvantage of this method is this that it does not specify the degree of difference between the first and the last rank.

IMPORTANCE OF MENTORING AND COACHING

In an organization, employees who work may have different levels of knowledge, competencies and experience. Some of them may be detrimental for the success of the organization. In human resource management, we need strong mentoring and coaching program for the employees career development, employees satisfaction, organizational success and reduction of turnover. Mentoring and coaching are not the same they are different.

What is Mentoring?

It is a collaborative process in which an experienced and skilled person referred as mentor establishes a coordinative partnership which is beneficial to a person who is looking to someone to help him to increase his skill knowledge and experience referred as mentee.

Mentoring is a partnership not a relationship between employee and his immediate supervisor. Both supervisor and employee agree to the relationship and both are responsible for the success.

Mentoring is a career development tool. Collaborative means the mentor and the mentoree have to work together to determine what the partnership aims to achieve and how it will be achieved.

Mentorship refers to a personal and developmental relationship that enables synergistic, and purposeful conversation to reflect on experiences make informed decisions and act upon ideas generated. It is a challenge, motivating and inspiring.

Mentor Concept

Manages relationship

Encourages

Nurtures

Teaches

Offers mutual respect

Responds to the mentor's need

(**Source:** http//synergy.edu.au/docs/choosing a mentor pdf)

Difference Between Mentoring and Coaching

Mentoring is a process of focusing on relationship between mentor and mentoree. The main goal is to ensure a therapeutic and a protective environment where the mentoree shares the problems affect his or her professional and personal career. Mentoring relationship focuses on job/life balance, self-confidence, self-perception, and how the personal life influences the professional life.

Coaching is a process of focusing on task, definite issues, such as managing patient care more effectively with available resources, interaction with patients and family effectively, and learning to think strategically. The coach is an expert who is capable of teaching these skills to coachee.

Mentoring is always a long-term process. If we want mentoring to be successful, both mentor and mentoree needs to understand and accept each other and build a trust. This relationship lasts from nine months to one year. This in turn develops an environment that ensures the mentoree feel secure in sharing the real issues to the mentor whereas coaching is short-term process. A coach is involved with the mentoree for a short period of time, just a few sessions of conversations. The coaching lasts for as long as is needed, depending on the purpose of the coaching relationship and the ability of the coachee to rectify the issue.

Mentoring is development driven process. Its purpose is to develop the individual's career for the current, and the future job. Since the immediate manager could be a mentor, it reduces the conflict between supervisor and employees because of the role change as a mentor.

Coaching is performance driven process. The main aim of coaching is to increase the capability and improve the individual's performance, skill, knowledge and experience on the job. This refers to either enhancing the existing performance skills or developing new skills. Once the coachee successfully develops performance skills, the coach is not required to coach further.

Mentoring requires a design that decides the mentoring plan and objective, the important areas of the relationship, the pertinent mentoring models, and the relevant components that will guide the relationship, especially the matching process.

Coaching does not require design. Coaching can be implemented immediately on any given subject. If a hospital seeks to provide coaching to a large group of nurses, then certainly an amount of design is involved in order to determine the competency area, expertize needed, and assessment tools used, but this does not necessarily require a long time to implement the coaching program.

In mentoring, the immediate manager is indirectly involved in the process. Though the immediate manager may offer suggestions to the employee on how to best utilize the mentoring skill, or may give a recommendation to the matching committee on what would constitute a good match, the manager does not has the connection with the mentor and he does not publicly inform during the mentoring relationship. This helps in maintain the mentoring relationship's confidentiality and integrity.

The mentoree's immediate manager is a partner in coaching. She or he often provides the coach with feedback on areas in which his or her employee is in need of coaching. This coach uses this information to guide the coaching process.

When to Consider Coaching

- When a company is seeking to develop its employees in specific competencies using performance management tools and involving the immediate manager
- When a company has a number of talented employees who are not meeting expectations
- When a company is introducing a new system or program
- When a company has a small group of individuals (5–8) in need of increased competency in specific areas
- When a leader or executive needs assistance in acquiring a new skill as an additional responsibility.

When to Consider Mentoring

- When a company is seeking to develop its leaders or talent pool as part of succession planning
- When a company seeks to develop its diverse employees to remove barriers that hinder their success
- When a company seeks to more completely develop, its employees in ways that are additional to the acquisition of specific skills/competencies.
- When a company seeks to retain its internal expertize and experience residing in its baby boomer employees for future generations
- When a company wants to create a workforce that balances the professional and the personal.

(**Source:** The Difference Between Coaching and Mentoring www. management-mentors.com/resources/coaching-mentoring).

Mentoring Cycle

Preparation Phase

In this phase, the mentor and mentoree establish mentoring relationship. This constitutes developing and facilitating well-defined objectives. Regular communications between them enhances effective relationships in which the mentor takes initiation to contact the mentoree regularly. By this process, the mentoree is encouraged to contact the mentor. The mentor strives to develop rapport. Thus in this phase, the mentor builds rapport and establishes practical goals. The mentor establishes a strategic plan that includes list of expectations such as when and where the they will meet time planning types of activities, maintain confidentiality the nature of giving feedback develop a timeline and topics of discussion.

Negotiation Phase

This is a phase of mutual satisfaction. Both mentor and the mentoree established a comfortable working relationship to achieve practical goals. They meet periodically to assess the progress made and quality and quantity of behavior change between the mentor and mentoree.

Enabling Phase

The mentoree achieves the goal under the guidance of the mentor. The mentor evaluates the mentoring program and its cost.

Closure

At this phase, the mentor and the mentoree summarizes what has been mutually agreed. They both keep their relationship strictly professional.

Evidence Speaks

Mentoring is widely recognized today as an extremely beneficial career development tool. Studies have shown that mentored employees perform better on the job, advance more rapidly within the organization, express lower turnover intentions than their non mentored counterparts. Report more job and career satisfaction (Poe, 2002).

The Business Case for Mentoring, 35% of employees who do not receive regular mentoring plan to seek other employment within a year and 16% of employees with good mentors planned to leave their companies. More than 60% of college and graduate students listed mentoring as a criterion for selecting an employer after graduation. Training alone increased managerial productivity by 24%, but jumped to 88% when mentoring and coaching were combined. (Lockwood, 2004) (APQC, 2004)

Coaching

When the performance appraisal of the employee is not satisfactory, the supervisor arranges for coaching the employees.

Coaching is a collaborative relationship undertaken between a coach (supervisor) and a willing individual, the client (employee). It is time-limited, focused and uses conversations to help employees to achieve their goals. It demands skill on the part of the supervisor (coach) in facilitating meaningful conversations and letting the client lead. Learning starts when the coaching conversation begins with new actions with new practices, are always the final stage of a successful coaching conversation.

What are the Advantages of Coaching?

- It enhances the learning of the employee
- It helps to motivate the employee to improve his/her performance
- The employee and the supervisor are willing to take risk
- Ensures deeper commitment to the job
- It gives opportunities to collaborate with peer group
- It gives chance to the employee to learn from each other

Grow Model of Coaching

There are four steps in this model:

G — Goal setting
R — Reality
O — Options/Obstacles
W — Wrap-up/Way forward

- **Establishing goals:** The employee should be very clear about his immediate and long-term goals. They needs to be defined well and should be well-understood by the employee. For example, the midwife wants to assess the newborn as she felt. She is not confident in performing the task. By coaching, the midwifery supervisor and the midwife agrees the topic for learning and establishes learning objectives for each session. A long-term aim also discussed and agreed upon by the midwife that she will be able to perform the task confidently to all normal newborns till their discharge without any mistake.
- **Reality**: The coach (supervisor), in this step identifies the current reality of the topic. She, through conversation identifies what are the issues and the challenges. How far the employee is away from goal? From the above example, the midwifery supervisor finds out from the midwife from herself assessment why she is not confident or not able to perform the task, what are her reasons. The supervisor discards the irrelevant causes and her assumptions.
- **Options/obstacles:** Sometimes there may be some obstacles to achieve the goal. Sometimes there may not be obstacle. When there are no obstacles, the supervisor discusses many options to achieve the goal and ensures that the employee is very clear about the option accepted. In the above example, the midwife expresses no hindrances. However, the midwifery supervisor discusses wide range of options like demonstration and return demonstration. The midwife ensures the supervisor that she will perform newborn assessment under supervision on 40 normal newborns.
- **Wrap-up/ way forward:** After the option is selected and agreed upon the supervisor needs to make action plan to achieve the goal. As discussed in the above example, the midwifery supervisor selects a postnatal ward and helps the midwife to learn and do newborn assessment. She perceives any obstacle while helping the midwife and ensures that she achieves confidence by assessing 40 normal newborns. A feedback from the midwife is taken and the supervisor follows her further performance.

Role of a Nurse Administrator in Mentoring and Coaching Nurses

- The nurse administrator should know about importance of mentoring and coaching in nursing
- Identifies the needs and documents a need for the program
- Establishes specific organizational needs
- Gets top administrative level support and involvement for the program.
- Establishes, philosophy, vision, mission, outcomes, guidelines, and design for the program
- Establishes a reliable matching procedure
- Understands the match between mentor and the mentoree is the basic principle of success of the program

- Recruits and trains mentors, nurses and supervisors and communicates with them about mentoring
- Acts as a sponsor that helps increase exposure of the nurses in sharing
- As a teacher helps to solve nursing care problems and creates further learning opportunities
- Her role as coach is advisory that advises nurses on how to accomplish their goals. Nurse administrator always speaks for nurses and nursing, and protects them when they make mistakes by prompt corrections
- Ensures a safe environment in which the coachee can make mistakes without losing credibility
- As a counselor enhances the nurses self-esteem through supportive, nonjudgmental discussions
- She is a role model and demonstrates the behaviors necessary for success. (Adapted and applied in nursing from Digh, 2002)

DISCIPLINE

Discipline of the employees is the backbone for effective and smooth running of any organization. When the employees carry out the task within the framework of organizational goals, adhering the norms, rules regulations and policies of an organization that enables the employees improved performance and organizational success. One method by which a nurse administrator can control subordinates behavior is to invoke official disciplinary procedure. Discipline can be self controlled by which an employee brings his or her behavior into agreement with the agency's official behavior code, or it can be a managerial action to enforce employee compliance with agency rules and regulations.

Concept of Discipline

Discipline is the regulation and modulation of human activities to produce a controlled performance. It is to encourage employees to conform the established standards of job performance and to behave sensibly and safely at work.

Meaning of Discipline

It is derived from the Latin word ***disciplina*** it means learning, teaching and growing.

According to Webster's dictionary, the meanings of discipline are the following:

- It is a training that corrects, moulds, strengthens and perfect.
- Control gained by enforced obedience.
- Punishing.

Definition

It is defined as a procedure that corrects or punishes a subordinate because a rule of procedure has been violated (Dessler 2001).

It should be viewed as a condition within an organization whereby the employees know what is expected of the organization's rules, standards and policies and what the consequences are of infraction (Rue and Byars 1996).

From the above two definitions, the following elements of discipline could be observed: The main aim of discipline is an orderly behavior that helps to achieve organizational goals. When employees behave in an appropriate manner and is called self-discipline. When employees violate rules and regulations of the work place punitive actions are needed against those employees. In other words, discipline is defined as a training or molding of the mind and character to bring about desired behaviors. Discipline refers to working in accordance with certain recognized rules, regulations and customs, whether they are written or implicit in character.

Major Aspects of Discipline

- **Negative discipline**: It is a force or an external influence. It is a traditional aspect of discipline when the employees do not adhere to the norms, standards, rules and regulation of an organization, and punishment is given for disobedience or indiscipline. The employee develops fear of getting punishment and performs the task. However, this approach does not show effectiveness of performance. It creates an emotional conflict.
- **Positive discipline:** The employees adhere to the norms, standards, rules and regulation in an organization. It is not because of fear of punishment, but the employee willing to abide with the rules and regulation for his success as well as to achieve organizational goals. The employee experiences a psychological satisfaction. It develops self-discipline among employee.

Purposes of Discipline

- To encourage employees to behave sensibly at work where being sensible is defined as adhering the rules and regulations (Dessler 2001).
- To improve work performance
- To develop self-discipline among employees
- To eliminate non productive employees from the organization
- To justify employment action (If the employee is terminated/demoted from job, the cause is justified as disciplinary action)

- To increase the working efficiency and morale of the employees so that their productivity is stepped up, the cost of production brought down and the quality of production improved.
- To create an atmosphere of respect for the human personality and human relations
- To give and seek direction and responsibility
- To develop among the employees a spirit of tolerance and a desire to make adjustments
- To impart an element of certainty despite several differences in informal behavior patterns and other related changes in an organization
- To obtain a willing acceptance of the rules, regulations and procedures of an organization so that organizational goals can be achieve.

Principles of Discipline

- It should be primarily positive, understanding not through fear
- It should ensure equal justice for all, respects for the rights
- It should be constructive and as per disciplinary policies. Discipline is not the end, it is rather a means for successful implementation of organizational program
- It should ensure respect the dignity of an individual employees
- It should be unbiased.

Causes of Misconduct

- Excessive tardiness
- Failure to report an absence from duty
- Insubordination
- Rude or using abusive language at work place
- Failure to follow departmental or unit policies, rules and regulation
- Dishonest
- Theft.

The role of nurse administrator in conducting disciplinary procedure.

- The nurse administrator identifies and ensures the misconduct occurs in work place
- Before conducting disciplinary procedure, she reviews the following:
  - Whether the nurse clearly understand for what purpose the action is taken. Ensures the rule/regulation/norms she violated
  - Ensures the administration has enforced that particular norms/rules/policy
  - Whether the nurse knows if she violates the norm/policy may lead to disciplinary action
  - Whether the nurse admitted the offence and apologized with the authorities
  - Whether the violation is caused by provocation
- **The nurse administrator proceeds with investigation (Investigation stage)–Collects pertinent data:** The nurse administrator collects all the information and evidences to make sure that what happened in the work setting. This information of evidences include statement from the witnesses, investigator's reports, documentary evidence, information from the witness who was present during incident, and the very pertinent information from the interviewing the employee involved in the misconduct.

  Where ever possible, two members from department of administration should be assigned to conduct the investigation and these two members also will conduct interview of all the witnesses together. Having two members in the investigating team to conduct investigation ensures the opportunity for better note taking and documentation of questions and answers during interviews. Sometimes the investigating manager may witness this activity. The nurse administrator should ensure that all investigating officers should be available at least for six months or more for future hearing. A manager who is expected to leave the hospital is not a good choice as an investigator.
- **Seeks outside help if needed to complete the data**
- **Interview the nurse**, and it should play a major role in management's decision to issue discipline. A nurse involved in misconduct should be provided an opportunity to explain herself/himself. The advantages of interviewing the nurse who is affected are:
  - It facilitates a chance for the nurse involved in the misconduct to explain his or her actions
  - To make her aware of her involvement if any in this misconduct
  - To gather direct evidence from the nurse involved in the misconduct
  - To gather evidence from third party witnesses about a misconduct.

When interviewing the nurse who is suspected in misconduct it is mandatory that all the evidences that the administrator has gathered during the investigation stage is clarified while interviewing the nurse. The administrator should maintain integrity and should not hide evidence that has proved against the nurse. The administrator should ask specific questions to the nurse, with emphasis on dates and approximate times that the events occurred.

After hearing from the nurse's explanation in the interview, verifications of the facts and gathering of all the evidences, the decision to discipline can be made after discussions with concerned officers in administration, and the case with the Human Resources (HR) Department. The basis for discipline should be decided on the factors i.e. the employee's previous record, the severity of the incident, the reason for provocation of the incident. After the investigation and interviews have taken place, decision to discipline should be issued in writing to an employee.

- **Decide for taking disciplinary action (Discipline stage)**
  After the interview is over, and the nurse administrator has gathered all available evidences, the decision to discipline is to be made. Before making a decision the nurse administrator should think whether the nurse's behavior could be corrected before sending her to the workplace or not. It is always good to discuss the type of cause for misconduct with the HR Department before finalizing disciplinary decision.
- **The nurse administrator ensures the evidences are of quality before issuing any decision to discipline.**

When the nurse administrator feels that the nurse has been involved in a misconduct, then discipline is certainly an option. If the evidence is weak, the administrator should not pursue decision to discipline Before issuing the disciplinary action, consultation with HR. Department will be very beneficial in disciplinary decisions.

To summarize the nurse administrator follows the following steps in sequential order of events to make disciplinary action when a misconduct occurs the department or nursing units of a hospital.

- Ensures a misconduct occurs in the workplace
- The nurse administrator collects data on investigated reports, documentary evidences of interview with the nurse with who affected with misconduct, and interview reports of the witnesses
- The nurse administrator interviews with the nurse suspected in the misconduct
- The nurse administrator reviews all the evidence and consults with HR management if requires before final decision
- Issues the letter of reprimand, letter of suspension, or termination.

DISCIPLINARY STRATEGIES

Verbal counseling is typically the first response to an infraction. A verbal warning must be administered to the employee in private and as objectively as possible. The presence of one management level witness, preferably an HR professional, is recommended. Any verbal counseling must be documented in writing in the employee's personnel file (**Source:** Boundless. Employee Discipline Boundless Management. Boundless, 21 Jul, 2015. Retrieved 01 Feb. 2016)

According to Lisa Mooney, some of the disciplinary strategies are given below:

Oral Warning

Usually, an oral warning is the initial step in disciplining an employee except in a very serious offence. The administrator finds a confidential setting preferably her office to meet with the employee who did not adhere to the organization's policy, call the employee with information about the offence, and asks him for his explanation and discuss ways to avoid further problems.

Written Admonishment

When an employee is fail to complete the job responsibilities, in spite of several warning, is termed as **acts of insubordination** or other violations of an organization that compels the administrator to issue a written warning to the employee. A written warning communicates the employee's adverse behaviors and gives a solution to address the problem by the administrator. She directly intervene with the employee to discuss the written warning and explains the behavior expected from the employee. The warning report to be filed in employee's personal file and an plan for remedial action.It is a highly confidential document.

Reassignment

Sometime the employee may not be able to cope up with the current role at the organization. This employee is relieved from the existing job position and given an alternative role in the job. This new role in the organization may reduce in pay or title demotion, but not always. The cause for changing the role position due to his inability to overcome the problems in the current role to be communicated to the employee. The change in responsibilities is likely to motivate the employee to commit towards the new assignment.

Suspension

A period of suspension is another disciplinary action with the intention to motivate the employee to change. This is considered as a last trial to get the employee to change his behavior. Sometimes, an immediate suspension is warranted due to a single serious offense. The suspension gives the worker enough time to think and reassess his position with the establishment so she/he can decide whether to abide by management's expectations or find another job.

Dismissal

When all the efforts found a failure, the management decides to terminate the employee who could not change his behavior in spite of several warnings. The administrator does this job with meticulous care, reassesses the reasons for dismissal, reviews documentation of employee infractions along and written accounts of disciplinary measures already issued from the management. Ensures the inability of the employee to comply with an improvement plan. She communicates the employee confidentially and personally of the decision by administrator. Sometime the employee may show adverse hostile reaction in this regard, and anticipating a hostile reaction, employ a security professional to escort from the facility.

Role of Nurse Administrator in Maintaining Discipline

- She informs the job expectations and organizational goals to all nursing personnel
- Ensures that all nurses know the policies, rules, regulations, standards of nursing, norms and other protocol of nursing service department
- Demonstrates a positive attitude and trust towards nurses that in turn will boost up their morale and motivate them to achieve goals
- Appreciates nurses who maintain self-discipline
- Arranges for informal gathering to encourage open communication
- Establishes a positive work culture
- Maintains objectivity in dealing with problems of nurses
- When disciplinary action is taken, maintains a complete record
- Takes constructive decisions and corrective action when managing discipline
- Utilizes mentoring, coaching, counseling. Teaching and guiding skill to develop nurses and avoid indiscipline
- Supervises the nurses effectively
- Formulates strong policies for disciplinary actions and revise periodically.

GRIEVANCE PROCEDURE

Human resource is a great asset to an organization. When employees are happy and satisfied in their work setting that increases the morale and efficiency of employees. However, when employees have problems and disputes in their work setting, and are not resolved by the management, such grievances results in frustration, dissatisfaction, low productivity, lack of interest in work absenteeism, discontentment and low morale in an organization.

Definition

Grievance may be any genuine or imaginary feeling of dissatisfaction or injustice which an employee experiences about his job, management policies and procedures. It must be expressed by the employee and brought to the notice of the management and the organization.

It is a complaint about an organizational policy, procedures or managerial practices or discomforts whether it is valid or not (Salipante and Rene Brownian)

According to Jucius, a grievance is any discontent or dissatisfaction, whether expressed or not, whether valid or not, arising out of anything connected with the company which an employee thinks, believes or even feels to be unfair, unjust or inequitable.

According to Fillipo, grievance includes any discontent and dissatisfaction that affects organizational performance. It can either stated or unvoiced, written or oral, legitimate or ridiculous. There is a difference between complaint and grievance. A complaint is a discontent but not believes as vital whereas a grievance is when the employee feels that injustice has been committed to him by the management.

Grievance procedure is a process in which a formal communication between an employee and the management takes place for the settlement of a grievance. The grievance procedures differ from organization to organization.

Types of grievance: A grievance may take from any one of the following forms if it is not addressed timely:

- **Factual grievance:** A factual grievance arises when the genuine requests of employees are not heard or addressed, e.g. confirmation on the job has been agreed by the management after performance appraisal, but the management did not adhere to it or not confirmed the post due to various reasons.
- **Imaginary grievance:** When an employee's has wrong perception about an information, he is dissatisfied without a valid reason and he develops a wrong attitude. Such a situation may create an imaginary grievance. Since, the management is not involved in it, still it has has a responsibility to clear the wrong perception of the employee immediately.
- **Disguised grievance:** Due to pressure from personal life or work setting, an employee may have

dissatisfaction for reasons that are unaware causes frustration. This employee develops disguised conflict against the administration. For example, if a new recruit is assigned as a class teacher of a group of students, this may become a frustration for the senior teacher who is supposed to get that chance and was ignored by the management.

Causes of Grievances

- Poor working conditions, unsafe working environment
- Poor employer-employee relationship
- Irrational management policies like overtime, transfer, and demotion
- Poor employment conditions like inadequate salary and benefits
- Ill-defined organizational policies
- When an employee suffers from feelings of neglect, victimization and becomes an object of humiliation in a work environment
- Policy issues with regards to promotions, transfer-disciplinary action
- Granting leaves–without medical certificates leave extended–medical facilities, etc.
- Poor, dispute-settling mechanism.

Objectives of a Grievance Handling Procedure (Jackson (2000)) discusses the following objectives of a grievance handling procedure:

- To help the employee to express his/her grievance
- To ensure the nature of the grievance
- To identify the causes for dissatisfaction
- To facilitate addressing of the problem immediately
- To ensure relevant actions and ensure that promises are kept by management
- To communicate the employee that on unsuccessful resolution the employee has every right to pursue the matter with grievance handling committee.

Advantages of grievance handling, the following are some of the clear cut advantages of having a grievances handling procedure:

- The management becomes aware of employee's perceptions regarding management policies and practices. It can reveal the opinion of the employees.
- Employees can express their feelings and opinion freely which is not possible through formal channel of communication by the virtue of the position, experience and expertize, the top level manager can deal the grievances better than the first level supervisors who lacks grievance handling skill.
- Supervisors are compelled to hear the grievance handling process sympathetically and patiently. It keeps a track on the supervisor's attitude and behavior towards their subordinates.
- If an organization has a proper grievance handling cell, it boosts up the morale of employees.
- Employees can get their grievances redressed promptly
- Ensures to foster good morale, and the employees maintain code of discipline
- Facilitates uniformity in handling grievances
- It develops trustworthiness of employees
- Minimizes personality conflicts and frustration
- It acts as a cushion to support employees at the time of problems
- Ensures judicial protection to the employees
- It provides a forum to express the problems
- Enables the employer and employees to resolve problems or grievances in a systematic and amicable manner
- Helps employer and employee to identify and discuss the problem

Principles of Grievance Handling Procedure

- The procedure should be explicit, relevant and timely.
- It should be clearly defined to both parties
- Helpful attitude of management towards the employees
- It should be based on facts and figures
- Respect for decisions taken
- Adequate publicity to be given
- Ensures periodic review

Grievance Redressal Procedure

There are two methods used in this procedure:

Open-door Policy

In this policy, the aggrieved employee is free to approach the top level manager to get his grievances resolved. There is a face to face discussion with management and this policy is possible only in a smaller organization. However, it may not possible in bigger organization as the top manager may be busy with other dealing of the organization.

Step Ladder Type Policy

In the 4 step ladder type, **the first step** is that the grieved employee submits his grievance report to the departmental representative who is a representative of the management and this representative is supposed to answer him within 48 hours of submission of report.

Step 2

The departmental head should address the grievance of the employee within 48 hours. Failing to which the affected employee can present his grievance to the head of the department. It is mandatory that he gives decision within 72 hours.

Step 3

When the aggrieved employee is not satisfied with the decision of departmental head, he can present his grievance to the Grievance Committee of the organization The Grievance Committee of the establishment, prepares recommendation to the manager within 7 days in the form of report. The final decision of the Grievance Committee is communicated to the aggrieved employee within three days of the receipt of the report.

If the employee is not satisfied with the decision by the Grievance Committee an appeal for revision of the decision could be requested by the employee within 7 days.

Step 4

If the employee is not agreeing for the decision, or unsettled, this case is referred to voluntary arbitration. Arbitration includes the settlement of the problem by a neutral party to both. This neutral party reviews and helps the employer and employee to settle the grievance. The use of arbitration helps to prevent the grievance from going to the Law.

Arbitration can be of two types:

1. Compulsory
2. Voluntary.

In compulsory arbitration, the parties involved go through the third party to settle their grievance. If an arbitration clause is included in a contract, and if the contract itself is valid, the parties must abide by the clause. Arbitration may also be ordered by a court as a means to prevent a situation from going to trial, and the parties must comply or face possible sanctions.

In voluntary arbitration, both the parties involved and agree on their own to use an outside party, like an arbitration attorney to help settle their differences. No contract or law requires this action, yet deciding to use arbitration can save money, time and maybe even good will. In business relationships, all of these are important. If the matter is personal, such as in a divorce proceeding, voluntary arbitration can be equally valuable. The aggrieved employee should be knowledgeable in matters dealing with arbitration.

Role of Nurse Administrator in Effective Grievance Procedure

Quick Action

The nurse administrator should identify and resolve grievance as soon as possible. Training must be given to the nursing supervisors and head nurses to effectively and timely manage a grievance. This will decrease the detrimental effects of grievance on the nurses and employees and their performance.

Acknowledging Grievance

The nurse administrator must acknowledge the grievance put forward by the aggrieved nurse as manifestation of true and real feelings of the nurses. Acknowledgement by the nurse administrator means that she is eager to look into the complaint impartially and without any bias. This will create a positive work environment with reduction of grievances.

Gathering Facts

The nurse administrator should gather appropriate and sufficient data explaining the type of grievance. A complete record of such facts must be maintained so that these facts can be used in later stage of grievance redressal.

Examining the Causes of Grievance

It is very important to identify the actual cause of grievance to make decisions and immediate action to prevent repetition of the grievance.

Decisioning

When the cause of grievance is identified, the administrator chalks out alternative course of actions to manage the grievance. The effect of each course of action should be analyzed based on the existing and future management policies and procedure and accordingly decision should be taken by the nurse administrator.

Execution and Review

The nurse administrator should implement the decision quickly, ignoring without hurting the feelings of aggrieved nurse. After implementing the decision, a follow-up must be done to ensure that the grievance has been resolved completely and adequately.

An effective grievance procedure ensures a conducive work culture because it redresses the grievance to mutual satisfaction of both the nurses and the administrator. It also helps the administration to frame policies and procedures acceptable to the nurses for the future. It becomes an effective medium for the nurses to express their feelings, discontent and dissatisfaction openly and formally.

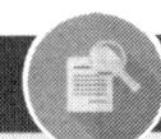

SUMMARY POINTS

- ✓ The modern management system gives more emphasis on employees performance appraisal that enables the administrator to facilitate the employees regarding job security, promotion, transfer training needs, rewards and punishment, retirement benefits, termination, etc. The feedback mechanism in performance appraisal communicates the employees to know their strengths and weakness constructive or adverse comments by the employer, and their performance level. This motivates the employees to work better to achieve the personal and organizational goals.
- ✓ Performance appraisal is a systematic and planned process to assess the performance capabilities of the individual on his job based on criteria, and serves as an effective control mechanism in organization.
- ✓ Performance appraisal is beneficial for both the employee and employer.
- ✓ Mentoring is relationship oriented, long-term, developmental driven, and well-designed program where employee's immediate supervisor takes important role whereas, coaching is task oriented, short-term, performance driven and does not require a planned design. The immediate employer may not be necessarily the coach for the employee.
- ✓ Discipline is a managerial tool to control the employees in an organization. It is the regulation and modulation of human activities to produce a controlled performance. It is to encourage employees to confirm the established standards of job performance and to behave sensibly and safely at work. It has both positive and negative aspects.
- ✓ When employees have problems and disputes in their work setting, and are not resolved by the management, such grievances results in frustration, dissatisfaction, low productivity, lack of interest in work absenteeism, discontentment and low morale in an organization.
- ✓ Grievance may be any genuine or imaginary feeling of dissatisfaction or injustice which an employee experiences about his job, management policies and procedures. It must be expressed by the employee and brought to the notice of the management and the organization.
- ✓ A grievance may take from any one of the following forms: (a) Factual (b) imaginary, and (c) disguised.
- ✓ A factual grievance arises when legitimate needs of employees remain unfulfilled, When an employee's dissatisfaction is not because of any valid reason but because of a wrong perception, wrong attitude or wrong information he /she has. Such a situation may create an imaginary grievance. An employee may have dissatisfaction for reasons that are unknown to him. If he/she is under pressure from family, friends, relatives, neighbors, he/she may reach the work spot with frustration this is referred as disguised grievance
- ✓ The nurse administrator has to play a vital role in handling grievances among nurses. An effective grievance procedure ensures a conducive work culture among nurses because it redresses the grievance to mutual satisfaction of both the nurses and the administrator. It also helps the administration to frame policies and procedures acceptable to the nurses for the future. It becomes an effective medium for the nurses to express their feelings, discontent and dissatisfaction openly and formally.

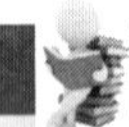

REVIEW QUESTIONS

1. Define performance appraisal. Describe the principles and advantages of performance appraisal.
2. Describe the importance of mentoring and coaching in nursing service administration.
3. What are the causes of indiscipline among nurses? Discuss the responsibilities of a nurse administrator in maintaining organizational discipline.
4. Discuss the causative factors for grievance among nursing personnel. Describe the advantages of grievance handling.
5. Describe in detail the grievance handling procedures.
6. Write short notes on the following:
   a. Performance appraisal tools
   b. Difference between mentoring and coaching
   c. Disciplinary strategies

d. Causes of misconduct at work place
e. Grow model of coaching
f. Qualities of a mentor.

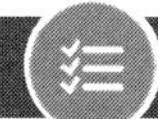

SELECTED READINGS

1. American Productivity and Quality Center (2004). Mentoring Digh, P. (2002)
2. Dolezalek. "Got High Potentials?" Training Magazine, January/February
3. Employee Discipline." Boundless Management. Boundless, 21 Jul. 2015. Retrieved 01 Feb. 2016 from https://www.boundless.com/management/textbooks/boundless-management-textbook/human-resource-management-7/employee-evaluation-and-management-in-detail-59/employee-discipline-301-4831/
4. Ganong.W.L. Grievance handling .Journal of nursing Administration, Jan/Feb 1974,4(1):11
5. Lockwood, N. (2004). The value of mentoring. Retrieved September 2, 2008, from SHRM Web site http://www.shrm.org/research/briefly_published/Mentoring
6. Mentoring to create a diverse pipeline for talent. Retrieved August 27, 2008, from SHRM Web site http://www.shrm.org/diversity/members/articles.novdec02/covstory.asp
7. Metzger, N. Handling grievances .Guidelines for RNHosp.Prog.1979 (Sept 60(9)69-71
8. Poe, A (2006). Launching a mentor program. Retrieved September 2, 2008, from SHRM Web site http://www.shrm.org/hrresources.whitepapers_published/CMS_000424.asp
9. The Difference Between Coaching and Mentoring www.management-Mentors.com/resources/coaching-mentoring.

UNIT VIII
MATERIAL MANAGEMENT

18

Material Management

LEARNING OBJECTIVES

This chapter imparts learning about:

- Concepts, Principles and Procedures of Material Management
- Planning and Procurement Procedures: Specifications
- Inventory Control
  - ABC Analysis
  - VED (Vital, Essential, Desirable) Analysis
- Condemnation
- Planning Equipments and Supplies for Nursing Care: Unit and Hospital

INTRODUCTION

Material management is an administrative function. It includes material planning and control, production planning, purchasing, inventory control, flow of materials of various departments, and waste management. Efficient management of materials in hospital is cost effective and at the same time it enhances quality patient care In other words the administrator is responsible for the coordination of planning, organizing and controlling materials efficiently with maximum utility to enhance quality care to patients at a minimum cost.

Material management is a systematic process referred as planning, forecasting, organizing and distributing and controlling the materials from purchase department to various internal departments with careful distribution. In hospital administration it is concerned with equipment, supply, drugs, linen and other materials needed for care of patient that are distributed to nursing service department. The administrator should keep in mind that the right quality of materials to be reached for patient care for safety of the patients.

CONCEPTS, PRINCIPLES AND PROCEDURES OF MATERIAL MANAGEMENT

What is Material?

Ballot (2006) defines that materials are physical items in nature that are purchased and used to produce a product. Bailey et al. (2009) describes that materials are items purchased from a source that are used to produce a final product. Stukhart (2007) states materials are raw items to produce a product such as equipment.

Definition

Material management is a process of planning, organizing, and controlling all those activities concerned with the distribution of materials into an organization to minimize inventory, purchasing, material handling and distribution costs.

Material management is a process consisting various steps like, planning, verifying, storage, and distribution of materials to the concerned units. The aim of material management is to ensure that the right materials are supplied to the right units and stored in the right place, and supplied in the right quantities when needed.

The responsibility of material management department for the distribution of materials from the time the materials are ordered, received, verified and stored and distributed.

Ballot (2006) explains material management as the process of planning, acquiring, storing, moving, and controlling materials to effectively use the resources.

Tersine and Campbell (2004) define material management as the process to provide the right materials to the right units at the right time in order to maintain quality outcome. It is cost effective.

According to LJ De Rose, material management is defined as the planning, directing, controlling and coordination of all those activities concerned with the procurement, storage and inventory control of equipments and supplies of the organization.

Aims and Objectives of Material Management

- To reduce the operating cost and improve profits for the organization
- To increase efficiency: Efficiency to handle materials among personnel.
- To ensure continuous supply of materials and prevent interruption of services.
- To procure of quality Materials to enhance quality outcome.
- To ensure efficient handling of materials by skilled professional.
- To improve interpersonal relationship with suppliers
- To identify and train talented future material managers from lower position
- To enhance coordination from various departments.
- To ensure adequate equipment and supplies to cater the patients at the time of need.
- To buy the material at minimum cost and get maximum benefits of quality and price.
- To reduce the inventory cost.

The Benefits of Material Management

Some of the benefits of material management are presented below:

- Reduction of the overall costs of materials used in hospitals
- Better handling of materials by skilled professionals
- Reduction in duplicated orders as it is a centralized system
- Accessibility and availability of materials as and when needed in quality and quantity
- Prevents waste of time when the stock is systematically preserved
- Quality control helps to discard out dated, obsolete and in-serviceable materials and replace by new materials
- Enhances good IPR with suppliers and departmental colleagues
- Prevention of overstocking and reduction of materials on surplus stock
- Ensures effective utilization of materials
- Inventory losses may be minimized

Principles of Material Management

- Before planning study all available system relationship of material management like current methods practices and problems.
- Planning should include need assessment, basic requirements, desirable alternatives and planning for contingency.
- Whatever system design selected for material management should integrate material handling and storage activities, which should be cost-effective.
- Handle product in a unit load as large as possible.
- Encourage effective utilization of all the space available in material management.
- Standardization of equipment and supplies is one of the important principles of material management.
- Personnel's skills and capabilities and limitation should be considered while handling materials for effectiveness.
- It should ensure enviromental safety.
- Material handling incurs consumption of energy, hence it should be considered while procuring materials.
- Material management is a process. Technology and mechanization brings less time consumption
- Material management should be flexible in nature so that the patients receives services whenever is required and services should not be interrupted without material.
- The procedure should be as simple as possible to avoid unnecessary movement.
- It should ensure provision for safe handling equipment according to safety rules and regulation
- It must be updated with use of computers and gadgets for material handling and storage system.
- Ensures integration of data flow with physical material flow.
- There should be a definite operational sequence from planning to distribution.
- Another principle ensures cost benefit analysis of all solutions available.

- In order to keep the material serviceable for a longer period, preventive maintenance to be practiced
- In order to avoid stocking obsolete materials a policy of condemnation and discard to be followed.
- A stock book to be maintained that is updated and provision of periodical auditing bring better effectiveness.

PLANNING AND PROCUREMENT PROCEDURES

The following components are included in planning and procurement of materials.

Steps in Planning for Materials

- Need assessment and estimation of requirement of equipment and supplies
- Preparing purchasing order
- Inventory management
- Material planning based on the policies of the institution
- Reviewing feedback information from the departments
- While planning for material purchase the administrator should aim that:

1. Materials should be of right quality
2. Supply of materials should be in right quantity.The administrator should avoid under stocking or over stocking
3. The materials should be available when needed
4. Required materials should be distributed to the right departments
5. Procuring of materials should be at the right cost
6. The purpose of material management planning is to get the material at low cost by calling tenders and to meet the requirements and satisfy the needs during period of replenishment
7. To keep materials in reserve stock to avoid lack of availability of materials
8. To balance fluctuations in consumption of materials
9. To provide satisfactory services to patients.

The nurse administrator must identify the needs and specific items required for nursing service department, She should study the consumption rate in the past present and think for the future demands of materials for her unit. She needs to know the items which are scares in supply and calculate the materials required in quality and quantity. At the same time she must understand that availability of budget for the purpose before procuring materials for her unit.

PROCUREMENT

Procurement and purchasing refers to the intending of materials to meet the hospital needs of any health care facility: The major aim of purchasing and procurement is to acquire the materials at the lowest cost, with desired quality on time when they are needed. The administrator needs to ensure storage facilities, material handling requirements, flow of materials to various departments, inventory management and transportation of materials to the site with minimum cost prior to procure the materials. Thus, the major aims of procuring system is to get needed materials and supplies in minimum cost with desirable quality and quantity, within the specified time frame, and to distribute to the needed departments promptly and enhancing inventory management in a best possible manner.

Procurement Cycle

This cycle involves the following steps:

Identification of Need

The first step involved in procurement cycle is identifying the need for the materials to be procured. The nurse administrator to ensure whether the material is new or to be reordered for the department. She must also make sure that whether she will procure it from internal or external source.

Determining the Specific Need (Quality)

For ensuring the right material needed she may refer current catalogue or material standard hand book or past ordered requisition letter of the department for deciding the right material with specification for example Stainless steel Bowl with lid having 4 inches diameter. When buying items the administrator to see that it is of latest technology ,availability of maintenance and repair facility, with minimum time, postwarranty repair at reasonable cost, it is possible to upgrade them, should be from reputed manufacturer, with low operating costs and availability of installation guidelines

Determine Specific Quantity

This is calculated by developing of standards for a hospital/ward. Make specification of each item needs to be purchased.

Identify Suppliers

The administrator needs to decide from where the materials to be purchased. In government set up there is an approved agency to supply materials. The administrator has to purchase from those gazette notified agencies. In private sector there is no such rule. They will need to search for a supplier using purchase orders from other sources. Purchase can be done by, open tender, restricted or limited tender, negotiated procurement, direct procurement, spot purchase or purchase from many suppliers or few suppliers.

Ensure Financial Feasibility

The administrator has to search for the best product from the budget allotted from 3-4 suppliers before finalizing purchase.

Specify Contract Terms and Condition

The administrator negotiates with the supplier with purchase order that defines the item, specifications and terms and conditions of the product and the price. The following factors to be considered while making purchase order such as proper specification, invite quotations from reputed firms, comparison of offers based on basic price, freight and insurance, taxes, etc.,quantity and payment discounts payment term delivery period, and guarantee of the materials

Delivery of the Purchase Order

The administrator sends the purchase order by fax, mail, personally, or email and the receipt of the purchase order is acknowledged. Both supplier and the buyer parties keep a copy of the order on file.

Expediting

This step is referring to time frame for getting the materials. It is very important to avoid delay in delivery, payment dates and work completion of the product.

Receipt and Verification of the Items Purchased

As soon as the materials are delivered the administrator verifies each item for its quality and specification the cost is verified from the bills given. Accordingly the materials are accepted or rejected.

Invoice Approval and Payment

The administrator verifies and approves the very important three documents such as an invoice requests payment - the invoice itself, the receiving document and the original purchase order. Any discrepancies observed among three documents must be resolved before the payment of the bill. The administrator pays the bill in the form of cash, cheque, or any mode of money transaction as per policy decision of the hospital.

Record Maintenance

In order to conduct audit the administrator must present complete records. These include purchase vouchers, stock book, receipts invoice records to verify any tax information and purchase orders are required to confirm warranty information.

Storage

The following points to be kept in mind while storing the materials

- Ensure that a large store with adequate space is required to store all the purchased materials
- In order to furnish easy access the materials to be stored in pertinent place with correct order
- Most hospitals have a practice of storing materials group wise and alphabetical order for easy identification and replenishment
- As the material comes start storing and distributing based on First-in, first-out principle
- Monitor expiry date to avoid waste as well to avoid distribution of expiry date materials
- Follow two bin or double shelf system, to avoid stock outs
- Reserve bin should contain stock that will cover lead time and a small safety stock.

INVENTORY CONTROL

Inventory means a stock of goods. It is an ideal resource of any type of material having an economic value. Inventory control refers to the detailed list of articles stocking in adequate number, so that the materials are available whenever and whatever required by the unit. Scientific inventory control has the advantage of ensuring optimal balance between demand and supply. The main objectives of maintaining inventory are:

- To ensure maximum supply of materials, with maximum efficiency and optimum investment.
- To provide a balance between forecasted cost and actual demand for a material

The administration practices certain techniques and concepts to ensure the control of inventories. They are described as follows:

ABC Analysis (Always Better Control)

This concept is based on the criteria of cost of materials. This concept ensures a selective control when an establishment is in demand of large number of items .It justifies the number of orders, number of items and reduction of the inventory. In the principle of ABC analysis, a large amount of purchase of materials are bought in smaller percentage of cost and small amount of materials are purchased in large percentage of cost.

In ABC analysis, the administrator requires to list all the items in the store in quantity with the current amount

Table 18.1: ABC analysis of materials

S. No.	Item category	% of items	Cost in %
A	Category 1	10	70
B	Category 2	20	20
C	Category 3	70	10

Category 1: Needs close monitoring and control
Category 2: Needs moderate control category
Category 3: No need for strict control category

of consumption cost annually in rupees of each item. Then items are arranged cost wise in descending order. The highest cost will be entered in higher position and the lower cost will be put down in lower position. After rearranging the items they are categorized as A, B, and C.

- The B category of 20% materials consume 20% of budget resource
- The C category of 70% of materials consume 10% of budget resource
- The A category of 10% of materials consume 70% of budget resources (Table 18.1).

Therefore, the administrator must have in A items tight control on meticulous estimate of requirements, close monitoring, and storage is necessary and are managed by top level administration.

B items are intermediate in number must have: moderate control, purchase to be made based on rigid requirements, need close supervision and monitoring and are managed by middle level management like head nurses and unit managers.

C items are larger in number, but consume lesser amount of resources. These must have: ordinary control measures, purchase based on usage estimates always must be available in stock. They are vital for patient care ABC analysis does not stress on items those are less costly but may be vital.

VED (Vital, Essentials, Desirable) Analysis

The concept is based on critical value and shortage cost of an item It is a subjective analysis where the administrator in a hospital can decide from the record which items are vital, essential and desirable In this concept items are classified into vital (V), essential (E) and desirable (D).

Vital items are few in number and their shortage cannot be tolerated They consume large budget.

Essential items are moderate in number and shortage can be accepted for a short period of time.

Desirable items are larger in number and their shortage will not negatively affect the patient care however, they may consume more items. Therefore these must be strictly analyzed before purchase.

SDE Analysis (Scarce, Difficult, Easily Available)

The concept in SDE analysis is based on availability of the items. Those items which are **scarce** come in less number and consume more cost and these are managed by top level management. They maintain big safety stocks. **Difficult items** are moderately available, consumes moderate cost and monitored by middle level managers. **Easily available items** are in demand of larger number and consume less cost. Minimum safety stocks are maintained.

FSN Analysis (Fast Moving, Slow Moving, and Nonmoving)

The concept of FSN analysis is based on utilization of items for patient care. **Fast moving** items are consumed faster for care required large budget. Some items are slow **moving.** Which are moderately consumed whereas, **nonmoving,** are not used faster and they must be monitored for expiry date, obsolescence time to time.

HML Analysis (Highest, Medium, Low)

Based on the individual unit cost HML analysis is conceived. The cost per unit is calculated as highest, medium and low cost per unit and in HML system with the objective of controlling over consumption at unit or ward or departmental level for determining the frequency of physical verification.

CONDEMNATION AND DISPOSAL

Condemnation and disposal of items is one of the important functions of material management in any organization. Due to the continuous use of materials and other items become surplus, obsolete, in-serviceable, no longer required and become hazardous Condemnation of this type of materials need to be done periodically. Some hospitals there is a practice of doing it annually before the new stock arrives

Procedure of Condemnation and Disposal of Materials

- The administrator identifies the type of condemnation articles
- Categorize the such as surplus items, obsolete items, in serviceable items, hazardous items, etc.
    - Surplus items: These are items that are in working order but are not required for use in a particular setting. These are items lying in stores for more than five years and considered as surplus.
    - Obsolete items: These are items in working order but cannot be put into use effectively being outdated due to change in health care technology or procedure.

- In-serviceable items: These are items which are not in working order, had utilized for long period and are beyond economic repair.
- Scrap: Process waste, broken and any other item not covered above but has got resale value.
- Empties: These are items like empty containers, bottles, plastic jars, drums, etc.
- Hazardous items: These are items which are serviceable but hazardous to use for patients.

- Communicating to hospital standing disposal committee.
- Determination of date and timing for condemnation
- Circular sent to all nursing and other department units to display the articles for condemnation
- Inspection by the hospital standing Disposal committee
- Determination of mode of disposal of condemned articles
  - If there is surplus articles can be gifted to community health centers or could be sold
  - These article could be transferred similar institution.
  - Public auction.
- Fixation of reserve price and approval by the hospital authority
- Verify stock book. History sheet of equipment. Log book of maintenance and repairs.
- Enter in stock book the condemned item
- Bring the balance in stock and signature to be placed by the in charge of the stock and the authority who did the condemnation and disposal.

Maintenance of Hospital Materials Records

The following information to be completed while purchase and maintaining records of materials.

- Name of the equipment, specifications
- Code number
- Date of purchase
- Name of supplier and name of manufacturer
- Date and place of installation of equipment, date of commissioning
- Supply of spare parts, literature, technical manual cost
- The guarantee card, and warranty card
  - Life of equipment in years
  - Unserviceable date
  - Date of condemnation
  - Date of replacement
  - Balance stock in hand
  - Signature of the concerned officer with date.

Preventive Maintenance of Hospital Equipment

Preventive maintenance ensures efficiency, economy and effectiveness.

- All items purchased should be with warranty and spare parts.
- Protect all the electronic equipments as per guidelines given in the manual (Voltage stabilizer, UPS, automatic switch over generator, ventilator, incubator)
- Requirement of electricity, water, space, atmospheric conditions, etc. Must be taken into consideration while stocking the equipment
- There should be a technical person to be responsible for monitoring the maintenance in 24 × 7 days
- Monitoring annual maintenance contracts. (AMC) and renewal of AMC accordingly communicate the same to the supplier timely
- There should be a work shop in the hospital for repair and exchange of materials
- Follow-up of maintenance and repair services could be done from outside agency if the hospital has no facility.

PLANNING EQUIPMENTS AND SUPPLIES FOR NURSING CARE: UNIT AND HOSPITAL

One of the functions of administration is planning and establishing material for patient care. Hospital materials includes equipment and supplies. Equipments are items which are permanent in nature and are classified as fixed and movable. Fixed equipments are attached to the walls or floor of the hospitals like fans, sterilizers' cupboards, etc. which has a life of more than five years. Movable equipments are furniture instruments, etc. Supplies are consumable items like stationeries, drugs, chemicals, antiseptics food materials, etc.

When we aim to purchase supplies and equipment for hospital, we must know that they are available from general store, pharmacy store and dietary department. The central sterile supplies department supplies linen and instruments for patient care. The budget planning is important for getting these materials. The budget should include the actual cost of the materials, transport charges to bring from the source to the hospital, incidental charges, the cost for accessory materials along with the equipment (For example: scan machine include the graph paper, lubricant materials) cost for technical assistance, servicing charges as per policy, (usually 10%), etc.

When we purchase equipment for hospital we need to see that the equipment are according to the standards. In India in order to meet the standards of the materials for the hospitals, the Government has set up. Indian Standards Institution (ISI) as the national agency monitor the standards. The articles are certified as ISI mark. The ISI certification ensures safety to the patient and the health care providers, hazardous and faulty equipment can harm to patients.

Factors to be Kept in Mind While Purchasing Articles to a Hospital

- The equipment should be safe to use by patients and handling by health care providers
- It should be certified by ISI standard
- It should be long lasting durable in nature
- Specifications should be according to the type of services rendered
- Very often, spare parts will be available of the material that should be collected from the purchase agency
- All surgical instruments used in a hospital should be sterilizable and they should stand the tests for leakage, hydraulic pressure tests for bursting and thermal capacity, etc.
- Accurate in measurement
- Simple to operate.

The Central Sterile Supply Service

According to current trends most hospitals possesses a central sterile, supply department (CSSD) where equipments and supplies are sterilized, stored and distributed to the service units. They are linen, diagnostic procedure trays with sterile. Instruments, sterile syringes, etc. According to the needs of the ward unit, linen and other items are distributed and the same amount of materials used from the wards are collected, cleaned, laundried and sterilized for next use as exchange basis.

General Utility Services in the Hospital

- Electric supply and installations
- Water supply
- Disposal of waste—liquids and solids.
- Refrigeration, air conditioning, ventilation and environment control.
- Transport
- Supply of medical gases, compressed air, hot water, vacuum suction and gas plants
  - Uninterrupted supply of safe water
  - Fire extinguishers and training for fire extinguishing to prevent hazards
  - Maintenance of services without disrupting hospital services.
- Hospital laundry
- Fire extinguish unit
- Telephone booth
- There should be a workshop to ensure repair and maintenance of equipments used in the hospital.

ESSENTIAL EQUIPMENTS FOR A FIFTY BEDDED DISTRICT HOSPITAL (WHO)

Scope of Services

Safety of equipment for anesthesia

Safety of equipment for radiology department, pathology, clinical laboratory, rehabilitation unit and physiotherapy. to be ensured

Essential Medical Equipment

Diagnostic imaging equipment include X-ray and ultrasound equipment. X-ray

Electrical Medical Equipment

Portable electrocardiograph, Defibrillator (external), Portable anesthetic unit—two small aesthetic units, respirator.

Dental chair unit: Delivery table—it should be standard and manually operated. Diathermy unit.

Other Equipment

Autoclave—for general sterilization and small sterilizers. Small, inexpensive equipment and instruments, such as BP apparatus, oxygen manifolds, stethoscope, diagnostic sets and spotlights.

Responsibilities of Head Nurse in Maintaining Equipment and Supplies

- The head nurse should ensure adequate equipment and supplies for patient care in her unit.
- All equipment and supplies should be available in quality and quantity, accessible and conveniently located.
- According to the type of patients, age of the patients, and the type of service unit (maternity/paediatric/medial/surgical unit) and number of patients, she should develop a standard of equipment and supplies for her unit.
- Sometime the item become unserviceable before discarding or purchasing the new one, she must see that whether it can be sent to hospital workshop for repair and get an exchanged one like. Wheel chair, trolley, etc.

- The head nurse must maintain an inventory control of items in her unit. Inventory is a detailed list of articles with their specification and number. Currently used in the ward.
- She should plan and help in condemnation and disposal of items time to time with the concerned authorities
- Maintains stock book updated
- Monitors the various articles used in the wards for their effective use
- Verifies the ward stock periodically
- Delegates the responsibility of inventory to one of the senior nurses
- Educates nurses regarding importance of keeping equipment and supplies for safe patients care and their economic utility
- For safe patients care and their economic utility ensures that each staff nurse aware of cost of each item used in the ward
- Maintains policy for loss, theft, pilferage of the materials
- Practices preventive maintenance of equipment used in the ward.

One of the criteria of maintaining standards of the hospital is material management. Hospital administrators and nurses should aware of the materials used in the hospital. Good material management ensures quality patient care and brings efficiency, economy and effectiveness in hospital administration

The quality of health care services are based on materials used in quality and quantity for patient care. As hospital administrators nurses should also know about the terminology of materials used in the hospital, their classification, category such as perfusion materials, surgical disposables, instruments, electrical, civil and engineering items for maintenance, housekeeping materials, linen, biomedical equipment drugs, food items, etc. pay an effective role in improving the quality of health care services.

SUMMARY POINTS

✓ Material management is an administrative function. It includes material planning and control, production planning, purchasing, inventory control, flow of materials o various departments, and waste management.

✓ Materials include equipment and supplies.Equipments is permanent items classified as fixed and movable items. Fixed items are permanently fixed on walls and floor whereas movable items are equipment can be moved from one place to another like furniture.

✓ Supplies are consumable items like stationeries, food items medicine, chemicals and antiseptics.

✓ Material management is a process of planning, organizing, and controlling all those activities concerned with the flow of materials into an organization to minimize the costs like inventory, purchasing, material handling and distribution costs.

✓ Material planning is the scientific way of determining the requirements that goes into meeting production needs within the economic investment policies, It is done at all stages and all levels of management. Material planning is based on certain feedback information and reviews.

✓ Procurement and purchasing refers to the acquisition of materials to be Utilized in hospital or in any organization. The first and foremost function of purchasing and procurement is to get the materials at the lowest cost possible, with desired quality on time when they are needed.

✓ Inventory control refers to stocking adequate number and kind of stores, so that the materials are available whenever required and wherever required. Scientific inventory control results in optimal balance between demand and supply.

✓ Condemnation and disposal of items is one of the important functions of materials management in any organization. Due to the continuous use of materials and other items become surplus, obsolete, unserviceable, no longer required and become hazardous.

✓ Preventive maintenance ensures efficiency, economy and effectiveness in material management.

✓ The head nurse has a responsibility in material management for her unit. Setting standard, requisition, exchange, inventory control and condemnation and disposal are important function in material management.

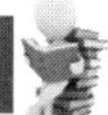

REVIEW QUESTIONS

1. Define material management. Describe the aims and objectives of material management.
2. Describe procurement cycle.
3. What is inventory control? Describe various techniques used in inventory control.
4. Describe the process of condemnation and disposal in a hospital.
5. What is the responsibility of a hospital administrator in planning and maintaining material management in a hospital setting?
6. Write short notes on:
   a. Benefits of material management
   b. Purposes of material planning
   c. Preventive maintenance in material management
   d. ABC and VED analysis
   e. Role of ward sister in material management
   f. Procurement of material.

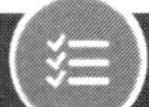

SELECTED READINGS

1. Barriet J .Ward management and Teaching. 2nd ed. Delhi: EBS Publishers; 1967.
2. District hospitals- Guidelines for development. WHO. Geneva: HTBS publishers; 1994.
3. Gopalakrishnan, Sunderasan: Material Management, Prentice Hall of India Pvt Ltd. New Delhi, 1979.
4. Gupta S, Kanth S. Hospital stores management, an integrated approach. (First edn). New Delhi: Jaypee brothers; 2004.
5. Hospital Departments – SFH www.sfh.med.sa/.../Pages/HospitalDepartments.aspx
6. Hospital emergency response checklist ...www.euro.who.int/__data/assets/pdf_file/0020/148214/e...
7. Jha SM. Hospital Management. Ist ed. Mumbai: Himalaya publishers; 2007.
8. Koontz H, Weihrich H . Essentials of management an international perspective. (Ist edn). New Delhi: Tata Mc Graw Hill publishers; 2007.
9. Koontz H, Weihrich H. Management a global perspective. 1st edn. New Delhi: Tata Mc. Graw Hill publishers; 2001.
10. Kulkarni G R. Managerial accounting for hospitals. Mumbai: Ridhiraj enterprise; 2003.
11. Kumar R, Goel SL. Hospital administration and management. Vol 1 (first edn). New Delhi: Deep and deep publications;
12. Nursing Management: ABC, VED, HML analysis currentnursing.com/nursing management/planning...
13. Wise P S. Leading and managing in nursing. Ist edn. Philadelphia: Mosby publicatons; 1995.

UNIT IX
FINANCIAL ADMINISTRATION

19. Budget

19

Budget

LEARNING OBJECTIVES

This chapter imparts learning about:

- Budget: Definition, Concept, Philosophy of Budgeting
- Types of Budgeting, Plan and Non-plan, Zero Budgeting, Mid-term Appraisal, Capital and Revenue
- Budget Estimate, Revised Estimate, Performance Budget
- Audit
- Terms used
  - Cost Effectiveness
  - Cost Accounting
  - Critical Pathways
  - Health Care Reforms
  - Health Economics
  - Health Insurance
- Budgeting for Various Units and Levels–Issues and Challenges, Role of Nurse Administrator in Budgeting

INTRODUCTION

In the past, nursing service administration played a limited role in financial planning and management. Nurse administrators were given budgets without justification and were allowed very limited input. Because nursing was considered non-income-producing service, nursing input was under estimated and unrecognized. During the last three decades, health care organization have realized the importance of nursing input in financial planning and all middle level managers are also expected to be knowledgeable of budget preparation today.

Financial management includes a sequential steps of activities developed to allocate resources and plan for the efficient and effective functioning of an establishment. The major aim of financial administration is to meet the total financial needs of an establishment. Hence, all the establishments require to operate financial resources efficiently.

Main characteristics of financial administration in nursing are:

- Financial administration is one of the non-clinical managerial task for nursing service administration
- The focus of financial administration is the allocation of scarce resources to bring maximum outcome.
- Financial administration aims to facilitate the efficient operation of nursing service department in an organization. Strategic planning in nursing influences financial outcome
- Nurses at all levels have a definite role in participating in financial administration
- Financial administration decisions may create legal and ethical dilemmas for nurses.

BUDGET: DEFINITION, CONCEPT, PHILOSOPHY OF BUDGETING

Budget

Meaning

Budget is derived from French word *Bugette* means a small leather bag that contains papers of plans estimate revenue, services, costs and expenses involved for a period of time. This leather bag or wallet is carried by the Chancellor or Exchequer in England to the house of commons. He would open it to place the papers containing financial plan before the house. So from that association the budget came to mean those papers which containing financial proposals for the year. Thus, the budget word is from British origin.

Concept

The budget in simple words refers to financial statement or the documents which contains estimates of the revenue and expenditure for a year. Budget is essentially the development of a plan for a given period in the future for specific numerical term. As such, budget is a statement of anticipated results. They are stated in financial terms as is the case with the expense, revenue or capital budget or they may be stated in non-financial terms as for human resources equipment and supplies or time.

The budget is a financial expression and simultaneously the means of implementing the functions of the department. The budget should be a dynamic plan of action reflecting the type, quality and quantity of the nursing service department as they are at present and as they are proposed for the future. It is the most important tool for management that connect future to past and present.

Definition

A budget is a written document that formulates plans for both income and expenditure. Income is needed to spend on an organizational activities and plans required to generate money to get the activities done. It is an estimate, about what an individual or organization will need in money terms to do the work (www.civicus.org). Budgeting is the allocation of scarce resources for the proposed activities of an organization based on the forecasted needs over a period of time. —**DN Gillies**

A budget is a written plan that utilizes numerical data to predict the functions of an establishment over a period of time and it provides a means for planning, control and enhances each unit needs and contribution for achieving the goals.

According to Gabriel son and Lund (1985), Nursing budget constitute one-third of total operating costs of most establishments. It is because of increasing health care cost and pressure to provide more skilled and comprehensive nursing care at low cost.

Thus, a budget is structured and a systematic plan of income and expenditure, that estimates the future needs of an organization arranged in an orderly manner. It is also planned in detail for a specific period of time. Before implementing the budget, a financial statement in quantitative form is prepared by the administrator. Being budget is a tool to control activities, the outcome achieved is measured by a standard criteria.

Purposes of Budget

- Translates financial objectives into projected expenditure
- Enhances financial planning and decision-making
- Clearly identifies controllable and uncontrollable cost areas
- Communicates financial objectives
- Allows feedback
- Measures and records financial success in relation to goals and objectives.

Budget Plan

According to the duration, budget plan can be divided into:

1. Short range budget is planned month-to-month for 12 months
2. Long range plan which is planned for a period of 3–5 years.

Factors Influencing Budget Planning

The following factors influence budget planning:

- Economic environment
- Client and providers
- Human resources (HR)
- Organization (type and complexity)
- Service costs/market price
- Organizational goals and strategic decision
- Plans and objectives of departments.

Philosophy of Nursing Service Budget

The nurse administrator is responsible to make budget for nursing service department. Since every departments of the hospital has a fair share of budget, it helps all round development of the hospital. The following are the sample philosophy of budget pertaining to nursing services.

PHILOSOPHY 1

We, the nursing service department believe that in order to provide quality nursing services to the patients and families, nurses working in all level should know budget planning and able to propose budget for their units.

Objectives

- To help nurses to develop skill in preparation and execution of budget
- To help them to establish priorities of activities.

PHILOSOPHY 2

We, the members of nursing service department recognize that staff development program is essential to enhance the quality of nursing services.

Objectives

To help, nurses to go for higher education or to provide for attending continuing education program sponsored by the institution financial assistance should be given from the budget allocated for nursing services.

PHILOSOPHY 3

We as members of the nursing service department accept the fact that a good work setting, service conditions and benefits enhances job satisfaction and improved performance that in turn will bring quality patient care outcome.

Objectives

- To provide adequate budget to improve working conditions by facilitating equipment and supplies needed for care
- To enhance service conditions of nurses by ensuring adequate salary benefits and other emoluments.

TYPES OF BUDGETING

Static Budgeting

This is also called **fixed type of budgeting.** This budget format is typically based on a single expected outcome, which can be extremely difficult to achieve. It does not fluctuate with volume of work or increase of staff members.

Zero-Based Budgeting

A zero-based budgeting is the fundamental technique of finance and accounting. In this method, all expenses are justified for each new year period of budget cycle. It starts from zero-based with scratch with no preauthorized funds. In this method, each function and its needs are analyzed and the cost is calculated in relation to the performance to be achieved. Then budget is prepared for the next year whether the budget amount is higher or lower than the previous year. The costs are grouped and measured against previous results and future expectations. This method ensures a systematic basis for resource allocation.

Flexible Budgeting

Flexible means able to adjust according to the changing situation. Flexible budget is that type of a budget which adjust for change in the volume of activities of an organization. It is more advantageous than fixed budget. It gives a set of income and expenditure projection at various volume of activities. The cost for expenses are able to vary as activities vary. It is based on actual output level during the budget period than is based on estimated output level like static budget. Flexible budget is difficult to prepare.

Incremental Budgeting

It is based on slight change made from the last year's budget outcome with an incremental amount which is added to the new budget period. This method is used by managers who are not interested to spend time in formulating budget or re evaluation of outcome. It is very simple and stable budget which can be prepared by managers of all levels. The allocation of resources is made is based on previous period. The impact of change is seen this type of budget

Rolling Budgeting

It is also called as **continuous budgeting**. It is an incremental extension of existing budget period. Since some of the activities are repeated every month, the manager needs to create budget on rolling basis. It provides constantly review of the budget and thus the organization have always budget for a specified future period in hands. This method provides budget for every three months to every 5 year period.

Performance Budgeting

It is a budget that gives the input of resources and the output of services for each unit of an organization. This type of budget is commonly used by the government organization to relate between the budget provided to the public sector and the outcome of these services. It focuses on outcomes of services than on decisions which made based on inputs. In this type of budget, allocation of funds and resources are based on their potential outcomes. Performance budgets place priority on employees' commitment to produce positive results, particularly in the public sector.

Mid-term Appraisal of the Performance

Mid-term appraisal refers to the performance assessment and feedback procedure which takes place at the end of the second quarter to know the employee is performing his/her tasks as per the planned performance standard of the organization. This is an important midway activity which can provide the adequate time to employee a chance for correction of his tasks to achieve the target.

Since a year is too long gap between appraisals. midterm appraisals can help in preventing that gap and provides an interim assessment. Accordingly, the employee is given corrective measures to improve in his job and need not to wait till annual appraisal.

Master Budget

A master budget is an overall financial and operating plan for a forthcoming calendar or fiscal year. It is usually prepared annually or quarterly. The master budget is really a number of sub budgets tied together to summarize the planned activities of the business. The format of the master budget depends on the size and nature of business. The annual financial estimates of a budget is the statement of receipts and expenditure of an institution.

Personnel Budget

Personnel budget estimates the cost of direct labor necessary to meet agency's objectives. such as cost for, recruitment, hiring, assignment, layoff and discharge of personnel training, salary, etc. According to Finkler (2001) Swans Burg and Swans Burg (1999), the following factors to be considered while planning for personnel budget:

- Decide type of services required
- Current staffing pattern
- Patient occupancy and general complexity of patients
- Seasonal fluctuations in admissions
- Personnel policies in terms of job benefits
- Status of turnover of nurses
- Recruitment and orientation costs.

The Operating Budget

According to Finkler (2001), operating budget is a plan to monitor anticipated day-to-day activities, resources, personnel, and supplies, typically over a one year period.

Steps in Preparing Operating Budget

- Collect past data
- Examine previous year objectives—achieved or exceeded
- Set objectives for forecast year
- State objectives in terms of production/service/ activities
- Consider salary and wage adjustments
- Prepare report of expense, e.g. tax, supplies.
- Prepare budget report. This include budget summary, budget statement and supporting schedules, and budget information—activities.
- Review of budget by administrator
- Evaluation of budget
- Modifications by finance committee
- Final approval by the board.

Capital Budget

A capital budget outlines the forecasted buying of large fixed assets ensuring necessary facilities for carrying out organizational activities. It includes the major equipment construction of new building, etc. Capital budget is an important component of plan to meet the organization's long-term goals.

The administration uses capital budgeting, i.e. a process of evaluating and ranking actual and potential expenditures or investments that are larger in amount. The large expenditures could include the purchase of new equipment, rebuilding existing equipment, purchasing delivery vehicles, constructing additions to buildings, etc. The large amounts spent for these types of projects are known as **capital expenditures.**

Revenue Budget

Revenue refers to income from sales of materials or services rendered to customers. These are business activities. In other words, the amount of money actually receives during a specific period of the year includes discount and deduction for return merchandise. When expenditure is deducted from the revenue we get net income or profit. Revenue budgets help the establishment to save time and effort by the proper allocation of resources for organizational activities.

Expenditure Budget

Expenditure means expending or spending out. It include paying out cash or credit for exchange of goods or services.

BUDGET ESTIMATE, REVISED ESTIMATE

A budget is a written plan for the allocation of resources that utilizes numerical data to predict the activities of an organization over a period of time and it ensures des a mechanism for planning, control and promote each unit needs and contribution.

Prerequisites of Budgeting

- An establishment must have a sound organizational structure with clear lines of authority and responsibility.
- Ensure that, all employees know their responsibilities, the person to whom they are responsible, the authority they have, what they are responsible for and are held accountable for their action. The establishment must have organization charts and all employees are given a clear, well-defined job descriptions.
- The establishment must have non-monetary statistical data, such as number of admissions, average length of stay of patients, percentage of bed occupancy and number of days the patients stayed are used for planning.
- A blue print of accounts are prepared that is consistent with the organizational plan. Revenues and expenses are reported by responsibility areas, which supplies previous years data that are significant for planning and provide budgetary control for evaluations because performance can be compared with plan.
- In every budgetary program, managerial support is very essential. Although, budgeting is done at the departmental level, it must be monitored and supervised by top level administration.
- The budget manual should be available at hand that include formal budgeting policies and procedures, the objectives of the budgetary program are defined, authority and responsibility for budgeting are clarified, and instruction for budget development are discussed in detail. The manual should include samples of standardized forms, a calendar of the budgeting activities with the schedule for each stage of the program and a procedure for review, revision and approval of budgets.
- The **budget calendar** should clearly states in three stages.
  - *Formation stage:* It includes developing objectives for management plan, gather pertinent financial, historical and statistical data and analysis of data.
  - *Review and enactment stage*: It include preparation of unit budgets, presentation of unit budget for approval, revise and combine into organizational budget and presentation to budget council of the organization.
  - *Execution stage:* It include direction and evaluation of expenses and receipts, and revision of budget as indicated.

STEPS IN BUDGETING

There are four steps in budget planning:

1. ***Assessment:*** It is the first step to assess what needs to be included in the budget. Unit managers develop goals, objectives and budgetary estimate with input from colleagues and subordinates. A composition of unit needs in terms of manpower, equipment and operating expenses can then be compiled to determine the organizational budget.
2. ***Planning:*** The second step is to develop a plan. A budgeting cycle that is set for 12 months is called a fiscal year budget (from April to March).This is then usually broken down into quarters or subdivided into monthly, quarterly, or semiannual period. A perpetual budget may be done on a continual basis each month so that 12 months of future budget data are always available.
3. ***Implementation:*** In this step, ongoing monitoring and analysis occur to avoid inadequate or excess fund at the end of the fiscal year. In most health care institutions, monthly computerized statements outline the each department's projected budget and any deviations from that budget. Each unit manager is accountable for budget deviations in his or her unit. Most units can expect some change from the anticipated budget, but large deviations must be examined for possible cause, and remedial action must be taken.
4. ***Evaluation:*** The budget must be reviewed periodically and modified as needed throughout the fiscal year. With each successive year of budgeting, managers can more accurately predict each unit's budgetary requirements.

The annual financial estimates of a budget is the statement of receipts and expenditure of an institution.

PREPARATION OF INDEPENDENT BUDGET

The estimates are divided into three parts:

- **Receipts**—deals with the receipts from the institution
- **Nonplan**—expenditure (operating budget) deals with expenditure connected with the normal functions of the institution. The major chunk of the non-plan expenditure is set apart for the payment of salary and other allowances of the staff, supplies, repair and maintenance, etc.
- **Plan expenditure (capital budget):** It deals with expenditure of the developmental activities of the institution. Capital expenditures include purchase of land or building or major equipment that has a

long life. Capital budgets are composed of long-term planning which has a major acquisition component and a short-term budgeting component.

The long-term major acquisitions budgeting component outlines future replacement. It also refers to organizational expansion that may to exceed to one year. The short-term component of the capital budget nclude purchase of equipment within the annual budget cycle.

Budget Cycle

A budget cycle describes the activities time frame that a budget covers. This is used in establishments who prepare monthly, quarterly and/or annual budget cycles to control costs and bring regularity in administrative duties. Understanding the purpose of a budget cycle and the types used will help the nurses to decide how to implement one or more in hospital administration and departmental units budget.

Purposes

Purposes of budget cycles include:

- It helps in control costs
- It makes it simpler for a finance department to prepare reports
- It allows management to respond to performance problems.

For example, if we know that how much money we can spend on stationary in a three months, we can plan how much stationeries to be supplied to each ward based on the availability. Then, the administrator can evaluate at the end of three months whether she needs to raise the supply of stationary to the departments. If it is to be raised, the budget proposal also should be increased to the departments. In terms of stationeries' variance analysis will be helpful to compare the expenditure in each three months. It gives the nurse administrator more information before she makes a financial decision and help her to supply the stationeries according to variation compared to projections.

Budget Cycles versus Periods

A budget cycle includes the time during which budgets are planned, discussed, approved and analyzed for a year whereas budget period covers the dates from it is allocated to the end in which the date ends. Thus, a quarterly budget cycle covers a three-month budget period, will start before those three months and end afterward.

Monthly Budget Cycle

When the budget period starts on the first day of the month and ends on the last day of the month is called **monthly budget cycle**. The daily average total expenditure vary from months to months according to the changing number of days in a month. This type of budget is used at the departmental level with regards to few items not for all items used in the department.

Quarterly Budget Cycles

A quarterly budget cycle covers the plan of budget for three months. Usually from January to March month, April to June, July to September and October to December. Most organization functions on quarterly budget. Because of the amount of work is more in monthly budget cycle than in quarterly budget cycle with regards to preparing, monitoring, analyzing and reporting for that period. It is helpful when there is seasonal variation in expenditure.

Annual Budget Cycles

It helps to monitor the financial year data of income and expenditure and the establishment's profits based on projections at the beginning of the cycle and actual performance at the end of the cycle. Most establishments utilize an annual budget cycle to assess the overall performance of the organization. Annual budget periods usually calculated from April 1st to March 31st or according to the policy of the establishment.

Lapsed budget

Both government and private sector organization use lapsing budgets. It refers to a department or organization that must return any unspent budget funds to the authority (Usually the state's Treasury in Government sector) that issued them at the end of the budget period. Lapsed budget indicates the incapability of the administrator who could not utilize the sanctioned budget for the department.

States government-funded hospitals often use budget lapsing because as per government policies require them to return their unspent government allowance at the end of the budget year (Usually on or before March 31st).

Negative Aspects of Lapsed Budget

Some of the administrators use the lapse budget for other items than on allowed for prescribed head. For example, if the fund is allotted to linen for the patient (Under Linen Head), it cannot be used for heads like furniture or equipment. An organization or department facing the loss of unspent budget funds at the end of the year often results in wasteful spending, stockpiling or spending the funds for another department or program like mentioned above. But it does not show any relationship with original purpose for which it was sanctioned for. They use lapsed budget because of the fear that next year they may be sanctioned with less amount of budget.

Positive Aspects of Lapsed Budget

A lapsing budget can have some benefit. It ensure the administrators on planning long-term programs, rather than shortchanging those programs to fulfill more urgent needs. It also prevents managers from building up a cash pile to spend when their term of office is about to end.

REVISED BUDGETS

Sometimes the budget year finds unanticipated needs that may influence the central government budget. In such situation, when an agency requires more funding, the Government can revise the central government budget by an increased budget proposal. This is referred as a revised budget and these revised budget proposals are submitted by the Government in April and September. It may be revised and sanctioned or it may borrow from next year's sanction of budget. This is practiced in government agencies. Revised budgets usually mean that some appropriations are increased and others are reduced by a corresponding amount.

Government agencies are obliged to monitor carefully the ongoing budget year and notify the Government in advance its utility if a budget appropriation looks exceeded then the Government on quarterly basis decides the measures to handle such situations.

The Government normally submits revised budget proposals in April and September of a year.

PLAN AND NON-PLAN EXPENDITURE (INDIA)

Plan and non-plan are two components of expenditure. In the year 1951, India has envisioned and established Five Year Plans aimed to rapid economic development. Eleven Five Year Plans have been implemented so far and at present the Twelfth Five Year Plan (2012–2017) is running. Reference to the Five Year Plans the Government of India. classified in budget as plan and non-plan expenditure.

Plan Expenditure

Plan expenditure refers to the expenditure that is focused for current programs which are presented under the current (Five Year) plan of the center and is referred as the expenditure estimated for different sectors of economy. It includes both income and expenditure. Plan expenditure is further sub-classified into Revenue Expenditure and Capital Expenditure. In plan of expenditure, assistance is given by the Central Government for the plans of States and Union Territories (UTs), e.g.:

- Expenditure on electricity generation
- Irrigation and rural developments
- Construction of roads, bridges, canals
- Science, technology, environment, etc.

Non-plan Expenditure

Non-plan expenditure is all expenditure other than plan expenditure of the government. For example;

- Protecting the lives and properties of the people
- Protecting the country from foreign invasions. (police, judiciary, military), etc.
- Expenditure on normal running of government departments and on providing economic and social services
- Non-plan revenue expenditure is accounted for by interest payments, subsidies mainly on food and fertilizers
- Employees salary, wages and pension,
- Expenses incur on economic services in various sectors
- Expenditure of services such as tax collection, social services, and grants to foreign governments.

AUDIT

The word audit is derived from a Latin word '*audire*' which means to hear:

- ***Auditing*** refers to a thorough and sequential way of examination of books, accounts, documents and vouchers related to money or budget of an establishment to ensure the accuracy of the financial statements presented and are properly maintained according to the legal requirements. As a result of an audit, the management effectively evaluate and improve the effectiveness of risk management, control, and the governance process over the budget of their establishment.
- ***Financial auditing*** refers to an accounting process that comprising of using an individual body (Auditing group/auditors) for assessing the financial transactions and statements of an establishment. The major objective of financial audit is presenting the managerial transactions amount of an establishment accurately and that the accounts presented to the public and shareholders are accurate and justified. The results of financial audit are useful for banks, health care institutions shareholders, and anybody else with an interest in the establishment aid to foreign governments and establishment.

Basic Steps in Auditing Process

Generally, four key phases are outlined for financial audit process. These phases include:

1. Planning the audit
2. Determining the working of internal control
3. Testing significant assertions about the data and evaluating compliance,
4. Reporting the evaluations.

- ***Planning phase*:** The process of financial audit begins with a plan that involves the method of collecting data to form an opinion about the organization's financial status. A way is planned to collect a sample reflecting a point in time in the life of the company or organization. The financial transactions and documents are then looked at. It is noteworthy that the sample should show compliance with audit standards.
- ***Internal control phase:*** The next step involves giving a look at the internal controls. The auditor demands information, looks closely at the records, and watches financial procedures in action. Without these steps, the auditor cannot give a statement about the financial status of the organization.
- ***Testing phase:*** Testing implies checking whether the internal controls are working or not. An auditor requests more information, returns to the company for more inspections, and watches how financial procedures are being performed. If the evidence demonstrates standards compliance, the auditor determines that the company successfully detects and prevents the errors.
- ***Reporting phase:*** The final step in financial audit involves giving a conclusion on how the company adheres to accounting standards. The audit ensures the organization an unqualified approval, a qualified approval, a disclaimer, or an adverse finding. The unqualified approval is considered as the best result and the adverse finding is considered to be the worst result.

The audit cycle is a continuous process. It has five components Fig. 19.1. They are:

1. Setting standards for auditing
2. Measure current practices
3. Compare the results of practice with standards set
4. Reflect, plan, change and implement change
5. Re-audit.

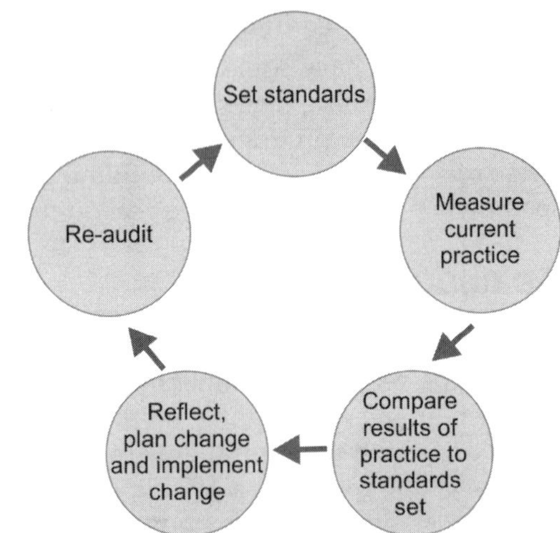

Fig. 19.1: Audit cycle

TERMS USED IN BUDGETING

Cost-effectiveness

According to Business dictionary, cost-effectiveness is referred as the correlation between the financial inputs and the desired outcome, such as the relationship between quality nursing services and increasing patients satisfaction. Today we are experiencing a worldwide crisis in health care delivery system because of economic recession. This compels all health care organizations to re-evaluate the existing health promotion strategies and its relationship to cost-effectiveness. When we want to bring desirable changes for adequate, efficient and cost-effective system, the we need to develop constructive strategies and implement them for desirable change. Health care professionals, including nurses, must change their strategies and vision of education both in classroom and clinical practices. All academic and clinical program must concentrate on health promotion and illness prevention and to strengthen primary health care strategy that in turn may bring cost-effectiveness in health care.

Cost Accounting

Cost accounting is a financial concept. It is referred as the function of collecting, analyzing, summarizing and evaluating various courses of action underwent by the organization in terms of finance. It's aim is to advise the administrators on the most appropriate course of action based on the cost efficiency and capability. It ensures the detailed cost information that the administrator needs to control current practices and accordingly plan for the futuro.

In this method, there is no comparison of information of cost which is required because it is an unique decision made by the individual organization only. However, whatever information regarding the cost to be communicated that should be relevant to the particular setting. The main purpose of cost accounting information is to help the managers to make financial decision.

There is a difference between cost accounting and financial accounting. Cost accounting is a collection of information regarding the cost incur in carrying out an activity or achieving a purpose. After the data is collected, categorized and recorded. Then the data is summarized, and analyzed to determine for a selling price keeping in mind saving of money also. Cost accounting is used as a financial tool for management in budgeting and in setting up the cost control programs, which can improve net margins for the organization in the future whereas financial accounting considers money as a measure of economic performance. Financial accounting represents assets and liabilities of the organization apart from financial performance.

One key difference between cost accounting and financial accounting is that in financial accounting the cost is classified depending on the type of transaction while the cost accounting classifies the costs according to information needs of the management. Cost accounting, is used as an internal tool by management, because it does not have to meet any specific standard.

Types of Cost Accounting

- *Standard cost accounting:* This type of cost accounting uses ratios and variance analysis to compare efficient uses of labor and materials to produce goods or services under standard conditions. Some of the issues associated with cost accounting is that this type of accounting emphasizes labor efficiency despite the fact that it makes up a comparatively small amount of the costs for modern companies.
- *Activity-based cost accounting:* This type of cost accounting based on activity-based costing developed out of a survey to employees who will then account for the amount of time they spend on different tasks. This gives management a better idea of where their time, task and money is being spent.
- *Lean accounting:* This is a Japanese concept. This is a value-based cost accounting in terms of pricing and lean focused performance measurements. It does not believe in traditional mass production. The method brings changes in company's accounting, control, measurements and managerial process. The main strategy is with the assumption that cost increases as a result of labor and overhead cost. It gives better information regarding financial decision-making.
- *Marginal costing:* It is also referred as cost-volume profit analysis It is a simplified model of cost accounting. Marginal costing is described as an analysis of the relationship between a product or service's sales price, the volume of sales, the amount produced, expenses, costs and profits. That specific relationship is called the **Contribution margin**. It is calculated by dividing revenue minus variable cost by revenue. This type of analysis can be used by management to gain an idea on potential profits as influenced by changing costs like fixed costs, variable costs, opening costs and direct costs.

Critical Pathways

Critical pathways, also referred as care pathways, critical pathways, integrated care pathways and care maps in literature. This is one of the main tools used to manage the quality care in health services. It's aim is to standardize the care processes. Various literature supports that implementation of critical pathways reduces the variability in clinical practice and improves patient care outcomes. Clinical pathways promote organized and efficient patient care based on the best practices evidence informed. Use of clinical pathways help to improve the outcomes of patient care admitted in the acute care and home care settings. Clinical pathways refer to medical guidelines. However, a single pathway may refer to guidelines on several conditions and the situations. Critical pathway in budgeting aims to create a schedule that minimizes the total execution time of a work-flow, such that the total execution cost does not exceed the user specified budget. This process has two phases: in the budget distribution phase, it recursively assigns sub-budgets to the tasks on the partial critical paths ending at previously assigned tasks, and in the planning phase it assigns the fastest service to each task while meeting its sub-budget. The simulation results show that the performance encouraging or discouraging. (The concept of critical pathway is discussed in Chap 6 Innovations in nursing service administration)

Health Care Reforms

It is very widely accepted fact that health is wealth of individual and empower individuals . Empowered people enjoy freedom from poverty, hunger, and malnutrition, and freedom to work and lead a healthy life **—Sen, 1999**

For empowering a person access to health care, good health is necessary. Ensuring access to health care helps to minimize absenteeism, enhance labor productivity, and prevents illness. Though there is a regional imbalance observed in health care delivery system in India, the government has taken lot of initiatives to improve the health of the population of the country implementation of various Health Committee Reports, Five Year Plans, National Health Policies, National Population Policies, AYUSH plans, enactments to improve health of all walks of life from newborn care to geriatric care, implementing primary health care, and Millennium Development goals, etc. are some of the strategies and reforms made by the Government in health.

Throughout the world, Governments demonstrated a significant role in providing and best possible health services to the people of developing countries especially focused on poor people. The 58th session of the World Health Assembly held in 2005 defined universal health care as providing means to have access promotive, preventive, curative, and rehabilitative health interventions for all at an affordable cost.

However, most low- and middle-income countries find this a major challenge because they have scarcity in health care resources and inadequate budget allocated for health-related activities.

The National Rural Health Mission (NRHM), established in 2005, and the recent introduction of Rashtriya Swasthya Bima Yojana (RSBY), a national health insurance scheme for people below the poverty line are the two most important initiatives taken by the Central Government. Several state governments also come up with their own insurance schemes. In spite of these initiatives, taken by the Government of India, the actual allocation of budget for health sector has not been increased.

Health Insurance

India health care today is in high rocketing cost. It is very essential that every Indian should be covered by health insurance as country like India that ranks very low on human life index. Health insurance should cover medical costs, hospitalization costs, treatment and diagnostic test costs and all types of critical illness.

Types of Health Policies in India

There are various plans readily available in India to cover every aspect of a medical emergency. Some popular types of policies are explained below:

- *Individual health plan:* This type of plan covers an individual against various illnesses with cashless hospitalization.
- *Family floater mediclaim:* With this one, individual can cover his family members against diseases under a single insurance plan. This needs to a fixed sum insured for the family members that can be availed either by an individual member or as a sum total for treatment of one family member.
- *Surgery and critical illness policy:* This is a plan policy in case of treatment against cancer, kidney failure, heart attack, paralysis, etc. As the treatment of such diseases is expensive so the premium is also go on a higher rate.
- *Pre-existing disease cover:* Pre-existing disease plan covers the diseases or illness that the policyholder had before buying the policy. For example, diabetes, hypertension, kidney failure, etc.
- *Senior citizen health plan:* This offers to protect senior citizens from health issues during their old age.
- *Preventive health care:* This policy includes preventive care treatments like regular checkups, consultation charges and other tests or X-ray fees concessions. The idea is to assess one's health at timely intervals and provide overall health care benefits.

Advantages of Health Insurance Policy

- *Cashless treatment:* Every insurance provider will have a list of hospital under its network. When a person is hospitalized in these hospitals he or she, does not need to pay cash. According to the type of plan, the agency will rectify the expenditure and payment is made by the insurance agency to the hospital expenses. The documentation should be complete while proceeding to the payment.
- *Pre- and posthospitalization:* This plan of insurance take care of both pre- and posthospitalization charges for a period of 30–60 days depending on the plan purchased and the disease condition.
- *Ambulance charges:* The insurance agency will pay for the ambulance charges and ensure it is in the purchasing of the plan.
- *Medical check-up:* Free medical checkup is provided by some of the insuring agency when a person has a good history of no claim bonus.
- *Tax benefit:* According to India's tax system if you are paying a premium amount then you are liable to get tax rebate under section 80 D of Income Tax Act for a maximum value of ₹ 25000 for Indians in the age group of 18–50 years and ₹ 30000 for senior citizens.

Health Economics

We are experiencing shift in demographics advancing medical and health care technology, and increased consumer expectations, scarce resources allocated for health care and distribution of scarce resources for health care.

If we want a comprehensive health care service to be provided to the society, we need a system that enable us to provide the same efficiently and effectively

Definition

Economics is a special field of discipline. Health economics is a branch of economics deals with application of economics to health care. Economics is a study of allocation of scarce resources among alternatives by the individual or society. Health economics deals with issues related to utilization of scarce resources to efficient and, effective health services.

Purposes of Health Economics

- To ensure a way of thinking and techniques
- To assist in decision-making in health sector to provide efficiency and equity
- To optimize social benefits subject to the availability of scarce resources
- To study the pattern of allocation of budget for health services
- To study health care expenses versus health status of individual and community
- To prevent or minimize wasteful expenditure
- It facilitates a framework to formulate health policy
- To suggest course of alternative when there is scarce resources.

The main goals of health economics is help the administrators to allocate resources with various health activities. It suggests the quality of resources to be used in health care facilities and organization of health care institution with efficient and effective use of available resources that in turn will affect the health of the individuals and society.

Health economics functions at micro and macro level. This means that not only is it interested in how a whole health care system functions but also in how things work at the peripheral/unit level. (A subcenter to medical college hospital)

Health economics is concerned with the alternative uses of resources in the health services sector and with the efficient utilization of economic resources such as human resource, material and financial resources. Every health worker needs to acquaint him/herself with the basic concepts of economics and its application to the health sector in order to manage health institutions and health delivery system efficiently.

BUDGETING AT VARIOUS UNITS AND LEVELS

Budget planning will be successful when the unit managers involved in making the budget. The following are some of the responsibilities of unit managers in terms of budgeting:

- Managers must understand fiscal terminology
- Be aware of their budgetary responsibility
- Accountable to the organization for maintaining a cost-effective unit
- Forecast unit fiscal needs
- Articulate unit needs to ensure sufficient funds
- Monitor aspects of budget control
- Involve others in fiscal planning
- Be able to include flexibility, creativity and vision regarding future needs
- Anticipate budget constraints and act proactively
- Ensure that cost containment does not jeopardize patient safety
- Delineate unit budgetary needs in an assertive, professional manner so that they generally obtain a fair distribution of resources for their unit.

Who should be involved in budget planning ?

- Chief financial officer of the hospital
- Members of finance department
- Operating managers
- Unit managers at all levels of nursing hierarchy.

Prerequisites for Unit Budgeting

- Unit incharge must be forecasting of needs for the unit she works
- Must have a thorough knowledge of accounting system
- Knows various cost accounting system
- Aware of fixed lines of authority
- There should be a budget committee
- The unit must have budget policies
- Statistical information should be prepared prior to proposal of budget
- Support of top management will encourage nurses
- Budget period should be confirmed. **(Read apply steps in budgeting and budget cycle)**

Issues and Challenges in Budgeting: Role of Nurse Administrator

Issues:

- Changing health care costs
- Changing patient demands
- Rigid management philosophy
- Less opportunities for nurses to advance in budgeting
- Failure of automations
- Demotivated staff as no incentives given
- Lack of standards of practice
- Insufficient curriculum and lack of preparation
- Lack of organizational climate
- Autonomy crisis
- Under qualified administrators.

Role of Nurse Administrator in Budgeting

- The administrator should be a visionary with regards to developing nursing profession
- She requires to formulate philosophy, objectives and goals for nursing service budget

- She involves nurses in budget planning and encourages to participate in budgetary decision- making
- Collects pertinent data regarding staffing, equipment and supplies and uses the data effectively in proposing the budget
- Makes budgetary projection that ensures to meet the objectives of nursing service department
- Monitors revenues and expenditure throughout the time frame
- Monitors day today, monthly and yearly expenditure
- Makes budget calendar
- Participates in policy meetings in relation to finance
- Guides unit staff nurses to prepare standardization of equipment for their unit
- Conducts condemnation and disposal of items
- Organizes in-service education program on financial management for nursing personnel
- Conducts auditing for nursing service department
- Modifies budget priorities according to budget variation
- Maintains stock book
- The budget is reviewed, analyzed and modified on the basis of budget committee.

The success of nursing service department depend upon the leadership capability of the administrator, resources available in quality and quanity and proper control of budget.

Box 19.1: Sample budget particulars

Sl. No.	Particulars	Expense
I	**Personnel** A. Salaries and wages 1. 2. 3. } Different positions	
	B. Fringe benefits Training programs, health insurance, vacation, sick leave bonus, increments, etc.	
	C. Consulting and contract service (e.g. external faculty)	
II	**Non-personnel** A. Space costs Rent, sanitation, utilities	
	B. Purchase/lease/rent of equipment, e.g. desk, chairs, filing cabinet, include other equipments necessary for the units.	
	C. Office and house hold supplies, e.g. 100 ream paper, include other items as necessary, e.g. Linen).	
	D. Travel/transportation new vehicles, petrol/diesel repair/maintenance, insurance, etc.	
	E. Telephone new installation, monthly charges, etc.	
	F. Medical supplies medicines, dressings patient care supplies	
	G. Repair and maintenance equipments, building, library maintenance	
	H. Other costs/miscellaneous library, books, bindings, audio-visual aids, (an important head for educational institutions) postage, insurance for fire, liability, etc.	
	I. Contingencies	
III.	Other indirect costs interdepartmental charges (if any), meetings, administration charges, etc. (Pharmacy, CSSD etc.)	

Note: Items/particulars/details can be added or deleted as per specific unit requirement.

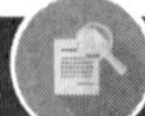

SUMMARY POINTS

✓ Financial management includes a sequential steps of activities developed to allocate resources and plan for the efficient and effective functioning of an establishment. The major aim of financial administration to meet the total financial needs of an establishment. Hence, all the establishments require to operate financial resources efficiently.

- ✓ The budget should be a dynamic plan of action reflecting the type, quality and quantity of the nursing service department as they are at present and as they are proposed for the future.
- ✓ Budget is a structured and systematic plan of income and expenditure that estimates of future needs of an organization in an arranged in orderly manner. It is also planned in detail for a specific period of time. Before implementing the budget, a financial statement in quantitative form is prepared by the administrator. Being budget is a tool to control activities, the outcome achieved is measured by a standard criteria.
- ✓ There are various types of budgeting. A capital budget outlines the forecasted buying of large fixed assets ensuring necessary facilities for carrying out organizational activities. It includes the major equipments construction of new building, etc. Capital budget is an important component of plan to meet the organization's long-term goals.
- ✓ Revenue budget refers to income from sales of materials or services rendered to consumers. These are business activities. In other words, the amount of money actually receives during a specific period of the year includes discount and deduction for return merchandise. When expenditure is deducted from the revenue we get net income or profit. Revenue budgets help the establishment save time and effort by the proper resources for organizational activities.
- ✓ Expenditure means expending or spending out. It include paying out cash or credit for exchange of goods or services.
- ✓ A budget cycle is the time frame a budget covers, with companies using monthly, quarterly and/or annual budget cycles to control costs and streamline administrative duties. Understanding the purpose of a budget cycle and the types used will help you decide how to implement one or more for your overall business or across your departments.
- ✓ Auditing refers to a systematic and independent examination of books, accounts, documents and vouchers of an organization to ascertain how far the financial statements present a true and fair view of the concern. It also attempts to ensure that the books of accounts are properly maintained by the concern as required by law.
- ✓ Cost-effectiveness is referred as the correlation of the financial inputs and the desired outcome, such as the relationship between quality nursing services and increasing patients satisfaction.
- ✓ Cost accounting is a financial concept. It is referred as the function of collecting, analyzing, summarizing and evaluating various courses of action underwent by the organization in terms of finance.
- ✓ Clinical pathways, are referred as care path-ways, critical pathways, integrated care pathways and care maps, are one of the main tools used to manage the quality care in health services.
- ✓ Health economics is the application of economics in health care. It studies the allocation of scarce resources among alternatives to bring desirable health outcome.

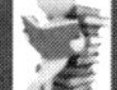

REVIEW QUESTIONS

1. Define budget. Describe the various types of budgeting.
2. Describe the various steps in budgeting.
3. Define audit. Discuss audit process.
4. What is cost accounting. Discuss its various types.
5. Discuss the issues in financial administration in nursing. Describe the role of nurse administrator in financial administration.
6. Write short notes on:
   a. Zero-based budget
   b. Budget cycle
   c. Lapsed budget
   d. Health economics
   e. Cost-effectiveness in nursing
   f. Health insurance.

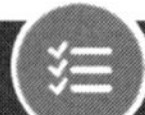

SELECTED READINGS

1. Dennis Arter, Quality Audits for Improved Performance, third edition, ASQ Quality Press, 2003.
2. HSRIC: Health Care Reform, Health Economics, and ...www.nlm.nih.gov/hsrinfo/health_economics.html
3. http://www.businessdictionary.com/definition/cost-effectiveness.html#ixzz40zVeuVm2
4. Huber, Diane.L 2006. Leadership and Nursing Care Management 3rd Edn., Saunders-Elsevier: Philadalphia Pages 757-788.
5. J.P. Russell, editor, The ASQ Auditing Handbook, third edition (formerly called The Quality Audit Handbook), ASQ Quality Press, 2005, p. 17.
6. Marquis , Bessie, L and Huston Carcol J 2006. Leadership roles and Management functions in Nursing, Theory and application 5th Edn., Lippincott Williams & Wilkins Philadelphia Pages. 215-237
7. National Health Insurance | policybazaar.com, policy-bazaar.com/nationalAd
8. Principles of Cost Accounting - Edward J. Vanderbeck - Google Books. Books.google.co.uk. Retrieved 2013-03-01
9. Second edition Health economics Supported by..www.medicine.ox.ac.uk/.../whatis/What_is_health_econ.pdf
10. Tomey. Merina .Ann.2009 . Guide to Nursing Management and Leadership 4th Edn., Mosby. Elsevier Missouri. Pages 241-271
11. Top #10 Health Insurance - Compare All Health Plans in 2 Mins easypolicy.com/health-insuranceAd
12. What is Health Economics | webcrawler.com www.webcrawler.comAd

UNIT X
LEGAL AND ETHICAL ISSUES

20

Law and Ethics

LEARNING OBJECTIVES

This chapter imparts learning about:

- Concept, Definition of Laws and Ethics
- Ethical Committee
- Code of Ethics and Professional Conduct
- Professional Responsibility and Accountability
- Legal System, Tort Law, and Liabilities
- Legal issues in Nursing: Negligence, Malpractice, Invasion of Privacy,
- Defamation of Character Patient Care Issues, Management Issues, Employment Issues Medico Legal Issues
- Nursing Regulatory Mechanisms: Licensure, Renewal, Accreditation
- Patient's Rights, Consumer Protection Act (CPA)
- Infection Control
- Standard Safety Measures
- Research Highlights

LEGAL AND ETHICAL ISSUES IN NURSING

Introduction

Nurse administrators are challenged with a health care system that has changed significantly in the recent years. The nurse managers experiencing pressure on providing quality care and patient safety and maintain cost effectiveness in caring patients. The expanded and extended role of the nurses warrants for knowledge, skill and decision-making capabilities in legal and ethical aspects of care at advance level which is mandatory for every nurse to safeguard herself and her patients and families from legal rights in relation to health. Therefore a nurse should know legal and ethical aspects of nursing, in her day to day practice.

DEFINITION OF LAW AND ETHICS

Definition of law

According to Creighton law refers to Standards of human conduct established and enforced by the authority of an organized society through its government.

Law refers to rules, regulation and conduct that guides individual's action it is established by a competent authority which each one of us needs to follow as a citizen of India.

Law is a basic and fundamental level of ethics of a community. There is a relationship with law and politics.

Law and ethics are related. Nurses may act in ways that are legal but not ethical. Both law and ethics are related to politics. Normally law follows ethical practice. As a matter of fact, laws are enacted to give formal recognition to ethics, which can then be enforced.

Sullivan and Decker, (2001) describe laws that are rules of conduct, established and enforced by authority, which prevents extremes in behavior so that one can live without fear for oneself or one's property.

Some the related terms used in law are:

- **Litigation:** It is the process of bringing and trying a lawsuit
- **Plaintiff:** A person bringing the lawsuit (the accuser) may be patients or family
- **Defendant:** The person accused example may be a health care professional
- **Trial court:** First level court
- **Appellate court:** Appeals court (where the case goes if the verdict in the trial court is appealed)
- **Bill:** A draft of an act presented to the legislative, but not enacted
- **Act:** It is a written law which has been formally passed by the Government
- **Certificate:** An instrument accorded by a competent authority which confers the right to perform some act
- **License:** A written permission by a competent authority to do some act without which such authorization would be illegal.

Types of law are described as follows:

- **Public law:** In this type government is directly involved and regulates relationships between individuals and government. It is designed to prevent harm to society and provide punishment.
- **Private law**: It is also referred as civil law. In this type, law regulates relationships among people. It is designed to protect the right of individuals and encourage fair and equitable treatment among people.
- **Criminal law**: This type of law is concerned with state and federal criminal statutes. It defines criminal actions, e.g. murder, theft.

What are the sources of law?

- **Statutory law:** Created by elected bodies state legislatures, e.g. The Bill of Rights; Nurse Practice Acts (In India is on the process of defining the boundaries of nursing practice act).
- **Regulatory or administrative law**: Created by state Boards of Nursing when they pass rules and regulations, e.g. regulations for nurses by Indian Nursing Council, State Nursing Council).
- **Common law:** Created by judicial decisions made in courts when individual cases are decided, e.g. Informed Consent, patients right to refuse treatment,

Definition of Ethics

Ethics is defined as a systematic inquiry into principles of right and wrong conduct, virtue and vices, good and evil. Ethics is different from religion, law, custom and institutional practices.

- The term ethics refers to a system of principles and rules of conduct. It says what is right and what is wrong. They guide our professional behavior/ practice.
- Ethics and law are interrelated, may go hand in hand and support each other.
- Ethics may address different questions than does the law. At times, individuals find that the law and their ethical beliefs diverge.
- For nurses and midwives, the code of ethics gives guidance for decision-making concerning ethical matters.
- Ethical and legal conduct of nurses and midwives assists to empower the clients to make informed decisions and choices.

Some of the related terms used in ethics

- **Value:** A belief about the worth of something, about what matters, a guide for behavior.
- **Value system:** An organization or ranking of values.
- **Ethical dilemma:** Occurs when conflicting courses of action are present.
- **Ethical distress:** When the nurse knows the right thing to do, but the situation makes doing that difficult.
- **Bioethics:** Concerns the life sciences. Issues regarding: Research conduct, environmental ethics, sustainable health care.
- **Clinical ethics:** Concerns issues at the bedside, issues regarding consent or refusal of treatment, assisted suicide, requests for futile treatment.
- **Nursing ethics:** Concerns clinical nursing issues. Issues regarding allocation of care and resources, confidentiality, unethical or incompetent conduct of colleagues.

ETHICAL COMMITTEE

We are living in the era of evidence-based practice. These evidences are derived from research findings. Medicine and nursing deals with human beings and the services provided by health care professional should be safe, effective and quality oriented. Health is a human right. Any intervention done on patients to improve quality patient care outcome, we need to respect bio ethics and human rights. If we violate human rights it is highly unethical.

Most of the hospitals are now establishing ethical committee where research is done on patients.

Due to globalization, rapid techniques of diagnosis and therapy, are now available through research. The advances in the area of genetics, genomics and molecular biology have grown rapidly with the resultant need to rein in these advances with sufficient safeguards to protect the rights and welfare of human participants subjected to biomedical research.

The Indian Council of Medical Research (ICMR) brought out the 'Policy Statement on Ethical Considerations involved in Research on Human Subjects' in 1980 and revised these guidelines in 2000 as the 'Ethical guidelines for Biomedical Research on Human Subjects'. Due to further rapid developments in science and technology in India after the release of the second version, it became necessary to update these guidelines to make adequate specific provision to meet ethical challenges led further revision at 2006. The ICMR is funded by the Government of India through the department of Health research, Ministry of Health and Family Welfare.

Functions of ICMR

- Formulation, coordination and promotion of biomedical research
- Establish research priorities on control and management of diseases
- Promotion of biomedical research through intramural and extramural research

The need for Institutional Ethics Committee (IECs) in medical and research organizations resulted from the realization that affirms human rights as a special right of all members of society. Health care professionals may not be able to do what is right in all instances as evidenced by the number studies.

IEC vary widely in their composition. It include multi-disciplinary membership. In addition to those with research and clinical experience, many committees include representation from psychology, human rights commission social work, and law backgrounds, and often a member with a more academic orientation. Moreover, most committees find it important to include individuals from the public representation to help to provide a patient's and public perspective.

Composition of IEC (Mala Ramanathan, ICMR 2006)

It is multidisciplinary and mulisectoral in composition consisting 5–12 members.

Chairperson (should preferably be from outside the institution and not head of the same institution to maintain the freedom of the committee)

- 1–2 basic medical scientists
- 1–2 clinicians from various institutes
- One legal expert or retired judge
- One social scientist/representative of NG/ voluntary agency
- One philosopher/ethicist/theologian
- One lay person (public representative)
- Member secretary (from the institution who will convene the meeting)
- If required, subject experts could be invited to offer views.

Functions and Responsibilities of Members of Institutional Ethical Committee

- To provide competent review of all ethical aspects of the project
  - Undergo appropriate training to enhance competence
  - To maintain confidentiality of documents obtained and discussions during the review process
  - To allocate time for reviewing the proposals.
- Undertake review free from bias and influence
  - Need to put on record various interests, financial or otherwise to avoid conflict of interest
  - Reflexivity about the nature of engagement with protocols
  - Nonjudgmental and unbiased decision-making.
- Provides advice to the researchers on all aspects of welfare and safety of research participants
  - Need to build capacity of researchers
  - Provide ongoing review
  - Monitor the taking of consent
  - Ensure that the guidance from the Institutional Review Board (IRB) is actually followed
  - Keep oneself informed of the research process and re-review whenever needed.

Functioning of Ethical Committee (EC)

The following describes the functions step-by-step to conduct ethical committee meetings:

Prefixed Dates for Routine IEC Meetings

The date and time including the venue for the meeting to be finalized in advance. This planning will help the research scholar to develop and finalize materials for presentation.

Submissions Made by Researchers in Keeping with the Requirements of the Ethical Committee

In this step the research scholar submit his project on time.

Finalizing Primary and Secondary Reviewers

The secretariat of the institution scrutinizes the project with other formalities, and send the proposal to the reviewers.

The Proposals Circulated to Members Giving Sufficient Time for Review

Receiving the projects from the reviewers the proposal is sent to all EC members so that they get enough time to go through the proposal before EC meeting.

The Members Undertake the Review

The EC members review the proposal keeping in mind the subjects (vulnerability), the process (consent, privacy, confidentiality), study requirements(risk and benefits).If necessary clarification is made.

The Meeting of the IEC

The president chairs the session, the secretary records the discussion, members clarify and discuss the proposal.

Discussions at the IEC

During this stage, many issues and problem arising from the proposal is clarified and discussed in detail. ICMR guidelines, Government regulation, professional regulations are referred in case of doubts. Sometimes members refer scholarly journals to support the decision made.

Documenting the Decisions Made

The secretary makes notes of each discussion, compiles them clearly record the decision. The decision is presented to the chairperson.

The Process and Decisions are Documented

In this step, the decision is communicated to the researcher along with the recommendation called for change of the proposal. Subject experts views are requested if needed.

The Following Decisions and the Reasons are Communicated to the Researcher

- Outright approval—means research approved only with minor changes
- Approval with modification—Research proposal is accepted with modification
- Re submit with more information
- Outright disapproval—the proposal is rejected due to ethical reasons.

THE CODE OF NURSING ETHICS AND PROFESSIONAL CONDUCT

The first code of ethics for nurses was developed by International Council of Nurses (ICN) in 1953 and revised in 2012. It was referred as a guideline for actions for nurses and was developed based on values and needs of the society.

According to the changing needs of the society, the ICN. revise the code of ethics regularly. Respect for human rights and dignity including right to life is the basic principles to be followed by nurses as per its code of ethics.

CODE OF ETHICS FOR NURSES IN INDIA (AS PER INDIAN NURSING COUNCIL)

The Nurse Respects the Uniqueness of Individual in Provision of Care

The nurse provides care to all patients irrespective of their caste, creed, religion, culture, ethnicity, gender, socio-economic and political status, personal attributes, or any other grounds and respects beliefs, values and cultural sensitivities. The nurse recognizes the respect of an individual in his family or community and ensures their participation in their care. The nurse believes that every patient is an unique individual, develops trustworthiness and accepts the patient as he or she is.

The Nurse Respects the Rights of Individuals as Partner in Care and Help in Making Informed Choices

The nurse recognizes that every individual has his right to make his decision related to his health and ensures that all information related to making decision is provided to him or her. The nurse appreciates the decision made by the patient. The nurse protects the individual, family and community from misinformation and misinterpretation especially of vulnerable group regarding their care.

Maintains confidentiality, and Shares Information Judiciously

The nurse respects and maintains the rights of the patient. To keep confidential regarding his personal information except in life threatening situation where the nurse uses her discretion in sharing information with concerned people. The nurse ensures informed consent and maintains confidentiality that is needed for legal/academic or quality assurance purposes. The nurse also maintains confidentiality of records and limits to exposure only to authorized persons if needed.

Nurse Maintains Competence in Order to Render Quality Nursing Care

The nurse gives care to patient is qualified and legally registered nurse certified from competent authority. The nurse maintains quality nursing care as prescribed in the standards of nursing practice. The nurse enhances her professional knowledge by attending in-service education and identifies opportunities for self-development. The nurse understands the value of nursing research to improve nursing practice, maintains ethical principles and participates in research.

The Nurse if Obliged to Practice within the Framework of Ethical, Professional and Legal Boundaries

The nurse always abides with the code of ethics and professional conduct and renders care within legal and ethical framework as prescribed Indian Nursing Council.

Nurse is Obliged to Work Harmoniously with Members of the Health Team

The nurse values team work in providing care to patients and cooperates, coordinates and collaborates with members of the health team to meet the needs of people.

Nurse Commits to Reciprocate the Trust Invested in Nursing Profession by Society

The nurse always demonstrates personal manners and professional attributes in dealing with patients and in all settings.

CODE OF PROFESSIONAL CONDUCT FOR NURSES IN INDIA

Professional Responsibility and Accountability

The nurse accepts a sense of self-value and nourishes it. The nurse's good behavior reflects on the profession and she continue her work within the professional boundaries. The nurse shows accountability in her practice and accepts accountability for her decisions and actions behavior. The nurse demonstrates compassionate and takes responsibility for continuous improvement in nursing practices. She demonstrates a healthy behavior and ensures information to patients to help them to make informed choices.

Nursing Practice

The nurse take care of all individuals and families with respect and dignity and provides a high standard of nursing care which is safe to patients. Accepts the health practices that are healthy and the nurse encourages the patient to practice and discourage unhealthy and harmful practices. The nurse facilitates autonomous decision- making by the individual and family and motivates the family members to involve in patient care. If needed and she feels, she is not competent enough to take care of the patients does not hesitate to consult, coordinate, collaborate and follow-up appropriately when individuals' care needs exceed the nurse's competence.

Communication and Interpersonal Relationships

The nurse develops effective interpersonal relationship and cooperate with patients, families and community and respect the dignity of team members. Maintains professional role of team members and accepts the team.

Valuing Human Being

The nurse protects the individuals from harmful and unethical practices and information. The nurse takes positive decisions for individuals regarding their care and supports the individuals and encourages them to use their rights to speak about their issues regarding their health and illness and supports choices made by the individuals.

Management

The nurse provides resources and utilizes them appropriately. The nurse as a teacher participates in educating and supervising students and other health workers. The nurse delegates responsibility to the appropriate person, communicates effectively with patients, family and members of the health team and ensures a work culture conducive to work and achieve organizational goals. The nurse participates in performance appraisal and evaluation of patient care given. The nurse participates in policy making and make the management sensitive to funding for resource allocation.

Professional Advancement

The nurse understands protection of human rights while advancing in education and contributes to the advancement of nursing practice. Ensures quality care demonstrates responsibilities to advance her knowledge and competencies contributes to the development of nursing knowledge by participating/conducting research.

LEGAL SYSTEM: TYPES OF LAW, LAW OF TORT, AND LIABILITIES

Tort and Liabilities

Tort is a legal system refers to a violation is made against a person or property causes damage, injury or harm to another person.

Tort: Unintentional

The violation may result from unintentional cause referred as unintentional tort that means the violation is caused by intentional actions, a breach of duty negligence or malpractice conduct which falls below the standard of care. So, there are four critical elements that must be proven in a malpractice case:

Example:

- The nurse owed a **duty** to the patient.
- There was a **breach of duty** because the nurse did not carry it out. (evident from expert witnesses, standards of care, hospital policy and procedure).
- The patient suffered **harm.**
- The nurse's failure to carry out the duty was **causation** of the harm.

Tort: Intentional

- **Assault and battery:** Assault is the threat to bring about harm; battery is any intentional touching without consent or any willful attempt or threat to harm another, coupled with the ability to actually harm the person. Statement of threat for eg. performing a procedure that the patient has not consented to.
- **Invasion of privacy**: Patient's right to protection against unreasonable and unwarranted interference with the patient's solitude e.g. release of medical information to unauthorized person, confidentiality of medical record is not maintained.
- **False imprisonment**: Example: Patient's right to leave LAMA (Leave Against Medical Advice).
- **Libel/slander:** False statements which damage a person's reputation (libel is written; slander is oral).
- **Fraud**: Intentionally misleading another person with the intention of causing legal injury or deprive the person of a right.
- **Patient's right to protection against:**
  - Appropriation of the patient's name or picture for institution's sole advantage
  - Publication of facts that place the patient in a false light
  - Public disclosure of private facts about the patient by the hospital or staff.

LIABILITIES

Liabilities referred as obligations that legally connects an individual or establishment to settle a wrongful act they may have committed. These are settled over a period of time with money, goods or services. The following are the various types of liabilities:

- **Personal Liability:** As individuals, nurses are responsible for their own actions or inactions
- **Vicarious Liability:** When the subordinates are doing some actions and the superior is held liable and this liability is because of association with the negligent person. For example, a charge nurse in the operation theater is liable when the floor nurse missed in counting sponges left in the abdomen of the patient.
- **Corporate liability:** Organization is responsible for the harm. The organization is held liable to hire, supervise and maintain skillful and qualified staff; to provide, repair and maintain adequate equipment; to maintain safety in the physical environment
- **Joint liability:** This is where several tortfeasors (the persons who commits offence) are held liable for a tort against one party. The tortfeasers are said to be jointly liable for the harm. The liability settlement depends upon the degree of harm done by the individuals and policies of the establishment or law.
- **Liability to/for third parties:** An individual may be held liable for injuries sustained by a third individual. For example, a landlord has a duty not only to protect the welfare of the person living in his house means their tenants are free from harm on the premises, but also that third party like family friends are safe as well.
- **Parent liability:** Parents may be held liable for the tortuous actions of their children.
- **Strict liability:** Strict liability means that the individuals may be held liable for a violation of law unknowingly a law. Examples of strict liability torts include like transporting hazardous materials in an off-limits zone.

LEGAL ISSUES IN NURSING

Nurse administrators today are confronted with number of legal issues in nursing. Our health consumers are more knowledgeable, about their rights and legal obligation of health care facility. For the last two decades, numerous lawsuits are being filed by patients against hospitals for the damages and injuries occurred during their hospitalization. Hospital administrators have great responsibilities in maintaining safe and quality environment including building, equipment, accessories for patient, employees, and visitors.

Today nurses role is expanding and extending. They encounter with various issues. In relation to nursing practice, they must have thorough knowledge on legal and ethical aspects of nursing care. They should abide with the code of ethics and professional conduct as per INC standard while caring the patients.

Some of the legal issues in nursing practice are described below:

Negligence

Nursing negligence is when a professional nurse who is fully qualified and capable to care does not use such capability as a skilled care nurse would use, and as a result the patient suffers from complication or harm. Negligence arises from:

- Failure to ensure patient safety such as patient falls due to failure to supervise, failure to assist, slippery floors
- Improper treatment/negligent performance of the treatment
- Failure to monitor the patient
- Failure to follow agency's policies and procedures
- Medication errors is very common
- Patient get injuries due to defective equipment (trolley, wheelchair, bed)
- Failure to communicate necessary information to patient/doctor or head nurse
- Failure to document, incomplete documentation, inaccurate documentation.

Malpractice

It is the failure of a nurse with professional education and skills to act in a reasonable and prudent manner.

Defamation

It is an act of holding up of a person to ridicule, scorn or contempt within the community. It is of two types:

1. Slander defamation-spoken words
2. Libel defamation-written words

Informed Consent

Authorization by the patient or the patient's legal representative to do something to the patient. like consenting for an operation/surgery. Based on legal capacity, voluntary action and comprehension is a must in informed consent. The consent should be valid.

Issues related to informed consent are:

- Nurses are witness to the signing
- Attesting only to the voluntary nature of the consent
- Inform the responsible person /health care provider regarding the inadequacy of comprehension if expressed by the patient.

EXAMPLES OF ALLEGATIONS IN LAWSUITS INVOLVING NURSES

As mentioned above the author has complied some the allegations and law suits against nurses from literature as follows:

- Failure to rule out potential health problems of patients
- Failure to convey discharge instructions to patient/ family
- Failure to follow nursing procedure with professional skill
- Failure to report questionable care or substandard nursing practices
- Failure to adequately document patient care
- Failure to monitor the patient in all conditions
- Failure to initiate treatment in an appropriate and timely fashion in spite of standing orders available in the unit
- Failure to follow physician orders
- Failure to notify the physician or senior incharge nurses as needed
- Failure to identify high-risk patients.

LEGAL ISSUES IN HOSPITAL NURSING ADMINISTRATION

- Failure to delegate the subordinate nurses.
- Failure to supervise nursing personnel in terms of patient care
- Failure to orient staff unaware of rules, policies and procedure
- Failure to educate staff nurses who do not perform well
- Failure to evaluate that leads to continue poor performance standards
- Failure to warn for repetition of errors, the administrator will not be able to justify their disciplinary action. The chance of correction and improvement among nurses is prevented
- Failure to maintain staffing norm, accreditation standards floating staff from unit to unit.

LEGAL ISSUES IN EDUCATIONAL ADMINISTRATION

- Failure to conform to norms of regulatory bodies
- Keeping false/duplicate records
- Production of fake certificates
- Acquisition of degree through non-attendance programs
- Malpractices during examinations
- Deprivation of students from benefits and facilities
- Utilizing students for service needs of the hospital
- Utilizing students for clinical trials

- Unauthorized presence of faculty in various institutions during inspection.

Medicolegal Case

Nurses are considered responsible and accountable for the quality of care of their patients and families. Nurses who are employed whatever health care facility, they are directly responsible to their immediate supervisors. The nursing standards are clearly defined, and legal documents to which nurses are considered accountable. Earlier days nurses seldom worried about medical malpractice lawsuits. They did not have any concern regarding their profession, which involves medico legal aspects. However today, a growing number of professional nurses find themselves involved in litigation These nurses end up losing their jobs and their licenses. as well as their assets. Nurses have found themselves in front of criminal charges and even jail terms due to medication errors that have led to patient death.

Today the role of nurses has undergone a paradigm shift, leading to the expansion and extension of their clinical roles in specialized settings. Mushrooming of hospitals, nursing homes and clinics have taken birth due to commercialization on one side and consumerism and knowledgeable patients on the other side.

The enactment of various legal provisions like Consumer Protection Act, India, 1986 (CPA), Right to Information Act, 2005 (RTI) and standardization of nursing procedures and practices has brought nursing care under the legal focus, more than ever before.

- **Medico Legal Case (MLC):** It is defined as a case of injury or ailment, where some criminality is involved or investigations by the legal authorities are required. In other words, it is a medical condition with legal implications for the attending doctor who assesses the patient, identifies the problem and decides the case is legally implicated and further investigation to be made by law enforcing agency. When it is a legal case where medical intervention is necessary. For example: suspected accident, poisoning, burns, comatose or brought dead persons admitted to the casualty are some of the medico legal cases.

The following are the initial responsibilities of a hospital when an MLC comes to causality department:

- All MLC cases should be admitted after verification with the police post of the hospital or after the police is informed.
- All medico legal papers must be stamped MLC for easy identity and alertness.
- In emergency, first aid treatment should promptly be given before documentation or other medicolegal procedures. All care given in casualty to be completed accurately.
- The medical officer in charge prepares two copies of the MLC report and in case of suspected poisoning he makes three copies. Original copy will be handed over to the concerned police officer and duplicate will be kept in safe custody of the hospital. Chief Medical Officer (CMO) is responsible to hand over the MLC report within 48 hours to the concerned police after the first assessment by CMO. No preliminary or interim report should be given to anyone. The MLC form should be duly completed by Chief Medical Officer (CMO) with special documentation like proper identification marks, consent, brief history general physical examination, specific comments like nature and stage of injuries, type of weapon used or nature of poisoning suspected. Investigations advised and material preserved and handed over to the police. All reports to be kept secretly in confidential form.
- The MLC should be handed over to police not to the relatives on discharge. MLC should be informed to the concerned police officer before discharge. In case of death of an inpatient MLC case, police is to be informed and the body handed over to them and written records to be kept.

NURSES ROLE IN A MEDICOLEGAL CASE

The nurses should be very alert and vigilant when an MLC is admitted in casualty or in ward.

- Do complete assessment of the patient and complete history either pateint or other relatives who brought the patient to hospital.
- The Bed Head Ticket (BHT) and all the other forms used in care of the patient should be stamped MLC.
- His BHT should not be left on bed like other patients before or after rounds of doctor.
- All records should be kept confidential and kept in duty room under lock and key.
- Avoid giving any information or statements regarding the patient's condition to police, magistrate or media. This responsibility is vested on the doctor to give information.
- When a patient has to be discharged, communicate the discharge of MLC to the police officer/constable on duty in hospital and/or the CMO.They are the final authority for discharging the MLC.
- The CMO or attending doctor to be informed immediately when the MLC absconds from casualty or from the ward. The nurse should count the patients in each shift while taking and handing over.

All the records of MLC who is absconded to be kept under lock and keys.

- MLC patients cannot leave the hospital against medical advice.
- Complete the documentation accurately, completely with relevance, and sign in care plan and nurse's notes
- Precaution should be taken while caring MLC including records kept and appropriate authority must be informed about MLC.
- Special care to be taken to hand over the MLC on parole to relatives. The patient on parole to be handed over to the relatives with the submission of relatives approved by CMO
- In case of death of MLC physician on duty must inform the CMO to withhold the body for postmortem examination according to hospital policy.
- Nurse must get instruction from the medical officer for handling over the body to mortuary/relative/ police officer.
- Protect the right of the female patient if she refuses to be examined by a male doctor discourage repeated examination of breast, abdomen and perineal part of patient specific to MLC.

LEGAL AND ETHICAL ISSUSES IN NURSING PRACTICE NURSING REGULATORY MECHANISMS LICENSURE, RENEWAL, ACCREDITATION

Laws and ethical practices had been in existence developed in the societies since beginning of civilization. Laws are changing constantly along with advancement in technology, modernization, subsequent social changes, and altering health care delivery system.

Globally, the nurses and midwives are governed by the laws and of the country, service rules and regulations of the central and state governments, standards of care and institutional policies.

There are Codes of conduct or ethical principles established by both International (ICN 1953) and National (INC 2006) bodies for Practicing Nurses and Midwives. Nurses and Midwives are also regulated under the Indian Penal Code (IPC) Act and Consumer Protection Act 1986.

The nursing practice in the state is bound by legal and ethical principles.

Nursing practice entails performance of acts requiring substantial specialized knowledge, skills, judgment and clinical decision-making. To practice legally, a nurse must possess genuine, valid and current registration issued by the State Nursing Council.

Indian Nursing Council ACT, 1947

- The Indian Nursing Council (INC) has the authority to control nursing education and what the Nurse is prepared to do.
- But it has delegated the authority for control of nursing practice to the state nursing councils (SNC).
- Each state nursing council has its' own Act. For example, The Kerala Nurses and Midwife Act 1953. The License to Practice in the State is issued by The Kerala Nurses and Midwives Act, 1953. Registration as Registered Nurse/Registered Midwife is mandatory to Practice in the State of Kerala per Section 20, 21 and 22 of the Kerala Nurses and Midwives Act 1953.
- Practice in Kerala without Registration from the KNMC is illegal and punishable as per Sections 33 of the Kerala Nurses and Midwives Act, 1953.

This act provides for Refusal to Register/Removal of name from the Register as per Section 69 to 82 in case of:

- Any offence that is committed including breach of regulations
- Legal responsibilities for safe nursing practice
- Professional incompetence/negligence
- Sentence by criminal court

Safe Practice Requirements

- Have current license to practice
- The nurse should know her job and job description well and update herself
- Follow policies and procedures and adhere to standards
- Have written orders, clarify orders and ensure the five 'Rs in medication procedure
- Protect the patients from injuries
- Respect the rights of the patients.
- Be alert
- Do not accept any money or gifts
- Obtain informed consent
- Maintain good IPR
- Report all unusual incidences
- Document well
- Maintain professional conduct.

Legal Liabilities

- Practice without state council registration
- Malpractice and negligence
- Unethical practices
- Witnessing a patient's will
- Incorrect identification of patients

- Medico-legal cases
- Environmental hazards (slippery floors, faulty equipment and electrical wiring, lack of bed rails when necessary, presence of inflammable substances, inadequate protection from stray animals, inadequate lighting and ventilation)
- LAMA (Left Against Medical Advice)
- Practicing medicine
- Advising contrary to physician
- Anything beyond the code of nursing practice laid down/level of comprehension.

Regulations for Nursing Practice

Indian Penal Code 1860

Section 88 of Indian Penal Code (IPC) says

'Nothing which is not intended to cause death is an offence, by reason of any harm which it may cause or be intended by the doer to cause, or be known by the doer to be likely to cause, to any person for whose benefit it is done, in good faith and who has given consent whether expressed or implied, to suffer that harm'. i.e. a person is not liable if he has done something in good faith for the benefit of somebody after obtaining his consent even if he dies.

Good Faith is Further Defined in Section 52 of IPC

Nothing is said to be done in good faith if done without due care and attention.

Due care and attention are not clearly defined but if due care and attention is given, a nurse is saved from punishment. Exercising reasonable skill and care, following standard protocols, guideline and regimes in treating a patient are examples of due care and attention.

Negligence—Failure to Attend

If death of the patient was due to the negligence or lack of due care and attention on the part of the nurse/doctor, she/he is liable *under Section 304 A of IPC* which says *whoever causes the death of any person by doing any rash or negligent act not amounting to culpable homicide shall be punished with imprisonment of either description for a term which may extend to two years, or with fine or with both.* During an emergency, the prime duty of the health team is to save the life of the patient. There will be no time to obtain the consent. Sometimes the patient, victim of a road traffic accident may be unconscious and in such a case, consent is not mandatory.

According to Indian Medical Council Act, 1956 all medicolegal procedures include not only actions performed by a medical officer, but also a nurse. [Ref. Indian Medical Council (Professional conduct, Etiquette and Ethics) Regulation, 2002] (chapter- 5.3)

Nursing Practice Act is Yet to be Enacted in India

- The Consumer Protection Act, 1986
- The Consumer Protection Act, 1986 passed by the Government of India protects the interest of the consumer.

Under this act, patients are considered consumers and can register complaints

As per a legal ruling in 1995, it does apply to hospitals, doctors, nurses and health care professionals.

Professional Malpractice

- Professional nurses have legal obligation to conform to standards of care
- The three ways of committing professional malpractice are
  - Performing a duty carelessly
  - Failing to perform a duty when it is indicated
  - Performing an unauthorized act.
- When the standards of care are breached causing injury to the client, there is professional malpractice. It is a form of negligence.
- Nurses are liable for the consequences of their action. Therefore conform to standards of care, policies and regulations while caring patients and families.

Ethical Considerations

Code of Ethics for Nurses in India (INC, 2006)

- The nurse respects the uniqueness of individual in provision of care.
- The nurse respects the rights of individuals as partner in care and in making informed choices
- The nurse respects individuals right to privacy, maintains confidentiality and shares information judiciously
- Nurse maintains competence to render quality nursing care
- The nurse ensures her knowledge with relevant laws and practices of the state where she is working and abides with code of ethics and professional conduct relevant to the country.
- Nurse works harmoniously with members of the health care team
- Nurse maintains ethical principles while working with individual, family and community.

Ethical Issues

- Rights of the individual versus that of society/state
- Patient decision versus family decisions versus institutional decisions.

Issues related to:
- Reproductive technology
- Organ transplants
- Research subjects
- Confidentiality
- Restraints
- Disclosure
- Informed consent
- Patient incapacity
- Court interventions.

Nursing councils have the power to recognize and derecognize the nursing educational institution which fails to comply with the regulations of the national and State Nursing Councils.

- Provision of a supportive environment that facilitates appropriate assignment and delegation
- Clear communication and documentation
- Adequate staffing and supervision
- Quality assurance
- Knowledge of disciplinary procedures
- Review nursing standards periodically and revise
- Display written instructions
- Performance appraisal
- Zero percent policy for all forms of harassment
- Speak for the nurses.
- Be advocates for the clients, subordinates and the profession.
- The consumers are becoming increasingly aware of their legal rights in health care. Safe nursing practice is absolutely essential for the nurses to safeguard self and the public from legal issues. One should be equipped to face the changes and challenges.
- Every nurse is liable for her/his own actions.
- Ignorance of law is not an excuse. Law governs man from cradle to grave. Therefore, it is better for men to cooperate with law to the best of its' intentions.
- Ignorance is not a legal defense (Latha K).

LICENSE

License refers to the permission granted by competent authority to exercise a certain privilege that, without such authorization, would constitute an illegal act. The certificate or the document itself that confers permission to engage in otherwise proscribed conduct. For example, for nurses license or registration certificate is given by the state. Nursing and midwives council when the nurses complete nursing course successfully from a recognized nursing school/college by the state and the country. A nurse without a registration certificate cannot practice nursing in India.

Sometimes, the terms license and permit are used interchangeably, whereas, a permit denotes a more temporary, form of permission with an expiry date. After it expirers the date the permit has to be renewed if the individual wants to continue the job. For example work permit.

Government Licenses

Some of the activities require license issued from the government. For example fishing; hunting; driving a motor vehicle; practicing law; manufacturing; engaging in retail and wholesale commerce; operating a private business, trade, or technical school; providing commercial services.

A license gives a person or organization permission to engage in a particular activity. If the government requires a license for an activity, it may issue criminal charges if a person engages in the activity without obtaining a license. Most licenses expire after a certain period of time, and most may be renewed. Failure to abide by certain laws and regulations can result in suspension or revocation of a license.

Procedure of Registration

The licensing process helps to control activity in a variety of ways. License application procedures allow government authorities to screen applicants to verify that they are fit to engage in the particular activity. For example, before any license is issued by the state nursing council, the applicant nurse must meet certain standards. She should submit two attested copies (Duly attested by Gazette officers) of following:

- Degree/provisional certificate
- SSLC
- Course completion certificate in nursing
- Mark lists
- Registration certificate from respective nursing council (if the nurse studied in Karnataka state, wants to get a registration from Tamil Nadu, she must attach Karnataka registration certificate along with the above certificates).

A DD or *chalan* for 1000 rupees along with ₹ 10/- as *chalan* fee (or as per policy of the council) should be submitted along with the certificates as fees. After completing the application form along with certificates and fees she should submit to the council's office and get the registration certification after verification. The council has all the power to withdraw the license if the nurse violates law.

RENEWAL OF LICENCE

Those nurses already registered with a particular state nursing and midwives council needs to renew their license or registration certificate once in 5 years. This has made compulsory from July 2013. It is possible to renew by online also.

Renewal of license is done for name correction, getting a duplicate certificate when the original is list or damaged, and for photo correction.

The renewal procedures are more or less same in state nursing councils.

Procedure for Renewing License

- They should obtain application form for renewal
- She/he should attach original registration certificate
- Appointment order from the current employer if she is working
- If she/he is studying a bonafide certificate from the principal
- Passport size photograph
- Renewal fees as levied by the council
- Keep an acknowledge form for future reference
- Complete address with phone number
- Online information is furnished according the cause for renewal
- Renewal certificate is obtained from the council in person or by post

ACCREDITATION

Accreditation is a recognition awarded by an authorized health care accreditation body to an institution when it adheres to the accreditation standards, demonstrated through an independent external peer assessment regarding its level of performance in relation to the standards.

PRINCIPLES OF ACCREDITATION

- **The activities of the health care facility should be patient care focused.** The health care providers should know the actual and potential needs of the patients needs and ensure that patients are very important for them. All the assessment should be done with respect of patients.
- **The activities of the organization are controlled by effective leadership.** The organizational leadership accepts responsibility and committed to provision of nursing care excellence, quality improvement and performance:

  This is ensured by excellent direction for the health service, pursuit of continuous development of strategies, systems and methods for achieving excellence of quality outcome, innovative and creative proposals and models of care, and motivating and encouraging employees for their self-learning and development.
- **The management and employees demonstrate continuous improvement** to **improve the quality of care**. The organization believes that improvement is an essential component of practice outcome and continuously it strives to achieve organizational goals and monitoring patient care outcome.
- **Evidence of outcomes:** Performance appraisal, and care based on best practices evidence informed are continuously practiced.
- **Striving for best practice:** The organization strives to achieve its best outcome by application of innovative techniques or models of care that results in efficiency and effectiveness of organization and enhanced patient satisfaction and outcome.

THE NATIONAL ASSESSMENT AND ACCREDITATION COUNCIL (NAAC) INDIA

In order to assess and accredit institutions of higher education in the country, the university grants commission constituted an independent body called National Assessment and Accreditation Council (NAAC) of India. It is an outcome of the recommendations of the national educational policy (1986)with the aim of addressing the issue of quality education in the country The Plan of Action (POA) 1992 advised to create an independent body at national level with the result NAAC was originated with its Headquarter at Bangalore in 1994.

This body is responsible to provide accreditation to educational institutions in India.

NATIONAL ACCREDITATION BOARD FOR HOSPITALS (NABH)

Definition

Due to expanding role of health insurance, rise in number of medicolegal cases, increasing knowledge of health consumers on their rights and medical tourism has resulted in need for accreditation of hospital.

Hospital accreditation has been referred as a self-assessment and external peer assessment process conducted by health care facilities to assess their level of performance in relation to established standards clearly, transparently and accurately and suggest to implement ways to continuously improve the quality of services.

In other words, hospital accreditation is a public recognition of health care organization by a national health care accredited body to ensure the achievement of accreditation standards by the health care organization demonstrated through an independent, external peer assessment of that organization's level of performance in relation to standard.

It is a transparent and accurate approach to improve the quality of the hospital. India follows National Accreditation board for hospital (NABH) standard and is recognized by international society for quality health care (ISQHC) that gives not only international recognition but also promotes international tourism.

Advantages of Accreditation to the Hospital

- Motivates to continued improvement of the organization
- Enhances commitment to quality patient care
- To provide opportunity to the hospital to benchmark with the best standard.

Advantages of Accreditation to The Hospital Employees

- To provide continuous learning
- To maintain a conducive work environment
- To facilitate leadership capabilities
- To enhance clinical care practices
- To promote professional development.

Advantages of Accreditation to the Regulatory Bodies

Accreditation of hospital provides a reliable information regarding facilities for care, infrastructure of hospital and level of standard of care.

Major Criteria or Standards Assessed in Accreditation of Hospital are the Following:

Patient Centered Standards

- Access, Assessment and Continuity of Care (AAC)
- Care of Patients (COP)
- Management of Medicine (MOM)
- Patients Rights and Education (PRE)
- Hospital Infection Control (HIC).

Organization Centered Standards

- Continuous Quality Improvement (CQI)
- Responsibility of Management (ROM)
- Facility Management and Safety (FMS)
- Human Resource Management (HRM)
- Information Management System (IMS).

Procedures for NABH Accreditation—Role of Administration

- Obtain a copy of the NABH standard tool from, NABH office
- Implement those standards in the hospital that requires accreditation
- From the website NABH obtain an application form for accreditation
- Fill the application form and submit the filled application along with fees to NABH secretariat including self assessment by the hospital
- Scrutiny of the application form by NABH secretariat
- Preliminary visit assessment by NABH team
- Final assessment of hospital by the committee members of accreditation
- Recommendation for accreditation by the committee
- Approval of accreditation by Chairman of NABH
- Issue of accreditation certificate by NABH
- Follow-up by the hospital administration as recommended by NABH. ("http://www.nabh.co/" \t "_blank"www.nabh.co)

PATIENT'S RIGHTS

The concept of patient's right originated from human rights, constitutional rights, civil rights, and consumer rights, codes of ethics of medical and nursing profession. Health is a human right and every individual in the country has a right to live. Since, health is a state subject, every state has a responsibility to ensure this rights to all individuals. The Government of India had enacted various laws to protect Indian citizens that include Consumer Protection Act, Medical Council Act, etc. The code of ethics for doctors and nurses provides duties and responsibilities of doctors and nurses. These forms the basis of patients rights.

Rights of the Patients

- Right to be respected
- Right to information on diagnosis, treatment and medications and all information related to care
- Right to maintain confidentiality regarding keeping patients records
- Right to privacy concerning medical care program
- Right to get prompt treatment in an emergency situation
- Right to refuse to participate in human experimentation, research, project
- Right to get copies of medical records

- Right to know hospital rules and regulations applied to patient and the facilities obtainable to the patient
- Right to get hospital expenses bill
- Right to seek second opinion of patient's disease.

CONSUMER PROTECTION ACT (CPA)

Definition of Consumer

In December 1986, the Indian parliament enacted Consumer Protection Act (CPA) and from 1st April 1987 it was implemented.

Any individual who avails services for which he has paid and is termed as consumer.

Aims of CPA

- To redress consumer grievances in a simple, speedy and inexpensive manner and the grievance caused by detective goods, deficient services and unfair trade practices.
- To include medical services under this act.

Patient Rights Under the Consumer Protection Act

- Right to protect the individual from hazardous goods and services.
- Right to get correct information about the quality and performance of goods and services.
- Right to be heard in matters pertaining to consumer where decision is taken regarding the consumer.
- Right for education of the consumer.
- Right to get quality medical services.

Grant of Reliefs Under CPA

- To replace the goods with new and undefective goods to the consumer
- The price to be returned to the consumer
- To give new good by removing the defect
- To refund the amount as a compensation to the consumer that has spent by the consumer for the loss he incurred
- To product should be barred from sale
- To stop the manufacture of hazardous goods
- To give correct publicity for avoiding the negative and misleading advertisement.

Forums of Consumer Protection Act: District forum, state commission national commission.

District Forum

The consumer can approach to district forum where the compensation price is ₹ 5 lakhs or less. In this forum, the decision is taken by district judge, two experts including one woman who are knowledgeable in economics, law, commerce, industry or administration.

The State Commission

The consumer can approach to state commission where the compensation price is more than ₹ 5 lakhs and less than ₹ 20 lakhs. This commission consisting three experts such as a person been worked as high court judge, who acts as a president of this commission. Two experts including a woman who are knowledgeable in economics, law, commerce, industry or administration.

National Commission

The national commission consisting of five members. The president of this commission is a person who is or has been a judge of the supreme court. Four experts including a woman who are knowledgeable in economics, law, commerce, industry or administration.

Consumer Protection Councils

This council is established by Government of India in which the minister in charge of the food and civil supplies of Govt of India and nonofficial members representing such interests selected by the government .

Responsibilities of Nurse

Ensure that the nurse is capable of doing competent and skilled care to patients. Otherwise she should not accept that assignment. She should be sensitive to the needs and problem of patients and demonstrate true concern for the patients. She needs to establish a conducive, therapeutic and trustworthy environment for patients and families. It is the responsibility of the nurse to communicate on the procedure she is going to do and the outcome of the procedure to the patient. Sometimes the patients may like to have a second opinion about their care, the nurse should facilitate or arrange for the same. The nurse should be available in the ward till the patient is discharged that give him confidence. Nurses need to enhance their professional knowledge, skills and attitudes through continuing education programmes.

HOSPITAL INFECTION CONTROL

Today, we are experiencing Hospital Acquired Infection (HAI) as a major problem worldwide. In spite of the scientific and medical advancement, antibiotic resistant organisms are growing very fast with emerging infectious pathogens with drug resistance. Outbreak of infections increasing. Alarming costs of antibiotics, irrational use of antibiotics by quacks pose a great problem.

Lack of proper legislation for implementation of best practice evidence informed, lack of specialized referral laboratory surveillance, lack of awareness among health care professionals and other employees of hospitals, are issues causing hospital infection. Adding to the above continuing education for health care professional also is not that encouraging.

There are three types of hospital infections:

- **Hospital associated infection:** When an infection occurs within 48 hours of admission of a patient. Patient is already having an infection and on incubation period. As per statistics as per the statistics it is predicted that 10–30% of patients admitted to hospitals having hospital associated infections in which 70% of organisms causing HAI are resistant to at least one antibiotic (www.biomerieux-diagnostics.com/upload/HAI)
- **Hospital acquired infection:** These are nosocomial infections that are acquired by the patient as a result of treatment or therapy in a hospital/ward. They are manifested infection symptoms within 48 hours or more after admission or 30 days after discharge from the hospital
- **Health care associated infection:** These are infections that patients get during hospitalization. There is an interaction of host (patient), agent (bacteria) environment (hospital ward in the process of infection).

The Role of Nurses in Prevention of Hospital Infection

Health Education

1. Communicate all health care providers about hospital guidelines for infection control
2. Ensure health education to staff, patient, and relatives regarding aseptic precaution and practices
3. Teach the mode of spread and mode of transmission of infection and prevention of transmission of infection
4. All employees in a hospital must undergo regular medical check-up
5. Proper disposal of solid and liquid wastes of the hospital to be maintained.
6. There should be a hospital infection control committee with following members:
   - Medical superintendent as a chairman of the committee
   - Nursing superintendent—member
   - In charge of CSSD—member
   - Sanitation/kitchen incharge—member
   - Microbiologist—member and secretary of the committee
   - **The major function** of hospital infection committee is to establish hospital infection control policies and guidelines that needs to be followed in all departments of the hospital. The guidelines in terms of:
     - Methods of sterilization of equipments and dressing to be monitored
     - Management of hospital waste should be done appropriately
     - Antibiotics protocol to be followed
     - Immunization of hospital staff to be facilitated
     - Pest control measures to be practiced.
7. There should be hospital surveillance system with a surveillance team headed by senior administrator, microbiologist. Incharge of hospital waste management and infection control nurse as members.
8. Functions of surveillance team are the following :
   - Implementation and supervision of infection control guidelines.
   - Collection of information about incidence of infection through departmental report.
   - Collection of lab reports.
   - Analysis of reports and communicating to the authority.
   - Ensure practices of prevention, promotion of healthy environment, appropriate hospital waste management and inducing aseptic procedures and practices.
9. **Provide environmental sanitation** include pest control and vector control measures. It should be done by:
   - Wet moping of floor
   - Proper hospital waste management
   - Disinfection and disposal of fomites
   - Facilitating safe drinking water
   - Providing clean toilets
   - Provision of CSSD supply department.
10. **Practice aseptic procedures and practices** include:
    - Handwashing before and after touching the patient and all procedures including handling fomites
    - Prevent from infection by wearing gowns, masks, gloves
    - Nontouch technique is good method to protect from infection
    - Carefully handle sharp instrument to prevent prick injuries

- All surfaces to be cleaned with antiseptic solution specially blood spilled area
- While doing dressing procedures, use sterilized cotton, gauze, instruments and dressing.

11. **Facilitate isolation of patient** for communicable disease:
    - Barrier nursing with minimum interference with the patient to be practiced.
    - Ensure restricted visitors
    - Individuals attending the patient should be immunized against preventable diseases
    - Use hyposolution for disinfecting fomites before disposal.
    - Patients should be encouraged to wear mask.
12. **Enhance health promotion strategies**
    - Increase host resistance and decrease suscepti bility.
    - Use of prophylactic therapy and passive immunization against infectious diseases.
    - Nutritious and balance diet.
    - Carrier detection and treatment.
13. **Prevention of nosocomial infections**
    - **Prevention of urinary tract infection**
      - It is better to avoid using catheter.
      - An intermittent catheterization could be better if it is essential
      - Use of catheter with lubrication to prevent injuries
      - When indwelling catheter is used use a close drainage system or condom catheter drainage to prevent infection.
    - **Respiratory infection pneumonia**
      - Proper tubing, respirator and humidifier to be used sterile
      - Frequent change of respiratory tubes may cause infection
      - Head up position to be made on suctioning the patient.
      - Prevent swallowing upper air way secretion in unconscious patients. Do not give liquids orally to unconscious patients
    - Practice sterile surgical wound management.
14. **Other responsibilities**
    - On suspicion of infection among patients send sample for culture and sensitivity with medical consultation
    - Investigate cause and prevent spread of infection
    - Ensure infection control guidelines followed
    - Restrict overcrowding and visitors to infected patient
    - Carriers must not be posted in sensitive wards
    - Immunize hospital staff against hepatitis B
    - Barrier nursing to all infected cases.

STANDARD SAFETY MEASURES

Standard safety measures are practiced throughout the world to reduce risks associated with health care delivery. According to World Health Organization (WHO), the management should create an institutional safety climate to implement recommended guidelines to improve health by reducing risk factors. It is mandatory that adequate nursing personnel, equipment and supplies knowledge on safety measures required by all workforce working in health care industry to enhance a safety climate for health consumers and health workforce.

Definitions

- **Standards:** A standard is a criterion based level of excellence that serves a guide for practice.
- **Safety:** Safety is the state of being safe, protected against physical, social, spiritual, financial, political, emotional, occupational, psychological, educational or other types or consequences of failure, damage, error, accidents, harm or any other event which could be considered nondesirable.
- **Safety measures:** They are measures or strategies taken to improve safety and reduce risk related to health.

STANDARD SAFETY MEASURES IN HOSPITAL

There are three standards of safety measures practiced in hospital setting. They are promotion of physical environment conducive to health, Biomedical waste management and standard precautions.

1. Promoting a Healthy Environment

The main aim of promoting a healthy environment in the hospital is to provide a favorable setting to recovery, to promote comfort of the patients, destruction and control of vermin and preventing mechanical injuries, fire and chemical injuries to patients.

2. Biomedical Waste Management (BMW)

It refers to proper handling and disposal of any solid, liquid waste, that include container and any intermediate product, which is generated during the diagnosis, treatment or immunization of human beings or animals, in research or caring patients or generated in the production or testing of biological and the animal waste from slaughter houses.

Classification of waste

- **General waste:** These include waste from sweeping, kitchen waste, supplies, paper pieces waste water from laundry, human anatomical waste solid waste sharps hypodermic needles, stitching needles, needles attached with tubing, scalpel blades, razors, etc.

CLASSIFICATION OF WASTE CATEGORY–1

- Human anatomical wastes
- Animal anatomical wastes
- Microbiology and biotechnology wastes
- Waste sharps
- Discarded medicines and cytotoxic drugs
- Soiled wastes include items contaminated with blood, body fluids such as cotton, dressings, linen, beddings, etc.
- Solid wastes, i.e. waste generated from disposable items other than sharps such as tubing, catheters, IV sets.
- Liquid wastes (washing, cleaning)
- Incineration ash
- Chemical wastes (disinfectants, insecticides).

COLOR CODING FOR SEGREGATION OF BMW

- **Yellow color:** Human and animal anatomical waste/ Microbiology and biotechnology wastes.
- **Red color:** Waste and deep burial soiled cotton/ dressings/linen/beddings, etc.
- **Blue color:** Tubing's, catheters, IV sets, autoclaving/ microwaving/chemical treatment waste sharps (needles, syringes, scalpels, blades. etc.) autoclaving
- **Black color**: Microwaving/chemical treatment and destruction/shredding discarded medicines/cytotoxic drugs, incineration ash.

Each institution should develop its own biowaste management policy and ensure that the health care workers are adequately trained to handle biological waste. All the employees should be encouraged to practice measures such as universal safety precautions, hand washing and proper segregation of waste material in their work settings. Proper house-keeping is very necessary and the hospital premises should be kept clean and well-ventilated. Use of disinfectants are beneficial in this regard.

Steps in the Management of Biomedical Waste

The management should see that all the waste generated are segregated and categorized. It should be put in appropriate color coded bins and should be disposed within 48 hours. These wastes are to be transported carefully and treated as per guidelines.

3. Standard Precautions

- **Standard precautions** are measures to reduce the transmission of blood borne or other type of pathogens. They are the fundamental level of infection control strategies used as minimum precautions which are to be used, in the care of all patients admitted in hospital or any health care facility.
- **Hand hygiene:** One of the important component in safety precaution is hand hygiene. It is the most cost-effective method to prevent transmission of pathogens associated with health care. The health workers should use personal protective equipment when they contact anticipated with blood and body fluids, or pathogens. Apart from the health workers, all individuals including patients and visitors should comply with infection control practices in health care settings. The control of spread of pathogens from the source is basic principle to avoid transmission. After the Severe Acute Respiratory Syndrome (SARS) outbreak, respiratory hygiene/cough etiquette, now included as part of standard precautions.

Hand Hygiene* (WHO Guidelines)

Handwashing (40–60 sec): Wet hands and apply soap; rub all surfaces; rinse hands and dry thoroughly with a single use towel; use towel to turn off faucet.

Handrubbing (20–30 sec): Apply enough product to cover all areas of the hands; rub hands until dry.

- Before and after any direct patient contact and between patients, whether or not gloves are worn.
- Immediately after gloves are removed.
- Before handling an invasive device.
- After touching blood, body fluids, secretions, excretions, nonintact skin, and contaminated items, even if gloves are worn.
- During patient care, when moving from a contaminated to a clean body site of the patient.
- After contact with inanimate objects in the immediate vicinity of the patient.

* WHO Guidelines on Hand Hygiene in Health Care (Advanced draft), at: http://www.who.int/patientsafety/information_centre/ghhad_ download/en/index.html.

Gloves

- Wear when touching blood, body fluids, secretions, excretions, mucous membranes.
- Change between tasks and procedures on the same patient after contact with potentially infectious material.
- Remove gloves after use, before touching non-contaminated items and surfaces, and before going to another patient.
- Perform hand hygiene immediately after removal.

Facial Protection (Eyes, Nose, and Mouth)

Wear a surgical or procedure mask and eye protection (face shield, goggles) to protect mucous membranes of the eyes, nose, and mouth during activities that are likely to generate splashes or sprays of blood, body fluids, secretions, and excretions.

Gown

- Wear to protect skin and prevent soiling of clothing during activities that are likely to generate splashes or sprays of blood, body fluids, secretions, or excretions.
- Remove soiled gown as soon as possible, and perform hand hygiene.

Prevention of Needle Stick Injuries* (WHO Guidelines)

When handling needles, scalpels, and other sharp instruments or devices, cleaning used instruments disposing of used needles.

Respiratory hygiene and cough etiquette (Persons with respiratory symptoms should apply)

Cover their nose and mouth when coughing/sneezing, with tissue or mask, dispose of used tissues and masks, and perform hand hygiene after contact with respiratory secretions.

Health care facilities should place acute febrile respiratory symptomatic patients at least 1 meter (3 feet) away from others in common waiting areas, if possible.

post visual alerts at the entrance to health care facilities, instructing persons with respiratory symptoms to practice respiratory hygiene/cough etiquette. Provide making hand hygiene resources, tissues and masks available in common areas and areas used for the evaluation of patients with respiratory illnesses.

Environmental Cleaning

Use adequate procedures for the routine cleaning and disinfection of environmental and other frequently touched surfaces.

Linens

Handle, Transport, and Process for used Linen in a Manner Which

- Prevents skin and mucous membrane exposures and contamination of clothing.
- Avoid transfer of pathogens to other patients and or the environment.

Waste Disposal

- Ensure safe waste management. Treat waste contaminated with blood, body fluids, secretions and excretions as clinical waste, in accordance with local regulations.
- Human tissues and laboratory waste that is directly associated with specimen processing should also be treated as clinical waste.
- Discard single use items properly.

Patient Care Equipment

- Handle appropriately equipment soiled with blood, body fluids, secretions, and excretions in a manner that prevents skin and mucous membrane exposures, contamination of clothing, and transfer of pathogens to other patients or the environment.
- Clean, disinfect, and reprocess reusable equipment appropriately before use with another patient.

The Role of Nurse Administrator in Facilitating Standard Safety Measures in Hospital

- Nursing administrators and managers have a vital role in assessing and monitoring the practice of nurses in different health care facility.
- Their role in policy and procedures development is immense in terms of providing safe care to patients.
- Providing the guidelines of standard safety measures to all nursing personnel and a copy of the same is available in all nursing units is her responsibility.
- The nurse administrator ensures that all nursing personnel are knowledgeable of standard safety precaution while caring patients.
- Organizes in-service education to all nurses and health workers in this regards

* The SIGN Alliance at: http://www.who.int/injection_safety/sign/)

- The availability of staff development departments is a critical factor in assisting the nurses to use these standard safety measures, policies and procedures in delivering safe and competent care.
- Nursing administrators and managers can also increase patient safety by fostering an environment in which nurses are in control of their own nursing practice.
- Ensure all the equipments/supplies available to practice standard safety measures.
- Hospitals that provide for professional autonomy for nurses and support control over nursing practice have better patient care.
- The nurse administrator also collects data with regards to any adverse event and participates in research activities.

Box. 20.1: Research highlights

Hemani Kumar et al. conducted a cross sectional randomized study on Legal awareness and responsibilities of nursing staff in administration of patient care in a Trust Hospital, Pune. The main aim was to ass the legal awareness and knowledge on basic nursing procedures. The sample size was 443 nurses comprising 304 GNMs and 139 ANMs. The GNM and ANM nursing staff deployed at the nursing home and general wards only were randomly screened and specialty nurses were exempted.

An open ended questionnaire was used to assess the level of legal awareness among the nursing staff. The researchers observed that the knowledge on various legal provisions, as was applicable to nursing, across all categories of nurses which were under review, was found to be poor. The nursing staff had poor knowledge on patients' rights and also on their legal obligations towards patients. The GNM nurses fared better than ANM nurses. However, 46.67 % of nurses were found to be aware about cases of omission or commission.

The study concluded that nurses had poor knowledge on the law that governed their profession and that in days to come, it would become increasingly difficult for them to avoid law suits which were prepared against them, unless remedial actions were taken.

Box 20.2: Research highlights

INFLUENCE OF STATE REGISTRATION COUNCIL ON QUALITY CLINICAL PRACTICE*

The public has a right to expect registered nurses to demonstrate professional competence throughout their careers. In all the activities of professional bodies, there needs to be a balance between professional bodies and public so as to promote nursing care. The statutory body has specific roles in clarifying and disseminating documents, lobbying and regulating and advocating for education and issues. Shija Binoy and Jaya Bijoy conducted a descriptive study aimed to assess the knowledge and opinion of staff nurses regarding the influence of state registration council on clinical practice and to recommend strategies for enhancing the roles of state registration council and nursing personnel on clinical practice.

Hundred staff nurses working in selected hospitals of Bhopal, Madhya Pradesh were selected by Stratified Random sampling technique. The tool used for the study was structured questionnaire and opinionnaire. Majority of study participants (90%) were females and were between the age group of 36–45 years (82%). Majority (87%) of staff nurses did not possess knowledge on role and responsibilities of state registration council, continuing professional education, special certification. The role responsibility known to the staff nurses was issue a licensure for practice. Majority (94%) of study participants opinioned that state registration council has no influence on clinical practice. This study concluded that state registration council has a pivotal role in setting standards for clinical practice. It exists to safeguard the health and well being of the society. Council needs to act with integrity, accountability, exhibit professionalism, look for innovative solutions and positive responsive feedback mechanism. The state registration council and nursing personnel work together to embrace excellence.

(*Sija Binoy and Jaya Binoy, faculty Pragyan College of Nursing Bhopal)

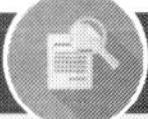

SUMMARY POINTS

- ✓ The expanded and extended role of the nurses warrants for knowledge, skill and decision-making capabilities in legal and ethical aspects of care at advance level which is mandatory for every nurse to safeguard herself and her patients and families from legal rights in relation to health, therefore that a nurse should know legal and ethical aspects of nursing, in her day to day practice.
- ✓ Law refers to rules, regulation and conduct that guides individual's action. It is established by a competent authority which each one of us needs to follow as a citizen of India.
- ✓ The Indian Council of Medical Research brought out the 'policy statement on ethical considerations involved in Research on human Subjects' in 1980 and revised these guidelines in 2000 as the 'ethical guidelines for Biomedical research on human subjects'. Due to further rapid developments in science and technology in India after the release of the second version, it became necessary to update these guidelines to make adequate specific provision to meet ethical challenges led further revision at 2006. The ICMR is funded by the Government of India through the department of Health research, Ministry of health and family welfare.

The need for Institutional Ethics Committee (IEC) in medical and research organizations resulted from the realization that affirms human rights as a special right of all members of society. Health care professionals may not be able to do what is right in all instances as evidenced by the number studies.

- ✓ All nurses are required to follow code of ethics and professional conduct formulated by Indian Nursing Council (INC).
- ✓ The violation may result from unintentional cause referred as unintentional tort that means the violation is caused by intentional actions, a breach of duty,: negligence or malpractice–conduct which falls below the standard of care. So , there are four critical elements that must be proven in a malpractice case.
- ✓ Liabilities referred as obligations that legally connects an individual or establishment to settle a wrongful act they may have committed. These are settled over a period of time with money, goods or services.
- ✓ Medico legal case: It is defined as a case of injury or ailment, where some criminality is involved or investigations by the legal authorities are required. In other words it is a medical condition with legal implications for the attending doctor who assesses the patient, identifies the problem and decide the case is legally implicated and further investigation to be made by law enforcing agency. It is a legal case where medical intervention is necessary suspected accident, poisoning, burns, comatose or brought dead persons admitted to the casualty are some of the medico legal cases.
- ✓ License refers to the permission granted by competent authority to exercise a certain privilege that, without such authorization, would constitute an illegal act. The certificate or the document itself that confers permission to engage in otherwise proscribed conduct.
- ✓ A ccreditation is a recognition awarded by an authorized health care accreditation body to an institution when it adheres to the accreditation standards, demonstrated through an independent external peer assessment regarding its level of performance in relation to the standards.
- ✓ Health is a human right and every individual in the country has a right to live. Since, health is a state subject, every state has a responsibility to ensure this rights to all individuals. The Government of India had enacted various laws to protect Indian citizens. That include Consumer Protection Act, Medical Council Act, etc. The code of ethics for doctors and nurses provides duties and responsibilities of doctors and nurses. These form the basis of patient's rights.
- ✓ Any individual who avails services for which he has paid and is termed as consumer.
- ✓ According to World Health Organization, the management should create an institutional safety climate to implement recommended guidelines and to improve health by reducing risk factors. It is mandatory that adequate nursing personnel, equipment and supplies knowledge on safety measures required by all workforce working in health care industry to enhance a safety climate for health consumers and health workforce.

REVIEW QUESTIONS

1. Enumerate various legal and ethical issues in nursing. Describe the role of nurse administrator in maintaining legal and ethical standard among nurses in hospital.
2. Define medico legal case. What are the responsibilities of nursing personnel in relation to caring Medico legal cases?
3. Describe the code of ethics and professional conduct for nurses in India.
4. Discuss the role of nurse administrator in prevention of hospital infection.
5. Describe the standard precautions to be practiced by nurses in infection control.
6. Write short notes on the following:
   a. Relationship of law and ethics
   b. Liabilities
   c. National accreditation board for hospitals (NABH)
   d. Consumer protection act and health
   e. Patients rights
   f. Biomedical waste management (BMW).

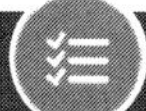

SELECTED READINGS

1. Bramhe R, Mehendale S. Profile and role of the members of ethics committees in hospitals and research organizations in Pune, India. Indian J Med Ethics. 2009;6:78–84. [PubMed]
2. Hemant Kumar,1 Gokhale,2 Kalpana Jain, 3 and D.R. Mathur4 Legal Awareness and Responsibilities of Nursing Staff in Administration of Patient Care in A Trust Hospital J Clin Diagn Res. 2013 Dec; 7(12): 2814–2817. Published online 2013 Nov 18. doi: 10.7860/JCDR/2013/7737.3886
3. Hospital Administration Made Easy http//hospiad.blogspot.com An effort solely to help students and aspirants in their attempt to become a successful Hospital Administrator. hospi ad DR. N. C. DAS
4. http// HYPERLINK "http://www.nabh.co/" \t "_blank"www.nabh.co re/ghhad_ download/en/index.htm
5. http://www.legalmatch.com/law-library/article/tort-law-
6. Jesani A. Ethics in ethics committees: Time to share experiences, discuss challenges and do a better job. Indian J Med Ethics. 2009;6:62–3. [PubMed]
7. Kaur Harbinger. Legal Aspects of Nursing, Nursing Journal of India- Centennial Issue, 2010
8. Kumar N. Bioethics Activities in India under ICMR. [Last accessed on 2011 Nov 11]. http://icmr.nic.in/bioethics/cc_biothics/presentations/haryana/activity.pdf .
9. Mala Ramanathan. AMCHSS, SCTIMST Functions and responsibilities of Functions and responsibilities of Institutional Ethics Committees Short Term Training Program 'Ethics in Social Science Research Related to Health'ICMR, New Delhi and CSER, Mumbai 27 Nov – 1 Dec 2006,
10. Nadig P, Joshi M, Uthappa A. Competence of ethics committees in patient protection in clinical trials. Indian J Med Ethics. 2011;8:151–3. [PubMed]
11. Pandiya A. Quality of independent review board/ethics committee oversight in clinical trials in India. Perspect Clin Res. 2011;2:45–7. [PMC free article] [PubMed]
12. Srinivasan S, Nikarge S. Ethical concerns in clinical trials in India: An investigation. [Last accessed on 2011 July 25]. Available from:http://www.cser.in/Publication .
13. Tharyan P. Ethics Commitees and clinical Trials registration in India: Opportunities, obligations, challenges and solutions. Indian J Med Ethics. 2011;8:1689. [PubMed]
14. The Govt. of Kerala. Kerala Medicolegal Code,2010.
15. The Indian Nursing Council Act 1947.
16. The Indian Nursing Council, Code of Ethics and Professional Conduct.
17. The Kerala Nurses and Midwives Act 1953.
18. Thomas G. Institutional Ethics Committees: Critical gaps. Indian J Med Ethics.2011;8:200. [PubMed]

UNIT XI NURSING INFORMATICS

21

Introduction to Nursing Informatics

LEARNING OBJECTIVES

This chapter imparts learning about:

- Current Trends in Nursing Informatics
- General Purpose of Nursing Informatics
- Use of Computers in Hospital and Community
- Patient Record System
- Nursing Records and Reports
- Management Information and Evaluation System (MIES)
- E-nursing, Telemedicine and Telenursing
- Electronic Medical Records
- Research Highlights

CURRENT TRENDS IN NURSING INFORMATICS

The technological advancement has made tremendous impact on health care delivery system. Nurses are using technology for the past several decades in nursing care. We are living in digital era today and the advances in information technology have created new roles for nurses, and stressed the need for all nursing personnel irrespective of their position to become more knowledgeable about health information concepts and the technology. The Indian Nursing Council (INC) has already introduced information technology in nursing curriculum i.e. designed to manage and process information in their seminars and research conducted at undergraduate, postgraduate and doctoral level.

Telemedicine and telenursing are coming up to exchange information from one place to another with the purpose of improving the patient's health condition. Nurses are able to access the patient's electronic health records, and able to provide the patients with health care information and also with education and other technologies.

Concept of Nursing Informatics

Informatics comes from the French word *informatique* which means computer science. Informatics is referred as a combination of computer science and information science, it further explains as an application of computer science and information science to the management and processing of data, information, and knowledge in a particular discipline like medical informatics, nursing informatics, health informatics, etc.

According to Hebda (1998), nursing informatics refers to the use of computers technology to support nursing, including clinical practice, nursing administration, nursing education, and nursing research.

American Nurses Association (ANA) (1994) has explained nursing informatics as the development and evaluation of applications, tools, processes, and structures which help nurses with the management of data in taking care of patients or supporting the practice of nursing. ANA, (2015) states Nursing Informatics (NI) is a specialty that combines nursing science with various information management and analytical sciences to identify, define, manage, and communicate data, information, knowledge, and wisdom in nursing practice.

Nursing informatics (NI) is the synthesis of nursing, its information, and management with information processing and communication technology, to support the health of people worldwide (IMIA-NI Strategic, July 2007).

GENERAL PURPOSES OF NURSING INFORMATICS (NI)

- The purpose of informatics aims to develop nurses, as well as to benefit from integrating computer technology into everyday nursing practice.
- NI supports nurses, consumers, patients, the interprofessional health care team, and other management personnel in their decision-making in all roles and all settings to achieve desired patient care outcomes. Effective utilization of information structures, information processes, and information technology support nurses and health care team to achieve goals.
- NI ensures nurses basic information selection and utility of information systems and information management in all aspects of nursing practice.
- NI helps to apply the vast technological advances in health care, including Health Information System (HIS), internet usage and their relevant integration.
- NI ensures nurses on how to use computers and information management systems in their clinical, and administrative practices.
- NI imparts guidance to nurses on implementing computerized solutions for information management strategies.

USE OF COMPUTERS IN HOSPITAL AND COMMUNITY

The application of Information Communication Technology (ICT) in various fields especially in health care system is very common today. Increasing use of computers in hospitals is one of the examples for it. Technology has replaced many manual strategies of daily activities of the hospitals, and has encouraged nurses and doctors to work more efficiently with patients and families.

To increase the efficiency of working is the main objectives of use of computers to the health care system. Computers are supporting nurses and doctors keep online with various activities starts from admission to discharge procedures and their follow-up in scheduled appointments. The advancements that computers have brought to hospital setting can be applied in four different areas like clinical nursing and medical procedures, administration, research and community settings.

Clinical Nursing Procedure

In clinical application, computers are used for:

- **Assessment:** The computers are used in assessment of patients. It helps to collect relevant data and preserve them in patient's record.
- **Patient monitoring:** In special health care units like casualty, neonatal intensive care unit (NICU), intensive care unit (ICU), pediatric intensive care unit (PICU), and intensive coronary care unt (ICCU) computers helps in monitoring vital sign, calculations of cardiac output, and pulmonary artery pressure. This helps to compare the current health status with the past condition of the patient.
- **Documentation:** Nurse's observations entered in the computer specially in nurses notes and patients records. Computer programs helps nurses as a library with common terminology and questions pertinent to care that they can select appropriately to describe the patient's condition, or answering the questions to describe patients status. There is also documentation on the computer that lists on a patient's discharge sheet about all the personnel that worked on their case.

First personal digital assistant a hand-held computer was used in 1996. According to ANA (2001), all nurses need to use nursing informatics.

In teaching hospitals, video conferencing and web based conferencing connects students and educators across distance and connects diverse student groups. Many nurses use hand-held computers such as personal digital assistants to communicate with physicians about the patients in their care.

Thus, clinical applications of computers in nursing are so many. Physicians prescribe medications and treatments on the computer, and the nurse can either transcribe those orders onto paper tools or print the paper documents for use in patient care. Staff nurses can order medications or supplies on the computer to look up drug interactions or research medical condition.

Telemedicine

The internet is used to transfer medical instruction, or consultation, examinations, and small medical procedures to patients or health care professionals.

Electronic Medical Records (EMR)

EMR is an emerging technological application of information in hospital today. It has increased the efficiency of health care facility by providing patient information easily available. It helps to save space comparing the occupation of space for huge volume of paper-based hospital records. It eliminates illegible handwriting, decreases errors on data-entry, and connects related records automatically. It can be opened by selected authority with passwords and thus it maintain security of records. The computer keeps track of the individuals who have visited certain records. It reduces paper and storage services in hospitals.

Nursing Service Administration

Computers are used in the administrative areas of nursing for basic tasks that once were done on paper. Staffing and scheduling systems are used to construct daily, weekly or monthly. Many scheduling systems also collect data on individual employees such as the amount of sick time used or vacation hours accumulated. Staffing and scheduling systems often provide a variety of reports to the administrative nurse. Budgeting and financial tracking are another way in which computers are used in nursing administration. The performance appraisal report of nurses are prepared using computers.

Nurse administrators use computers for financial administration such as to monitor the cost of nursing services and to compare the expenses between the past and the present. Computers help in the calculating of salary and benefits and tax calculation for all nurses and health workers. At the same time, it helps to assess the bills of the hospitals paid. It ensures the administrator that the health care given to patients are cost-effective and efficient. Computers evaluates the quality assurance program of the hospitals and the utilization of available resources appropriately. Computers helps to justify new roles and job description of nursing personnel.

Nursing Research

In research, we can use computers for:

- Preparation of a research protocol
- Review of related literature
- Identify various research approaches and designs
- Data gathering by developing research instruments
- Preparation of computer assisted teaching as nurse led intervention instruction
- Statistical analysis using various software packages like SSPS
- Computing data and data presentation by charts and diagram including tables.

The application of computer technology is widely used in medical research. These databases gathered from computers allow the doctor to search of relevant literature and abstracts and standardized tools pertinent to his study. This saves the time of the researcher. Online journals are available in internet for references. Web based instruction is very common now-a-days where the teacher can teach the student without direct or personal contact. Computerized video system takes online classes, tutorials and simulated real life situation makes learning more easy today with computers.

Community Settings

In community settings, we use computers for collecting statistics, community diagnosis, patient-appointments, home care management, and remote patient monitoring. Computers are used in gathering statistics accurate documentation in a compiled, summarized, and meaningful form. The information is presented in table, chart diagram and graph for better understanding. The patient appointments-identification system of the hospital is a means to increase efficiency in areas such as waiting rooms. The advantages include minimizing waiting time, smoothing the load of appointments, and establishing patient priority. The computer also assists in home care management. This includes personal medical plans for the patients that are stored in computer memory banks. These plans assess the personal care the patients would do for themselves such as monitoring prescriptions and other activities. The computer is helpful in the area of automated remote patient monitoring. It is most often used on patients with pacemakers.

An example of this system is an electrocardiogram (ECG). Use of computer kiosks for teaching community is used in villages where the villagers can feed their questions and the computer where the network is connected with a doctor in community health center can give them answer or direction.

The application of computer systems to hospitals has many advantages:

- It provides clinical information in an easy and simplest manner
- The application of technological information system has enhanced health care system efficiency
- The abnormal speed and efficiency of computers has resulted in better care for population
- The fear of loss of information from paper based record is reduced by online medical record system
- Computers enhances the accuracy of the information resulted in the best-equipped medical plan for each patient
- Advanced systems are bringing more advanced care resulted in saving lives of patient with prompt intervention. (Ashutash K)

PATIENT RECORD SYSTEM

Maintaining patient record is one of the major functions of hospital administration. Records are permanent items which are kept in hospital for minimum of 15 years in earlier days. Because of complexity of the organization, increasing activities of the hospital and increasing diagnostic and treatment modalities as well as increasing number of in-patients in the hospital the administration is compelled to store a large volume of records that occupies a major share of space in the hospital. To overcome this issue, most of the hospitals have switched over from paper based medical record system to electronic record system.

The patient record is the very important document for information concerning a patient's health care. It has an impact on everyone associated with providing, and receiving, health care services. Though many technological advances in health care has been implicated the patient record system in recent years, patient record in the government hospitals of some of the states in India remains unchanged.

Present Scenario of Patient/Medical Records

At present, the condition of patient record system, in the public hospitals is quite discouraging. The clinicians record patient information, diagnosis and treatments in paper in a free style manner, which is called the **case Sheet.** There have been some attempts in the recent past to standardize the manual forms, but there is still a long way to go. The paper medical records remain the legal and official record of patient care. Although, some super-specialty hospitals have started using computer-generated information as part of the medical record, file folders full of slips of paper and massive file rooms are still the norm in the public hospitals.

Purposes of Management of Patients Records

Accurate and relevant documentation enhances better communication as well as continuity, consistency, and efficiency, and reinforces professionalism within nursing. For the sake of patients and professionals as well as nurses' legal protection, they should record their observation accurately and professionally. The ultimate aim of record management is to store, to protect, preserve and provide records to the administrator or nursing personnel as and when they require them. It also helps to remove the obsolete and old records so that space for storing new records could be made available.

There should be ideal control system of managing records with following key features:

- There should be clear cut policies for managing hospital records.
- All health care personnel must be aware of the objectives of keeping records.
- There should be sufficient equipments and design of filing system of records to maintain current and future needs of the hospital.
- There should be clear cut policies to discard records which are no longer required.
- There should be policies for retaining some of the specific records which are needed for legal transactions, assets, liabilities, making decision for future of the organizational activities, etc.
- There should be a good filing system with the principles of availability when needed, carefully stored and protected, and properly arranged so that it could be located easily when needed.
- There should be policies to handover the records to patient or referred doctor when requested.

Characteristics of Good Filing System

- **Compactness:** It means it should occupy minimum space.
- **Accessibility:** It means the file should be easily available if they are not confidential records.
- **Economy:** It means it is cost-effective in terms of installation and operation.
- **Simplicity:** It means it does not require complex skill to operate.
- **Flexibility:** It is not a rigid system as and when needed we can switch over to other system.
- **Easy to locate** the records for health care professionals.
- There should be **a cross reference number** if the file number is changed or if the file is closed.

MEDICAL RECORDS

Medical records and reports are very important documents used in health care delivery system. These are documentation of an individual patient's medical history and medical care during his hospitalization maintained by the attending physician or surgeon in an orderly and systematic manner. It is also termed as case sheet of the patient. The contents of the patients' records include complete history of the patients (past medical history, surgical history, family history) present history of complaints, social history, immunization history, medication if any, allergies, habits diagnostic investigations and reports, that include X-ray reports if needed, vital signs including blood pressure, diagnosis, prescription of treatment, (drugs and therapy) nurse's notes, progressive notes by attending physician/surgeon.

Many other information are kept within the medical record are digital images of the patient, flow sheets from operations informed consent, ECG report, intake and output chart and other important information based on his/her case.

A discharge summary is written when the patient is discharged from the hospital.

The unit incharge nurses and doctors has a great responsibility to maintain complete and accurate records of patients. Signature of the physician/surgeon and in nurses notes, the nurse's signature to be must for the completion of records.

Medical records should be complete, adequate and accurate.

Significance of Medical Records

- It is useful for nurses and doctors to provide a comprehensive and informed care.
- It is a channel of communication between doctors and health care team for planning everyday care.
- Keeping medical records are essential for the hospital for accreditation and to meet the requirements of regulatory mechanism.
- It is needed for completing hospital statistics such as admission, discharge, transfer, death, Left Against Medical Advice (LAMA), abscond of patients, morbidity and mortality pattern, calculation of bed occupancy, calculation of staffing, etc.
- Medical records are good educational resource for teaching doctors, nurses and allied health workers.
- Medical records observations are utilized by researchers to conduct research in their specific area.
- It is an authentic document that protects legally doctors and nurses.
- Medical records meet the patients need also. It is very essential to get a medical certificate, insurance claim, claim for financial support from other agencies, and the discharge summary and investigation reports given to the patient helps to avoid duplicate investigation.
- Medical records meets the physician's needs also. It helps to maintain continuity of care, communication with other members of the health team, demonstrates the capabilities of the physician and ensures practice of scientific medicine. The physician can refer the records for medico legal purpose.
- The hospital or health care facility is benefitted from medical records. These records are useful in generating statistics, teaching for medical and nursing students and allied health professionals, can control admission, helps in planning for resources and other services, improve quality patient care for better outcome and protect the institution law suits.
- Public health authority is also benefitted by medical records. Medical records ensures reliable information regarding morbidity pattern, causes of mortality, births, infection diseases, notifiable diseases, and prevalence of diseases that is very essential to know the health status of the population of that particular region.
- It demonstrates quality assurance.

Thus, medical records serve as a clinical document, scientific document, administrative and legal document relating to patient care written in sequence of events justifies diagnosis and treatment and the patient care outcome.

Types of Records Maintained in Hospital

- Outpatient records: Each type of outpatient has their registers that is compiled with special out patient wise and overall OPD statistics at the end of the day
- Inpatient records-case sheet, or bed head ticket (BHT)
- Consultation sheets
- TPR chart
- Intake output chart
- X-ray, ECG and scan physiotherapy request sheets
- Laboratory form
- Diet intend sheet
- Medication intend sheet
- Laboratory reports
- Consent form
- Procedures protocols
- Various registers:Admission and discharge, ward inventory, stock register, CSSD and linen register, exchange register, ward indent, patient reports book, attendance register, daily duty assignment register. etc. It depends on the type of service unit.

NURSING RECORDS AND REPORTS

Nursing is a practice discipline. Nursing professionals are accountable for the services rendered to their patients and community. One of the important functions of nurses is documentation or record keeping.

Documentation in nursing is a key factor in our role and responsibility as a patient care provider. It is very important for assessing the standard of care was rendered to a patient in quality. Failure to chart, incompleteness, and poor communication are hard to defend.

A record is a written document that communicates information relevant to a patient's diagnosis, treatment and other intervention. It is permanent in nature. A nursing record is a clinical tool describes the nursing care given to the individual family or community. It is more scientific, legal and administrative tool. However, reports are oral or written exchanges of information shared between nurses and members of the health care team and family.

Each nurse uses her unique style in writing records However, it should be written clearly, relevantly appropriately and completely. Nursing record should comprising of relevant information based on observation, communication and services rendered. It should be neatly and legibly presented keeping in mind that this record is legally very important for a nurse, doctor, and the hospital. Nursing records are confidential documents accurately dated, timed and signed by the assigned nurse.

When the nurse maintains nursing record, the following factors to be kept in mind:

- The nurse should be very careful when she documents:
  - Abnormal vital signs
  - Codes
  - Transfers
  - Change of nursing shift or patient hand offs
  - Taking verbal orders
  - Noting physician's orders
  - Verifying medication orders.
- When the laboratory reports received, if the nurse finds a critical value, she should report within 15 minutes to the concerned physician for verification.
- When the physician is not able to reach within 30 minutes to see the critical value of lab report, the nurse should follow the standing orders or policy without fail as next step.
- While writing the report avoid using general statement.
- All nursing documentation should be legible, simple, objective complete and accurate written in black or blue ink. No grammatical or spelling mistakes are desirable.
- Allergies should be highlighted and flow sheets filled out completely.
- Avoid charting in advance that means after giving care or procedure, the nurse should chart in nurses notes not before giving care.
- All assessment procedures should be carefully done and recorded.
- The data should be analyzed and documented in DARE approach that means Document the data, Action taken by the nurse, Response from the patient and Evaluate the patient's condition Documentation should include staff notified and steps taken.
- Sometimes nurses use their own abbreviation in nurseing record. Only accepted abbreviation by nursing policy and procedures to be followed while writing nurses notes.
- Write exactly the patients responses and to be documented by time and date.

Advantages of Nursing Records

For the Individual and Family

- Records are useful to give information about the complete history of the patient and family.
- Records help in maintaining the continuity of care.
- Records provides evidences to defend legal questions.
- Records provides data on health needs and problems of patient and family that is need for research.
- Records facilitates for clinical teaching of nursing and medical students as an instructional aid.

For the Doctor

- Records are useful to diagnose, treat, follow-up and evaluation of patient care.
- Records facilitates continuity of care.
- Records demonstrates progress made in patient care.
- It acts as a tool for self-evaluation services by doctor.
- A record safeguards the doctor from legal problems and law suits.
- Records are useful for teaching and research.

For the Nurse

- Record ensures the nursing services rendered and the health status of the patient.
- Facilitates with data for future planning and allocation of resources.
- Provides evidences for the quality of the services provided.
- Records act as a tool for exchanging information among members of the health team.
- It is a managerial tool used for planning the future services. Indicate plans for the future.

For Authorities

- Records are required for gathering data for future planning, allocation of resources and organizational control.
- Records ensure the supervisor to monitor and evaluate the services provided by health care professionals including teaching and research.

Cumulative or continuing records are useful, time saving and economical and provides for the overall profile of the patients from admission to discharge period.

Family records gives information about the family members in both health and sickness situation, which are kept in family folder. It ensures an effective, economic service to the family as a whole.

Individual records are formats that are used for specific types of services such as TB, maternity, cancer, etc. all such individual records which relate to members of one family are secured in a single family folder.

Forms, case cards and registers. Family folder, eligible couple and child register, Sterilization and IUD (Intrauterine device), register, MCH card/register, child card/register, Birth and death register, Subcenters/ PHC/clinic register, stock and issue register, reports of blood test of malaria and filaria, malaria parasite positive case register and others.

The head nurse's responsibility for the clinical record are:

- **Protection of records:** The head nurse has a vital responsibility to protect and safeguard the patient's record from loss or destruction. Each patients record should be completed before it is send to medical record section of the hospital and none of the sheets from the patient's file to be removed. All the records to be kept safely in a cupboard after the discharge of patients till it is handed over to medical record section.
- **Safeguarding its content:** All the records should be kept confidential. The head nurse has a responsibility to take care of medico legal case records with special care.
- **Completeness:** The medical and nursing aspects of the care given (such as TPR chart, Intake-out chart, medication chart, observation chart if any, nurse notes and care plans) to patients to be recorded completely.No part of care or treatment should be missed from the records. Before submitting the records to medical record section, the ward sister should see that all aspects of care is written and completed with signature of the nurse/doctor and date.
- **Responsibility for nurses' notes:** Each hospital has its unique format for nurses notes. Nurses should write the notes in that format accurately and completely.
- **Get into the habit:** Nurse should record the information regarding the patient with accuracy, consistency, objectivity and without using unambiguous information.
- The nurse should be able to justify for any decision she records.
- Ensure nurses notes are accurately dated, timed, and signed, with the name of the nurse.
- When the care giver is involved in patient care, that should be mentioned in nurses notes.
- Errors should be corrected by putting a single stroke in the incorrect statement and signing and dating it. Do not overwrite the information.
- Be prompt in writing the record as soon as the event occurred and the care given. It is legally important and, by law, within 24 hours, making clear any subsequent change is needed.
- Nursing care plan should include assessment, nursing diagnosis, expected outcome, plan for implementing care, and implementation of care and evaluation of the outcome achieved or not. All column should be completed and the signature of the nurse and date of the care plan to be mentioned.

REPORTS

Definition

Reports are information or facts about patient communicated by nurse to health care team or patients and families. Both written and oral reports are used by nurses to exchange information.

Reports can be compiled daily, weekly, monthly, quarterly and annually.

Purposes

- It serve as a tool to communicate information among health care team members.
- It provides information regarding the patients' condition.
- It ensures the responsibility in carrying out assignment promptly.
- It helps the authority to whom the report is submitted to make decision for future plan.
- It brings quality care outcome.
- Report summarizes the services of the nurse and/ or the agency.
- It helps in efficient functioning of the ward.
- It eliminates duplication of effort and warrants the need for investigation to understand the fact in a situation.
- All relevant information are provided in a good report.
- Complete reports ensures security which is derived from correct information of the situation.

Salient Features of Reports

- Reports should be made on time if they are to serve their purpose well. Delayed report may interfere with the patients diagnosis and care.
- A good report is written in a clear, complete, and concise manner.
- Good report comprises of all pertinent, data such as date and time, the individuals related, the situation of the incident, the signature of the person making the report.
- Organization of the reports is very important in understanding the fact clearly.
- Only actual facts included in the report, avoid irrelevant information.
- All oral reports should be concise and communicated well.

Types of Report

- Oral reports
- Written reports
- Situational reporting
- Change-of-shift reporting
- Transport report
- Structured report
- Incidental report
- Census report
- Birth and death report
- Accident report.

Oral Reports

Oral reports are given when the information is for immediate use and not for permanency. It is an exchange of information verbally from nurses to members of the health team, a patients and families. It is more informal, unstructured and situational need to be shared immediately.

Written Reports

These reports are referred as formal, communication of information in written form used by many health care professionals. It has a permanent value like patients night report, hospital census report.

Change-of-shift Reports or 24 hours Report

In this report information is exchanged with nurses. These reports are given when handing over and taking over the nurses moving bed to bed, showing the patients and the written report regarding, diagnosis and medical treatment routine care given during the shift issues and problems and related causes. The report also explains what is to be done during next shift period like drug, diet or any therapy which is due to patients.

Transfer Reports

A transfer reports refers to communication of information about the transferred patient from one unit to other. The report is given by a nurse who is responsible to transfer the patient to the nurse who is going to receive the patient. This report consists of the information regarding. patient's name, age, physician incharge, medical diagnosis summary of medical progress up to the time of transfer, current health status, current nursing diagnosis or problems, etc. and the care plan is attached with the report While transferring the patient the nurse communicates any due medicine or therapy to be given to patient with timing including any special observations need to done.

Incident Reports

It is a report when the nurse who witnessed the incident and found the patient at the time of incident needs to file the report. The nurse describes the incident in brief without any interpretation, cause or judgment. The nurse maintains objectivity in reporting the incident. She reports any activities taken by the nurse, other nurses, or doctors at the time of the incident are reported. The report is submitted as soon as the incident occurred to the concerned authority.

Census Report

This is a compilation of report of patients admitted in the ward. It is calculated at midnight and are collected by the night supervisor. The report highlights the total number of patients, the number of admissions, discharges, transfers, births and deaths. The nurse accurately maintains the census report.

Birth and Death Report

The nurses are responsible for sending the birth and death reports to governmental authorities for registration within the specified time. It is a routine practice in maternity hospitals where deliveries are conducted.

Accident Report

An accident report refers to concise report of accidents like burns, falls and head injury that are legal in nature occur in ward or hospital. They are reports of legal importance. This report include Name, Age, Address, Bed no, Ward no, Date and time of accident, Description of accident occurred, Safety precautions, Condition of the patient before and after the accident, Doctor's examination and his findings, Treatment ordered, witness to accident, Signature of the doctor, Signature of the nurse unit, Date of report, etc.

Factors to be considered while writing a good report:

- Organize the information in mind before writing the report.
- Avoid writing reports which has no relevant information.
- While writing report principle of conciseness, accuracy and completeness are to be kept in mind.
- It is better to write more than one report when the information is different.
- Use terminology that is known to all nursing personnel. Short, simple, commonly used words to be used for nontechnical reports.
- Observe protocol of good writing with sensible sentences and paragraphs and margins.
- Avoid spelling mistakes and abbreviations. Use correct pronoun, punctuation and legibility.
- Write report in a conversational manner.
- The report should include date and time.
- It is always essential to read the report before signing when the report is written by somebody.
- A report should maintain objectivity. Avoid subjectivity.
- A reliable record and report ensures confidence among health care team members.
- A good report has complete information.
- Reporting should be recent. Delays in recording or reporting can result in serious omissions and untimely delays for medical care or action. This is a part of negligence of nurse or doctor.
- The report should be well-organized. The nurse or nurse manager communicates information in a logical form or order. Health team members understand information better when it is given in a systematic and sequential order.
- Keeping patients record including diagnosis, treatment of patients needs, high degree of confidentiality. It is one of the legal and ethical responsibilities of nurses.
- Maintaining good quality records and reports has both immediate and long-term benefits for health care professionals. It increases nurses satisfaction and enhance morale of the institutions as well as legal protection.

MANAGEMENT INFORMATION AND EVALUATION SYSTEM (MIES)

Various Terms Used

Management Information System

It is an orderly arrangement of components of information system developed to change a collective set of data into knowledge item that is directly useful and applicable in the process of directing and controlling resources of an organization and their application to the achievement of specific objectives of administration. —**Hanson 1982**

Evaluation System

It is an ongoing and systematic assessment of a system to review its status periodically in term of original and current expectation and to forecast its future direction.

Health Information System

According to WHO, it is any quantifiable and non-quantifiable information that can be used by health decision-makers and clinicians to better understand disease processes and health care issues, and to prevent, diagnose or treat health problems.

Objectives of MIES

- To enhance communication among employs.
- To provide a system for recording and aggregating information.
- To reduce expenses related to labor-intensive manual activities.
- To support the organization's strategic goals and direction.

Importance of MIES

- Helps to plan and coordinate organizational activities in systematic manner.
- Ensures database on budgets, personnel, facilities and equipment.
- Provides direction in selecting entry points for program intervention.
- Promotes active partnership with other establishments.
- Provides information on the health status of the population served.
- Guides to set priority based on the problem identified.
- Provides criteria for monitoring and evaluation of performance.
- Assesses the impact of services on organizational outcome.
- Helps to forecast the future needs of the community served.
- MIES serves as a managerial tool for organizational improvement.

ADVANTAGES

The major problem in an organization can be easily identified and corrected before further complication arise.

1. MIES improves and supports the decision making process

2. MIES enhances job performance of all employees of an organization
3. It is a managerial tool through which the institution's activities are monitored and information is distributed to management, employees and customers
4. It evaluates the performance, and manage resources
5. It helps the management to provide feedback on the effectiveness of risk controls.

Disadvantages

- There is a possibility of error in reporting and decision-making.
- Since the data can be extracted by other units, it is difficult to control such factors.

NURSING MANAGEMENT INFORMATION SYSTEM (NMIS)

Nursing information systems (NIS) are computer systems that manage clinical data from a variety of health care settings and made available to nurses when they are in need of them that in turn help nurses in enhancing quality care to patients.

Applications

Fiscal resource management: NMIS helps the nurse administrator in financial administration. The data provided by the system can be used to monitor past performance or to predict future performance. The compiled information can be analyzed for the identifying trends by comparing the past and forecasting future expenditures. It enables her to make necessary reallocations and budgetary adjustments that is based on NMIS projection.

Workload measurement and staffing requirements: It helps the nurse administrator to store, manipulate and retrieve large volumes of data in planning, monitoring and evaluating use of nursing workforce resources on a daily basis as well as for a longer period yearly or 5 yearly calculation

Staff scheduling: Nursing managers are able to plan work, schedules in advance and nurses are informed well ahead of time. Staffing records, if maintained properly, provide useful information for monitoring absenteeism, scheduled time off, and turnover. It is time saving also.

Personnel management: A nurse administrator can identify the competetent nurses from the data provided. This can be used for nurses' promotion, sponsorship for higher education and deputation. It will also help the administrator to give assignment to nurses.

Advantages

In Nursing Administration

- It helps to evaluate quality assurance in nursing
- It helps to justify resource allocation to nursing service department
- It demonstrates the contribution of nursing services to bring quality patient care outcome
- To explore staff educational needs based on follow-up care and outcomes.

In Nursing Practice

- It improves documentation by nurses
- It provides data to enable research directed at examining the interrelationships between data elements and nursing outcomes
- It ensures development of the nursing process
- It develops body of knowledge with focus on nursing process
- It improves student nurse's accurate skill in documentation.

Evaluation System

Every organization needs to assess whether it has achieved the organizational goals or not. The management uses structure, process and product evaluation model based on the criteria laid down. Both formative and summative evaluations are conducted

In structure evaluation the management assesses the adequacy of environmental elements required to deliver nursing care such as policy, procedures, equipment, record keeping system, etc.

In the process evaluation the management assesses the professional elements required to deliver care.

In **outcome evaluation** the management focuses measurable elemwents demonstrating results of care. Patients fall, hospital acquired infection, bedsore, immunization levels, pressure ulcer prevalence, etc.

Thus, MIES helps a nurse manager to collect and use information to make management decisions accurately and promptly. Managers use MIS data to analyze, plan, make decisions, take actions and evaluate the achievement of the organization.

E-NURSING, TELEMEDICINE, TELENURSING

E-NURSING

Today, nurses are computer literate globally and are ready to meet the challenges confronted by health care technology. They have more access to internet, online libraries, and data bases of clinical nursing practice protocols from the computers that is facilitated at the work setting. They are competent to contribute in a variety of E-Health programs such as tele-triage. They interact with their colleagues through internet and discuss problems and interventions related to nursing patient care. Nurses are involved in standards development for the implementation of electronic health records and many other nursing educational packages with software engineers are now available at online.

Goal

The main aim of E-Nursing is to facilitate nurses from Information, Communication and Technology (ICT), that in turn will improve nursing and patient care outcomes.

Purposes

- Electronic health records, telehealth, databases, e-mail and internet resources are used by nurses to improve their decision-making capability. These information provides nurses timely access to the best practices evidence informed from the literature that in turn help them to make faster, better-informed decisions for patient care for quality outcome.
- E-Nursing ensures use of advanced technology to nurses' daily practice. Many health care facilities have already installed such program for nurses as they recognized the necessity to support nursing care however, it is not yet practiced in many public sector hospitals.
- To enhance the application of ICT in nursing to enhance nursing and patient care outcome.
- If ICT is applied correctly it brings better practice of nursing.

Methods

E-learning methods include computer-based teaching, web-based lectures and presentations virtual classrooms in which patients are logged on to an online classroom environment at different times or at the same time as the learning activities are happening.

E-Nursing Application—Nursing Profession

Nurses in Clinical Practice

Nurses contribute in ICT initiatives, and focus on possible solutions for patients needs and health problems. It help nurses to increase skills in use of ICT. ICT helps nurses to identify the best practices evidence informed in nursing.

Employers and Administrators

Employees and administrators accept and recognize ICT as a managerial tool of professional nursing practice. They support nurses who involve in ICT initiatives. They also encourage other nurses to adopt ICT initiatives to improve standards of nursing practice.

Clinical nurse researchers liberally utilize ICT through internet and web for their research.

Nursing organizations facilitate leadership for nurses' involvement in ICT and recognizes ICT competencies as part of entry-level and continuing competence requirements through staff development program.

Regulatory bodies utilizes ICT starting from registration, credit system of nurses, manpower planning and other academic and clinical activities at state, national and international level.

Advantages

- ICT improves nursing practice through integration of information and knowledge related to health
- It helps in human resource planning
- It identifies new models of nursing practice and health services delivery.
- Nursing group will be well-connected by national and international network
- Improves the quality of nursing in various work settings.
- ICT contributes to the global community of nursing profession.

Disadvantages

- This system is highly expensive.
- Decreases manual contribution.
- Increases dependence on ICT.
- Misuse of the technology is possible.

TELEMEDICINE

Definition

According to WHO telemedicine is defined as the delivery of health care services, to remote population, (where reaching health facility is difficult for the people) by health care professionals using information and communication technologies. In this process, the exchange of important information for diagnosis, treatment and prevention of disease and injuries, research and evaluation, and for continuing education of health care providers, all in the interests of advancing the health of individuals and their communities are facilitated.

Telemedicine is defined as any health care provided to patients through technology to remote population. (Remmes, Thomson and Williams; 1996)

Types of Telemedicine

Telemedicine can be classified into three main categories Store-and-forward (asynchronous), remote monitoring, and interactive services (synchronous).

Store- and- Forward

This type of telemedicine involves gathering medical data including medical images, bio signals, etc. Then, the data is transmitted to the physician or medical specialist for evaluation or review. The patient and the doctor may not be together. In this specialized consultation from a specialist to patients are benefitted by rural population or the patients who are away from the hospital.

Remote Monitoring

In this type, the physician can monitor a patient who is in a remote place using technological devices through telemedicine. For example, the physician can manage noncommunicable diseases and asthma. This technology gives satisfaction to patients. It is cost-effective.

Interactive Services

Interactive telemedicine services ensures a real-time interactions between patient and health care provider. This technology include telephone conversations, online communication and home visits. Some of the examples are this technology conduct activities like history review, physical examination, psychiatric evaluations and ophthalmology assessments like traditional face to face method. It is cost-effective than clinical visits of patients in person.

Uses of Telemedicine

The first interactive telemedicine system, operating over standard telephone lines, for remotely diagnosing and treating patients requiring cardiac resuscitation (defibrillation) was developed and marketed by Med Phone Corporation in 1989 in the US served as receiving and treatment centers. Monitoring a patient at home using known devices like blood pressure monitors and transferring the information to a caregiver is a fast growing emerging service.

Telemedicine is most beneficial for populations living in remote areas. Specialties that use telemedicine often use a 'tele' prefix; for example, telemedicine as applied by radiologists is called teleradiology. Similarly, telemedicine as applied by cardiologists is termed as telecardiology, etc. Telemedicine, is also useful as a communication tool between a general practitioner and a specialist available at a remote health facility.

Advantages of Telemedicine

For the Patients

- People at remote areas get quality-oriented medical care from renowned hospitals.
- Telemedicine technology saves time and money of patients living in rural areas.
- By using this technology, many inconveniences related to care is minimized among rural population.

For the Hospitals

- Hospitals can do their outreach program to remote villages and serve people without much expenditure and infrastructure facilities.
- The hospitals get sufficient income from the reference made from the remote locations of telemedicine.
- After care or postoperative care patients need not to come to the main hospital for consultation for minor problems. The patients can come only when major surgical intervention is required.
- Through telemedicine approach, the hospital can organize CME and CNE program for doctors and nurses.
- A rare operation or a diagnosis can be informed to other hospital. Doctors and nurses can learn new techniques by connecting telemedicine technology eith foreign health care institutions.
- Live images like ECG, USG, CT scan, Echo, X-rays and any video output from medical instruments can be transmitted through computers. Screen captures software—use of graphic image and can be disseminated to audience.

APPLICATION OF TELEHEALTH CARE

- **Tele education:** It is the application of ICT for prevention of diseases, promotion of health and to provide health care facilities to the population residing in remote places. Tele consultation and Tele-education are commonly used in distance education, that make interactive, flexible and accessible education to audience possible including any potential patient, nurse or any health care provider.
- **Disaster management:** Telemedicine can play an important role to provide health care facilities and health related information to the affected individuals by any natural calamity such as earthquake, tsunami, tornado, etc. and man-made disaster such as war, riots etc. Since , most of the communication links either do

not work properly or get damaged during disaster, a mobile and portable telemedicine system with satellite connectivity and customized telemedicine software can help in disaster relief.

- **Geriatric care at home:** Telemedicine technology can be applied to provide home health care to elderly or, home based patients with chronic illness. It allows community health care professionals or nurses and doctors specialized in geriatric medicine to monitor patients from a central station without going to remote areas. It is cost-effective, time saving, ensures patient satisfaction of care and efficient approach, Computer Telephone Integrated (CTI) system can monitor vital functions of patients 24 hours a day and give immediate notification if any.

Barriers in Application of Telemedicine

- Physicians and patients have unique technological resources available to improve the patient-physician relationship in these days. It has been observed that patients felt comfortable in accepting telemedicine program. However, in some hospital the telemedicine program is not available.
- Doctors in public sector view that telemedicine put additional burden on them. They are satisfied with traditional system of care.
- The private doctors are apprehensive that telemedicine is likely to increase their practice further.
- Though its technology is cost-effective, even then there is a false belief that telemedicine is very expensive.
- Because of poor infrastructure, communication and transport system, and frequent interruption of power supply, sometimes, it may be difficult to install this technology in rural Community Health Centre (CHC)/Primary Health Centre (PHC) or hospital.
- Health care professional are apprehensive about the reliability and quality of images and information transmitted for consultation and tele-diagnosis. Because if the system is not meeting the international standards, it is likely result for faulty diagnosis.
- Structural failure may result in delay in transmission of data that may cause delay in treatment and surgery.
- Inadequate trained professional to use this technology. Because it is a new venture, nurses and doctors should be aware of all terminology and functioning of telemedicine.
- Legal and ethical issues may be caused by poor maintenance of safety, privacy and confidentiality of patient data, and telemedicine consultations. There is a possibility that patient's rights of confidentiality of their personal data may not be secured and protected.

TELENURSING

Definition

Telenursing refers to the use of telecommunications and information technology for providing nursing services in health care facility whenever a geographical distance exists between patient and nurse, or between any numbers of nurses.

Applications of Telenursing

- Telenursing is applied in homecare management of patients who are immobilized, who have chronic ailments, such as chronic obstructive pulmonary disease, diabetes, congestive heart disease (CHD), disabilitating diseases, such as neural degenerative diseases, etc. may stay at home and be assisted by a nurse via videoconferencing, internet, videophone, etc.
- Other applications include homecare management of patients in immediate post-surgical situations, the care of wounds, ostomy, care, etc. Using telenursing, one nurse can visit 12–16 patients than visiting 5–7 patients in person by home visit.
- Telenursing is also benefited by call centers operated by managed care organizations, which are staffed by registered nurses who act as case managers or perform patient triage, information and counseling as a means of regulating patient access and flow and decrease the use of emergency rooms.
- Telenursing involves activities such as patient education, nursing teleconsultations, and assistance to physicians in the implementation of medical treatment protocols.

Legal, Ethical and Regulatory Issues

Like telehealth, telenursing is also not free from legal, ethical and regulatory issues. In some countries, telenursing is not permitted legal issues such as accountability and malpractice because of possibility of legal issues are still unsolved and difficult to address when telenursing is practiced.

ELECTRONIC MEDICAL RECORDS (EMR)

High volume of hospital paper based records, illegible hand written information about patients, records prepared on format which lacks standards, duplication of records, delay in retrieving records, inability of part of patients to preserve medical reports, missing records are facts about traditional recording system, strongly suggests the necessity of a computerized patient record system for the health care facilities today. The health care delivery system is changing, and today's health care facilities need to develop and share integrated patient information within their own establishments as well as across the countries.

If we want to improve efficiency, improve quality and patient safety, quality assurance and quality care improvement, evaluate the performance of health care professional and hospital, increase accountability of care, it is high time that we need to have standardized and computerized format for patient's health related information records, and that can be used as a managerial tool to assess quality patient care outcome.

Concept of EMR

Electronic medical record (EMR) is an organized systems, used by health care organization comprising of health related information on an individual patient that can be developed, gathered, managed, and consulted by authorized clinical experts and health care professionals.

It has potential benefits to physicians, management and all health care providers. The system also facilitate work flow to enhance quality patient care and patient safety

An EMR is a computerized medical record developed in an organization that delivers care, such as hospital or health center. It tends to be a part of a local stand-alone health information system that allows storage, retrieval and modification of records.

The information stored in EMR is not easily shared with providers outside of a practice. A patient's record might even have to be printed out and delivered by mail to specialists and other members of the care team.

Other Advantages of EMR

- It improves Physician's access to patient information, such as diagnoses, allergies, lab results, and medications.
- It helps to identify and compare the present and past test results of patients.
- Computerized decision-support systems helps nurses to prevent drug interactions and improve compliance with best practices in medication.
- Ensures electronic communication among providers and patients.
- It helps the patient to access health records, disease management tools, and health information resources.
- It helps in administration a computerized scheduling systems.
- It promotes standards-based electronic data storage and reporting for patient safety and disease follow up.
- It can track patient or hospital data overtime
- It helps to identify patients who are due for preventive visits and screenings.

Limitations

- It is not cost-effective.
- To switch over from traditional method to computerized records, will take time.
- Health professional demonstrates concern that systems will become obsolete.
- To implement and support EMR skilled resources are required.
- Sometimes, it may result in negative unintended consequences of care.
- Difficult to implement in rural areas.

Information technology helps nurses with unprecedented capacity more rapidly, generate and disseminate new knowledge. Service delivery in which nurses can expect to play a key role.

Box 21.1: Research highlights

'Designing and studying the utility of internet modular materials on teaching competency for nurse educators.'*

In view of the rapid changes in health care system and advancement in technologies, it is essential for nurse educators to keep improving their skills of teaching to fulfill the need of their students.

Sunita Lawrence conducted a non-experimental descriptive evaluative study on designing and studying the utility of internet modular materials on teaching competency of nurse educators as a part of continuing nursing education with the use of cost-effective, time saving and self-directing internet modular materials. Specifically the objectives of the study were: (1) to identify the training needs of the nurse educators regarding teaching learning process through the internet modular materials; (2) to develop internet modular materials on teaching competencies; (3) to validate the quality of internet modular materials by website experts; (4) to validate the teaching competencies content of internet modular materials by experts; (5) to evaluate the acceptability of newly devised internet modular materials on teaching competencies by nurse educators; and (6) to associate acceptability of newly devised internet modular materials with the selected demographical variables of nurse educators.

The study was undertaken within the conceptual framework of modified model of Stuffle Beam's evaluation Model describe as 'CIPP Model'.

Contd...

Contd...

The setting used for the study was Nursing Training Institute of Madhya Pradesh and Chhattisgarh states. There were 150 samples of nurse educators with degree in nursing, working in various nursing training institutes. Convenience sampling technique was used for sample selection.

Internet modular materials on teaching competency for nurse educators include: concept module; aims of module; definition in terms; basic assumptions of teaching competency; competency profile of nurse educators in teaching domains; competency profile in clinical domains; summary; and references.

Findings of the study shown that there was high acceptability of internet modular materials by 60.4% nurse educators; 54.5% of nurse educators preferred internet as a choice of continuing education; 64.8% experts given consent that content was adequate; 46.6% website experts classified the internet modular materials on teaching competency under excellent quality and overall the internet modular materials utility proved a good choice of CNE by nurse educators. Implementation of findings were applicable in clinical practice; nursing education; Indian Nursing Council (INC) and planners of nursing services.

(Dr. Sunita Lawrence, Principal, Pragyan College of Nursing, Bhopal, M.P.; India)

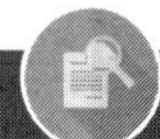

SUMMARY POINTS

- ✓ We are living in digital era today and the advances in information technology have created new roles for nurses, and stressed the need for all nursing personnel irrespective of their position to become more knowledgeable about health information concepts and the technology. The Indian Nursing Council (INC) has already introduced Information Technology (IT) in nursing curriculum that is designed to manage and process information in their seminars and research conducted at undergraduate, postgraduate and doctoral level.
- ✓ Nursing informatics (NI) is a specialty that combines nursing science with various information management and analytical sciences to identify, define, manage, and communicate data, information, knowledge, and wisdom in nursing practice. NI is the synthesis off nursing, its information, and information management with information processing and communication technology to support the health of people worldwide.
- ✓ Computers are supporting nurses and doctors keep online with various activities starts from admission to discharge procedures and their follow up scheduled appointments. The advancements that computers have brought to hospital setting can be applied in four different areas like clinical nursing and medical procedures, administration, research, and community settings.
- ✓ The patient record is the very important document for information concerning a patient's health care. It has an impact on everyone associated with providing, and receiving health care services. Though many technological advances in healthcare has been implicated the patient record system in recent years patient record in the government hospitals of some of the states in India remains unchanged.
- ✓ A nursing record is a clinical tool describes the nursing care given to the individual family or community. It is more scientific, legal and administrative tool. However, reports are oral or written exchanges of information shared between nurses and members of the health care team and family.
- ✓ Reports are information or facts about patient communicated by nurse to health care team or patients and families. Both written and oral reports are used by nurses to exchange information.
- ✓ Management information system is an orderly arrangement of components of information system developed to change a collective set of data into knowledge item that is directly useful and applicable in the process of directing and controlling resources of an organization and their application to the achievement of specific objectives of administration.
- ✓ Nursing information systems (NIS) are computer systems that manage clinical data from a variety of health care settings and made available to nurses when they are in need of them that in turn help nurses in enhancing quality care to patients.
- ✓ The main aim of E-Nursing is to facilitate nurses from Information, Communication and Technology (ICT), that in turn will improve nursing and patient care outcomes.
- ✓ Telemedicine is used to transfer medical instruction, or consultation, examinations, and small medical procedures to patients or health care professionals through Internet. Telemedicine is defined as the delivery

of healthcare services, to remote population, where reaching health facility is difficult for the people by health care professionals using information and communication technologies. In this process, the exchange of important information for diagnosis, treatment and prevention of disease and injuries, research and evaluation, and for continuing education of health care providers, all in the interests of advancing the health of individuals and their communities are facilitated.

✓ Telenursing refers to the use of telecommunications and information technology for providing nursing services in health care facility whenever a geographical distance exists between patient and nurse, or between any numbers of nurses.

✓ Electronic medical record (EMR) is an emerging technological application of information in hospital today. EMR has increased the efficiency of health care facility by providing patient information easily available. EMR helps to save space comparing the occupation of space for huge volume of paper based hospital records. EMR eliminates illegible handwriting, decreases errors on data-entry, and connects related records automatically. It can be opened by selected authority with passwords and thus it maintain security of records. The computer keeps track of the individuals who have visited certain records. EMR reduces paper and storage services in hospitals.

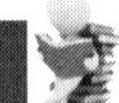

REVIEW QUESTIONS

1. Define Nursing Informatics (NI). Discuss the general purposes of nursing informatics.
2. Describe the use of computers in health care delivery system.
3. What are patient records? Discuss the responsibilities of a nurse in maintaining patients record.
4. Describe management information and evaluation system (MIES). Discuss its advantages and disadvantages.
5. Differentiate records and reports. Explain the facors to be considered while writing a report.
6. Write short notes on:
   a. Medical record
   b. Nursing Informatics System (NIS)
   c. Electronic Medical Record (EMR)
   d. E-Nursing
   e. Telemedicine
   f. Telenursing.

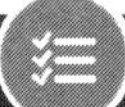

SELECTED READINGS

1. Anale. Seria Informatica. Vol. X fasc. 2 – 2012
2. Annals. Computer Science Series. 10th Tome 2nd Fasc. – 20
3. Ashutash, Dr K How the Computers Are Useful in Hospital and Community? Doc2doc. BMJ Group, 6 Jan. 2012. Web. 5 Sept. 2014. www.doc2doc.bmj.com/forums/open-clinical_general-clinical_computers-useful-hospital-community.
4. Coriina Verniic, Nursing Informatics. Current and Future
5. Dick RD, Steen EN, Editors The computer-based patient record. An essential technology for health care. Washingon, DC : National Academy Press; 1991.
6. Electronicmedicalrecords : cited on on 9 Feb 2013:available from:http://en.wikipedia.org/wiki/Electronic_medical_record
7. Garrett, LE, Hammond WE and Stead WW, The effects of computerized medical records on provider efficiency and quality of care. Methods of Information in Medicine1986; 25: 151-7.
8. http://www.scribd.com/doc/6120543/Nursing-Informatics
9. KosterA, Waterstraat FL, and Sondak N, Automated and ambulatory record systems: A comparative cost analysis. Journal of American Medical Records Association 1987 58:26-31.
10. Mahapatra P, Berman P, Using hospital activity indicators to evaluate performance in Andhra Pradesh, India. International Journal of Heath Planning and Management 1994; 9 ; 199-211.
11. Management information system: cited on 10 Feb2013: available from :http://en.wikipedia.org/wiki/Management_information_system

12. Management information system: cited on 9 Feb 2013: available from :http://www.instahealthsolutions.com/modules.html
13. Management: cited on 10 Feb 2013:available from http://www.slideshare.net/Jyothi19587/management-pptgifty
14. Metzer, J.B., the potential contributions of patient care information systems.
15. mis: cited on 11 Feb 2013: available from 4:http://nmis.sourceforge.net/nmis-features.html
16. Nis : cited on 13 Feb 2013: available from http://www2.pathfinder.org/site/DocServer/MIS.complete.pdf
17. Nursing Informatics: Scope and Standards of Practice, 2nd Edition, ANA 2015
18. Raja, E.E.J., Mahal, R. and Masih, V.B. (February 2004). An Exploratory Study to Assess the Computer Knowledge, Attitude and Skill Among Nurses in Health care Setting of a Selected Hospital, Ludhiana, Punjab, India. Online Journal of Nursing Informatics (OJNI). Vol. 8, No. 1. [Online]. Available at http://ojni.org/8_1/raja.htm
19. Rogers JL, Haring OM, Wortman PM, Goetz JP, Medical information systems: Assessing impact in the areas of hypertension, obesity and renal disease. Medical care 1982; 20 : 63-74
20. Senior Faculty, Health Care Management, Institute of Health Systems. HACA Bhavan, Opp Public Gardens, Hyderabad 500004, AP, India
21. TRENDS Anale. Seria Informatica. Vol. X fasc. 2 – 2012 Annals. Computer Science Series. 10th Tome 2nd Fasc. – 2012
22. www.ahrq.gov AHRQ National Resource Center; Health Information Technology: Best Practices Transforming Quality, Safety, and Efficiency

22. Introduction to Ward Management

UNIT XII
NURSING UNIT MANAGEMENT

22

Introduction to Ward Management

LEARNING OBJECTIVES

This chapter imparts learning about:

- Planning Physical Facilities, Floor Space
- Time Planning Daily/Weekly Plan
- Factors Influencing Ward Management
- Maintaining Therapeutic Environment
- Role of a Head Nurse in Student Education—Nursing Rounds, Nursing Care Conference

Hospital is a place where patients come for consultation, investigation and diagnosis, admission, treatment and follow-up care. These treatments include preventive, promotive, curative, restorative and rehabilitative services. The role of hospital in providing clinical experience for medical and nursing students are very significant. Clinical research and innovative intervention carried out by the hospital is one of the very important functions of all health care facilities today.

All the above functions are carried out by various wards or nursing service units of a hospital. The ward sister or head nurse has a very important role to play in ward management.

The main objectives of ward management are:

- To provide quality care and patient's safety.
- To educate patients and their families.
- To facilitate good clinical field for medical and nursing students for their clinical experiences.
- To provide patient satisfaction.
- To promote job satisfaction among health care professionals.
- To enhance professional development.

The head nurse occupies a very important position in hospitals. She is the manager of her nursing unit or ward and is responsible to the nursing superintendent of the hospital. She is responsible for:

- Participating and implementing policy decision.
- Delegating responsibilities to subordinates.
- Maintaining equipment and supplies.
- Supervising and monitoring patient care.
- Assigning duties.
- Planning and maintaining physical facilities and therapeutic environment for patients.
- Educating and supervising student nurses.
- Maintaining records and reports.
- Evaluating patient care rendered.

PLANNING PHYSICAL FACILITIES AND FLOOR SPACE

Planning physical facilities is one of the important functions of ward management. We are living in the era of consumerism and our health consumer (patient) has every right to have a safe, clean, noise free, spacious, fresh aired and restful environment for his speedy recovery from illness. Keeping these in mind many hospitals are constructed out skirts of the city.

Earlier hospital wards were built with large open wards with high ceiling. A modern hospital today focuses to provide more privacy by constructing individual rooms or cubicles for 2-3 patients. While constructing every ward needs a good planning designed in such a way that it is constructed with minimum cost with maximum functioning capacity with quality.

Objectives of Planning a Ward

- To provide quality care and patient safety.
- To ensure the best therapeutic environment for patient care.
- To provide facilities for visitors and attendants.
- To ensure job satisfaction to health care professionals.
- To ensure essential equipment, supplies, linen drugs, and other material required for patient care.
- To facilitate a conducive environment for speedy recovery from illness.
- To provide opportunity for education, training and research for medical, nursing and other allied professionals.

Before, we consider the physical facilities and floor plan required for a ward, we need to think the location and design of the ward.

Location of the Ward

The ward should be located away from crowded, noisy, and parking area. It should be situated away from hospital mortuary. The pediatric ward, antenatal ward and causality ward should be preferably located in ground floor. Labor room, operation theater, and diagnostic services to be located adjacent to the wards.

Design of the Ward

When designing a ward it should ensure that the nurses and doctors could observe patients from their station and it should take minimum walking time for nurses to reach the patients to avoid fatigue. From the period of Florence Nightingale many design has been developed and approved and some of the designs are given below:

Open Wards

In 1770, open ward was designed by Frenchman. After some years it was approved by Florence Nightingale and is known as Nightingale ward. In this type of ward, beds are placed in two rows facing each other in a huge hall (longitudinal) and the nursing station provided at the center. Other accessory rooms were provided on the sides of the hall like side rooms. The main advantages of this type of ward are to facilitate cross ventilation, patients could be observable and the construction is economically cheap. However, the major disadvantage of this type of ward demonstrates noise, lack of privacy and the space between the two rows of beds serves as a corridor.

Rig's Ward

In 1910 this type of ward was first designed in Rig Hospital in Denmark. Hence, the name Rig's ward was called, in this design ward is divided into small ward units or Bay ward separated from each other. Each unit consisted 4-6 beds arranged parallel to the longitudinal wall. Each such ward unit is separated by a small partition. Nursing station was located on side and side room also provided. The major advantage of Rig ward facilitated privacy, for patient, minimized the risk of cross infection, and was, less noisy. This type of ward was good to isolate infectious patients. This type of ward limits the communication between patient and direct observation of the patient is difficult for health care professionals. This design needs more nursing staff and costlier than open ward.

Unilateral Rig's Ward

This type of ward consists 6 beds in each Bay with single corridor. Nursing station is separated from each Bay and placed in a side. This design prevents noise and activities of doctors and nurses are assigned to each one Bay. Calling bells are fixed as the nurses cannot directly observe the patients.

Bilateral Rig's Ward

It is also called double corridor ward with central nursing station. It facilitates good observation of patients, cross ventilation, and the walking distance for nurses is minimum and it is widely accepted design.

T-shaped Wards

In this design the nurses' station is located at the center of the ward. Isolation patients are kept on the side bays of nursing station. Serious or critical patients are kept in front of nursing station and the other ancillary rooms are located behind the nursing station. Though it is a good design however, ventilation of the ward and communication system are to be taken care of **Y-shaped wards, circular and semicircular wards** are also designed like T-shaped wards.

Size of the Wards

The size of the ward varies from hospital to hospital. Normally it ranges from 20–80 beds. It should be kept to an optimum size because; the resources required are more or less same whether the ward size is 20, 30 or 40 beds.

The Factors Influencing in Determining the Size Depends upon the Following:

Type of Patients

The patients who are completely dependent and critical who requires close monitoring and supervision such as patients in ICU, CCU, ICCU, NICU, recovery room etc., can have 10-20 beds whereas chronic disease condition or nondependent conditions can have 40-50 beds ward.

Requirement of Nursing Personnel

When we calculate the nursing personnel in each shift that depends upon number of nursing hours required in each shift. It is observed that we need more nurses in morning from 7am to 12 noon, less in 12-7 pm am and very less nursing hours in 7-7 am night shift.

Availability of Head Nurse

As per recommendation by regulatory bodies, a head nurse is required for 50 bedded wards because she has more administrative responsibilities. If a head nurse is not available senior nursing staff with less than 50 beds to be planned as these nurses are required for more clinical nursing than administrative responsibilities.

Components of a Ward

- Primary accommodation or patient housing areas
- Ancillary areas
- Sanitary areas
- Auxiliary areas

Primary Accommodation or Patient Housing Areas: Floor Area

It means the place where patients are kept. In place of large longitudinal wards with 30–50 beds, nowadays, it is preferred to provide single bedroom or multiple bedrooms for 2–6 patients and a nursing station. The size of the single bed room should have 125 Sq. feet, 2 bedded rooms has 160 Sq, feet, 4 bedded room has 320 Sq. feet and 6 bedded room has 400 Sq. feet area is required. For ICU per patient 120–150–Sq. feet area and for maternity and orthopedic bed 120 Sq. feet per bed is required.

There should be sufficient space for nurses to do nursing procedures to patients and keeping equipment near bed side. In general ward, the floor area per bed is 70 Sq, feet, the space between the two rows of beds should be 5 feet, the distance, between the head end of bed and the wall should be 1 feet, the distance between the wall and side of the bed should be 2 feet and space between two beds should be 31/2 to 4 feet to prevent transmitting droplet infection.

Height of Ceiling

- Minimum of 3 meter recommended.
- For suspended ceiling fan a minimum of 2.6 meter. suggested.
- Windows should be built in 20% of floor area if there is one wall.
- When more than one window is required 15% of the floor area to be utilized.
- The width of corridor recommended is 2.4 meter to allow movement of trolley, bed, and stretchers.
- Door should not be less than 1.2 meter wide and 2.25 height.

Ancillary Areas

It includes services like nursing station, treatment rooms, clean utility room, pantry unit, store, dining or day room.

Nursing Station

Nursing station occupies a very important place in a ward. It should ensure adequate space, ventilation, light for nurses to work. There should be sufficient space or record cabinet for keeping records, stationeries, report forms charts, manuals and files and a computer table with computer. The medication unit is very important aspect of nursing station. A cupboard with lock and key is essential to keep medicine safe and out of reach to patient or other persons. The head nurse office with required furniture to be available. The size of nursing station should be large enough for the movement of nurses. A toilet should be attached with nursing station.

Treatment Room or Therapy Room

The room is used for examination of patient, dressing and procedures which cannot be conducted in ward. There should be an examination table and foot boards for patient, cabinets, dressing trolley and hand washing facilities with running water in this room.

Clean Utility Room

It should be equipped with cupboards, cabinets to keep procedure trays and other required articles for nursing procedures, linen, etc.

Ward Pantry

It is required to provide hot water , clean drinking water with filter facilities, heating facilities sink to wash vessels used, facilities to prepare therapeutic diet if there is no facilities to prepare therapeutic diet in hospital kitchen

Ward Store Room

This is a place some of the stocks and supplies are stored by the head nurse like linen.

In addition to the above dining and day rooms are provided outside of the ward for ambulatory patients with adequate facilities.

Sanitary Areas

Bath and Toilets

- If it is an open ward, there should be separate toilets for patients and male and female visitors and employees of the ward.
- One bath room for 8 patients and one toilet for 5 patients is considered normal requirement. If, it is a single room bath and toilets are usually attached with the room or cubicle.
- Bath rooms and toilets should cleaned and dried as and when needed to prevent slip or fall of patients
- Deodorants to be used to avoid bad smell.

Dirty Utility Room

This area is very important place in a ward. This is used to wash bedpans, urinals, sputum cups specimen bottles, bedside bowls, and soiled mackintoshes. Provision of running water is very essential in this area and facilities for drying them also to be ensured.

Store Room for Sweepers

This place is used for keeping cleansing materials, brooms, mops receptacles and hangers by sweepers

Wash Basins

There should be a separate wash basin for patients in the ward or Bay with 24 hours water supply. Wash basin to be washed and cleaned and the floor below the wash basin should be dried.

Auxillary Areas

In addition to the above a ward requires auxiliary areas for the education and welfare of the personnel working in wards for patient care. They are:

Changing Room for Nurses

This room is used for day scholars who come from outside and do not stay in hostel. Separate lockers to be provided in this room for keeping the nurses belongingness.

Attendant Room

These rooms are used for patients attendants, with locker facility to keep their things. For every 4 wards an attendant room to be facilitated

Duty Room for Nurses and Doctors

Separate duty rooms for nurses and doctors are useful to work during the day shift and can rest for a while during night shift. It should be furnished with a cot, table chair and attached toilet.

Clinical Side Room

In some hospitals clinical side rooms are provided to do laboratory test. It is available for every block or 3-4 wards or every floor.

Seminar Room

To educate doctors/ nurses without disturbing ward duty, this room is provided in each block/ floor. This room has seating facilities, and facilities to teach by projected aids and sometime patient care conferences also conducted here.

The nurse administrator has a role to ensure good physical facilities for patients and that is delegated to the head nurse or unit manager. The ultimate aim for maintain good physical facilities ensure quality care and quality ward management.

TIME PLANNING DAILY/WEEKLY PLAN

Good time planning is a managerial skill. The ward sister or head nurse has a responsibility to develop daily and weekly plan for nurses to utilize their precious time for patient care. The time planning refers to the plan of time in hours and days to be spend by nursing personnel for the activities for patient care. It helps in planning executing and evaluating the optimum use of time.

Objectives of Time Planning

- To provide nursing functions efficiently.
- To permit for optimum time to provide quality patient care.
- To improve morale and health with reduction in workload among nursing personnel.
- To impart good learning experiences for the student nurses and staff.
- To facilitate optimum use of resources to the care of patients.
- To enhance better communication between the staff to share reports and records.
- Maximize the control over time by the head nurse
- To prioritize care, of the patient, intervention and outcome.
- To find time to do research and work for professional development.
- To reduce fatigue of the nurses in the wards and critical care units.
- To develop leadership and administrative skills.

Principles of Time Management

- It should provide maximum coverage for nursing activities.
- To maximize the managerial time for all managerial activities.
- To maximize the organization time.

CAUSES OF TIME WASTING IN AN ORGANIZATION

The time of a person in health care system is wasted due to external factors, organizational structure, management factors and personal factors. The following causes are enumerated in relation waste of time:

Externl factors include

- Interruption due to failure of telephone communication,
- Sudden appearance of untoward event
- Sudden entry of visitors
- Noise

Internal factors include

- Failure to set vision, mission, objectives and priority
- Poor delegation
- Disorganized personality of the head nurse
- Indecisiveness
- Under staffing, underutilized nursing personnel
- Poor work culture
- Poor staff morale and IPR
- poor communication
- Delay in reporting and communicating
- Lack of trust
- Overworked subordinates

METHODS UTILIZED TO PLAN TIME BY THE HEAD NURSE

The following steps are used to optimum time management for nursing activities and to avoid wasting time.

Step 1 Planning Time of the Staff in the Ward

One of the responsibilities of the head nurse in time management. It means to distribute the nurses time within a week and also to distribute the time within 24 hour period for ensuring optimum staffing in the ward to meet the patients needs.

Distribution of Time Throughout the Week

- The head nurse assesses on which days of the week the nursing work load is heaviest such as admission days or operation days.
- She calculates the number of nursing hours which are assigned to the ward for the week by adding together the number of hours each nurse is assigned to work during the week.
- She identifies the daily average nursing hours by dividing the hours assigned for the week by the number of days in the week.
- It is very important to plan the days off duty to ensure the ward is staffed with professional and non-professional staff members on each day.

Distribution of Time Throughout 24 Hours

- The ward sister analyzes the activities that normally occur during the 24 hour period.
- She estimates the number and type of personnel needed at various times of day to carry nursing load.Usually in morning 8 am to 12 noon is the maximum nursing load observed
- Then she estimates the total number of nurses and aides needed to perform the ward activities and to permit time off duty for each person according to the hospital policy. Sometimes relieving nurses are available.

Step 2 Planning Time for Nursing Team

The time planning for the team members varies according the composition of the team. When team method of assignment is used to care for all patients in the ward , the teams should, if possible be so composed that members relieve one another for the days off. The day when two members are scheduled to be absent should be the day of the week presumed to be lightest i.e. Saturday or Sunday. Usually the functional methods are carried out in hospitals. Then the days off to be avoided in admission days, and operation days.

Step 3 Complying with Good Personnel Practices

All nurses have privilege to have off days to join their families in a week. Each hospital has its policy in providing duty off days as per personnel policy. A straight eight-hour day for all nurses instead of a day of split hours. The work day planned to fall within a 12-hour span such as 8:00 am and 8:00 pm. Regular day, evening and night periods for nurses and rotation through them. The arrangement of the work week, that is, the amount of consecutive off duty time that may be assigned. The advance time is to be planning—day to day or week or month ahead. In 8 hours shift one day off is given and if it comes to 12 hours shift two days off is given per week.

Step 4 Providing Coverage

As per regulatory bodies in nursing a trained staff should be available in each shift. It is important to provide the coverage of the ward in relation to the experience of individual nursing staff. The head nurse ensures that the ward is covered at all times with a sufficient number of nurses. This necessitates a professional nurse being charge of the floor every hour for 24 hours. Time is also planned taking over and handing over of patients with records and reports.

Step 5 Providing Best Experience to Student Nurses

There is close relationship with time planning and assignment planning. When the students are in the ward for their clinical experiences, the head nurse should provide experiences when such activity(procedure) occur in the ward. For example, if the first year student has to learn the procedure of enema for patients, it happens in the morning only. Therefore, the students are assigned at that time with their supervisors to learn the procedure and .to meet the educational needs. Some of the experiences are available only once a week. The student nurses should be assigned to be on duty at the hours when the experience is the best to meet their educational needs. The hours which the head nurse and staff nurses work may affect the experience of the student nurses.

Step 6 Preparing the Time Sheets

The time sheets can be daily or weekly. The time sheets show the distribution of work assignments. The weekly time-sheet with the time planned for each nurse is used by the nursing office to obtain an overview of the staffing situation. It is used by the clinical supervisor. The daily time sheet is considered important in order to keep track of absence and illness. The sheet is easier to use if evening and night nurses are listed separately from day nurses.

Step 7 Making Time Inventory/Schedules

The priority of time also can be used when listing the activities that are to be done first and later. The list is made by the ward sister weekly or monthly. It is a flexible planning tool.

Step 8 Use Advance Scheduling

The hours should always be scheduled at least a week in advance and if possible further ahead. The off – duty time, straight hour assignments and overtime are issues. The splitting of the hours of duty for comfort of the staff has been recommended. But, the work has to be distributed thoroughly and throughout the day for having more load during the day and less of it during the night.

Planning Schedules

Planning and scheduling is discussed in Chapter 12 in detail.

ROLES OF HEAD NURSES IN TIME PLANNING

Leadership Roles of the Head Nurses:

- Develop vision, mission and philosophy of nursing activities
- Encourage effective communication
- Enhance good IPR and improve staff morale
- Demonstrate as a role model
- Demonstrate flexibility in assignment
- Demonstrate as a transformational and transactional leader.

Managerial Roles of the Head Nurses:

- Understand routine work of the ward
- Aware of important and incidental activities
- Prevent interruptions
- Prioritize day today planning appropriately
- Analyze staff adequacy
- Utilize available resources including technology effectively
- Establish short-term and long-term goals
- Proper scheduling of workforce
- Conduct inventory activities that how the staff spent their time.
- Set goals and priorities helps resolve goal conflicts and directs how one will spend time
- Plan strategies or plan of operations to accomplish the goal
- The head nurses assess their peak and low times to plan a detailed schedule more effectively. A few minutes at the beginning of each day can be allotted for planning. Scheduled activities should be recorded.
- Learn to say no graciously, especially about low priority work
- Use transition times, e.g. incoming mails can be read, reports can be read while commuting to and fro work
- Improve reading-learn speed reading techniques.
- Assume the value by being attentive, delaying, judgment, maintaining eye contact and using attentive body language. Assess the content of the information by focusing on central ideas.
- Use telephone calls—instead of office visits or correspondence
- Schedule office visits
- Control visit time

- Use meetings effectively—key participants to be identified, agenda to be circulated before meeting, start the meeting on time with high priority items first control over interruptions, restate conclusions, make assignments and deadlines clear and end the meeting on time.
- Delegation—responsibility and authority to be delegated to a right person.

Educators Roles of the Head Nurses:

- Plan for student assignment in advance
- Provide enough time for supervision of students and staff nurses

The head nurse has a great responsibility in time management. When the time is wasted for un related work, the patient suffers and it decreases the morale of nursing personnel. Adequate staffing, time plan for day and week is very essential to avoid all interruption of activities.

FACTORS INVOLVED IN GOOD WARD MANAGEMENT

Quality of patient care depends upon not only the availability of resources and infrastructure, but the ability of the head nurse in managing the ward also. She should be aware the factors involved in good ward management They are the following:

Familiar of All Activities Performed in the Ward

To manage the ward efficiently the head nurse must have the knowledge of all the ward activities to be performed in the ward. Some of the activities are performed daily, some are performed in weekly and some activities performed under special circumstances. Those activities occur regularly in daily or weekly basis, she can plan them well in advance and communicate to the responsible subordinate staff.

Planning the Day's Program

A planned program for each day work prevents loss of time and helps in smooth running of the ward. The head nurse plans and assigns duties for staff nurses a day before and communicate the staff about their assignment, and asks them to read and sign in the assignment sheet. This helps the nurses to begin the day work as soon as they report on duty. If any changes in the assignment needed it is done and adjusted with other nurses. The ward sister reports to work earlier than her staff to see any change or adjustment needs to be done before the day duty begins In case of night duty, the night supervisor is responsible to solve the problem of change or adjustment.

Starting the Day on Time

Each nurse should start her day work on time. If one nurse is 10 minutes late for duty and the other is 5 minutes late, that means 15 minutes nursing care hour is lost which we cannot get again. From the head nurse to subordinate staff should practice punctuality and complete their work on time. When a night nurse is late to complete her work, the head nurse should solve such problem. A good ward management demonstrates timely taking over the patients and timely handing over to the night nurse so that both the parties have enough time to carry out their assigned work for their patients.

Preventing Interruptions

The cause for interruptions has already been discussed above. It is the duty of everyone in the ward to complete their activity before jumping to another activity. The head nurse should conduct inventory activities regarding how the staff spent their time and should set goals and priorities to resolve goal conflicts and directs how one will spend time. Many times it has been observed that ward boys spent lot of time in transporting patients or reaching the call book to call physician today we have technology available in hospital like cell phone, intercom, email. etc. The head nurse should use the availability of technology to prevent loss of time causing interruption in ward work.

Establishment of Ward Routine and Ward Policies

The head nurse should ensure that staff nurses and other workers working in her unit know the ward routine and ward policies and a copy of the same is available in the ward. Routine work such as bed to bed taking over and handing over of patients, and report, assigning duties like medication, vitals checking, morning and evening procedures, collection of specimen, preparation of patients for diagnostic investigation, doctors round and taking orders, carry out stat orders, cleaning and labeling of medicinal bottles, and cupboard, indent form, diet distribution ward inventory checking, etc. The head nurse should ensure that a procedure manual is available in the unit for nurse to refer like consent for operation, preparation for surgical intervention, collection of specimen etc. There should be a ward policy manual describing visiting hours, meal timing, visitors pass, doctor's round ward fire, theft or any intervention in emergency, etc.

Knowledge of ward routine, ward policies and procedure manual help nurse to develop confidence to do right things when needed.

Orientation of New Staff

It is one of the important functions of the head nurse. The main aim of this program is to familiarize the new staff nurses with the ward, policies and procedures and the job she or he is going to do. It is a planned activity. Before the arrival of the new staff, it is planned by the ward sister and communicated to all members in the ward who are assigned to do the job, areas where the new nurses are oriented and methods to conduct orientation. Usually it is planned for a week. An evaluation is done by the head nurse. An evaluation is done at the end of the program and recorded. The head nurse also introduces the medical team of her ward. Orientation helps the new nurse a sense of belongingness to the ward and that in turn motivates her/him to do a better job.

Maintaining a Conducive Environment for Patients

Patients admitted in ward require speedy recovery from illness. Florence Nightingale in her notes on nursing describes the importance of physical, psychological and social environment in providing quality patient care. Quality and patient safety is the bench mark of nursing. Providing safety and security, ensuring noise free ward, good light that should be soothing to eyes, ventilation, cleanliness, safe equipment and orderliness of the wards are to be considered while maintaining suitable environment to all patients admitted in ward.

Provision of Equipment and Supplies

One of the important functions of head nurse is maintaining equipment and supplies for the smooth administration of ward. Standardization of equipment needed for her ward, sending requisition, condemnation and inventory of articles in wards are main responsibilities in ensuring the availability and accessibility of equipment and supplies for patient care. She may delegate some responsibilities in this regard to her subordinates In this function she focuses on. controlling the pilferage, preventing waste and misuse of articles, and educating nurses regarding its maintenance and ensuring safe article for care are.

Clear and Written Orders of the Physician

The head nurse should be vigilant in getting written orders from doctor before it is implemented. She instructs the nurses regarding carrying out verbal orders only in emergency situation but it should be written by nurse/or other doctor and countersigned by the concerned physician who gave the verbal order. Clear and written orders are very important in terms of legal and ethical reasons.

Accurate Records and Reports

The head nurse has to see that the records are completed before it is sent to the medical record section and she has a responsibility to safe guard all the records and reports for legal and ethical reasons. (Refer Chapter 20 for details)

Establishing a Good Working Relationship

In order to run the ward satisfactorily, the head nurse ensures a good working relationship among nurses and with members of the health care team. A good work culture enhances patient and nurses satisfaction and improves staff morale.

Delegation of Responsibilities

The head nurse cannot function all the ward activities alone. She delegates some of the responsibilities to staff nurses who are competent and accept delegated assignment. However, the head nurse has the accountability of the work done (Refer Chapter 16 organizational behavior for further details of delegation)

Well Planned Assignment

Assignment of the patients depends upon the policy of the hospital as well as the availability of nursing staff for 24 hours in that ward. There are various traditional and modern methods of assignments. However, functional methods of assignment is very common in government hospitals. Each method has its own advantages and disadvantages. (Refer Chapter 10 organization of nursing services for patients care Section 1 methods of patients assignments for further detail)

Education of Nurses and Other Health Care Workers

Good ward management depends upon knowledgeable workforce caring the patients. The head nurse organizes planned and incidental teaching program to the nurses and others periodically without interfering the patient care to update their knowledge regarding new equipment, new procedures new policies and new disease condition to update their knowledge and document them.

Effective Supervision

Supervision of staff nurses and student nurses is an important function of head nurse. It enhances not only patient care but also improves the knowledge of nursing personnel. Earlier days the head nurse use to participate and supervise in students clinical experience and sent evaluation report to the principal school of nursing.

Evaluation

The head nurse evaluates the patient care rendered by nurses. She is also responsible to send the performance report of nursing personnel to the nursing superintendent periodically. Good evaluation helps to improve the standard of care and quality outcome.

MAINTAINING THERAPEUTIC ENVIRONMENT

One of the objectives of any health care facility is to ensure speedy recovery of patients from illness. This is achieved by facilitating patient safety, quality patient care, and maintaining a therapeutic environment. Therapeutic environment includes not only the physical structure of the unit, but also it envisages a psychosocially supported environment for patient, family and caregivers. In therapeutic environment the patient receives care that affects patient outcomes, patient satisfaction, patient safety, health workers efficiency, and satisfaction, and a positive organizational outcome.

The main objectives of maintaining therapeutic environment for patients are:

- To meet physical, social and psychological needs of patient, family and health care providers.
- To improve clinical excellence in managing the patients'.
- To promote quality effects on patients' clinical outcomes.
- To enhance employee and organizational effectiveness.

Therapeutic environment theory is originated from, psychoneuron immune theory that means the psycho social effects of environment on patients. When patients are admitted in hospital they are afraid of ward activities, ward routines their disease condition and prognosis. They are apprehensive about their safety and security because they are away from their families and friends. It creates stress, anxiety and tension in patients that results in depression of patient's immune system and adversely affects their recovery.

To create a therapeutic environment the doctors, nurses, architect, engineer, interior designer, site and landscape designer need to design a structure or design that will affect the patients and staff in a positive manner. It should be structured from entering of patients into the hospital to the patient's unit.

A good therapeutic environment can enhance patient care outcome, reduce or minimize stressors from environment, and promotes psycho social support for patients, family and health care providers

Other advantages of maintaining therapeutic environment are:

- Reduction of noise from the environment
- Provision of soothing light in patient unit
- Utilization of appropriate technology
- Enhances observation of patients
- Promotes patients' safety and security
- Improves Patients' satisfaction
- Enhances Nurses' satisfaction

Methods of Providing Therapeutic Environment

- Provide good physical environment **as discussed above**
- Facilitate Views of nature, from patient rooms, and wherever possible in lobby, waiting, and other 'high stress' areas.
- Access to nature, healing gardens.
- Chapel, meditation room, and meditation gardens.
- Artwork depicting nature, including back-lighted photographs of nature.
- Music; live piano in public area, recorded music in patient room when programmed specifically to create a healing environment.
- Facilities for mild physical exercise; corridors, public spaces, and gardens that invite walking when appropriate. **—Gary W Evans and Janetta MM**

Enable Social Support for the Patients

- Family zone in patient room; with furniture for sleeping, phone and internet connection, reading light with separate control, to be provided.
- Provide places where patients can engage socially with family and other caregivers, family kitchen on inpatient units where family members can prepare food for patients and families to eat together.
- Provide accommodation for accompanying family member to be with patient throughout the examination and treatment process.
- Organize family focus groups and patient and family advisory councils to be an active part of the design process, tuning in to the specific needs of the population and community to be served, as recommended by the institute for family-centered care. Ensure culturally appropriate environments. **—Geri Ann Galanti 2003**

ROLE OF A HEAD NURSE IN STUDENT EDUCATION—NURSING ROUNDS, NURSING CARE CONFERENCE

The head nurse plays an important role in clinical nursing education, helping to prepare nursing students for professional practice. A positive and enriched learning environment in the clinical setting has an impact on students perception of the ward unit as their future work is oriented to similar setting. Facilitating a positive clinical learning experiences to students can motivate students to translate theory into practice on real patients. Application of classroom or preclinical laboratory learning concepts to actual practice is an exciting and anticipated part of the curriculum for nursing students.

The interaction of nursing students with head nurse affects learning. Sometimes the head nurse's role as mentor is responsible for teaching and evaluating a student's clinical performance. The head nurse helps in the following manner in student's clinical learning

- Selects patients for learning experience according to the level of the students. For example, for first year students she assigns nursing procedures with consultation with the clinical instructor. For second year students she focuses on selecting students with illness and for third year onwards she assigns patients with difficult problems.
- Provides sufficient articles and supplies for caring patients.
- Supervises the care rendered by student nurses
- Counseling and guidance to students is one of the educative functions.
- Facilitates and participates when the student conducts health teaching and bed side clinic/nursing conference.
- The head nurse acts as a role model of practical nursing skills. A positive learning experience in the clinical site with a dedicated, kind, nurturing role model can promote student's learning.
- The role of effective mentoring behaviors as guiding, cooperating, supporting, and listening actively supports student's learning in the clinical setting.

The head nurse should accept and recognize their role in professional development of student nurses. The students develop a positive attitude from head nurses in caring patients The head nurse organizes bed side clinic nursing care conferences and nursing rounds to educate student nurses.

Bedside Clinic

Bedside clinic is always help to study the problems typically associated with a particular disease or disorder. It is one of the clinical teaching methods. Always ensure the presence of the patient while conducting the clinic. Either the group of students usually 6-8 visit the patient or the patient is brought to the conference room.

Patients with typical cases rather with unusual conditions are selected. During the clinic the patient may be asked to speak about himself, the course of illness, symptoms and involves the family members and plan for discharge. Brief history and therapy, nursing problems are presented along with the nursing care including physical, mental and social components during discussion.

Nursing clinic can be conducted by the head nurse or the clinical instructor. Before, the client's entry the head nurse points out the group the observations which should made while he/she is present. When the patient is no longer needed should send back to his bed. This is usually followed by a discussion and question and answer round. The teaching is summarized and the most important points are emphasized. The clinic lasts for about 30 min finally it is evaluated by the head nurse and the group members.

Advantages

The student nurse is getting an opportunity to observe, analyze and make-decision in nursing care. Remembers the nursing measures for longer time since directly they are involved in learning in actual situation.

Nursing Care Conference

Nursing care conference is same like a bedside clinic but the patient is not usually present for the class. This may be a method of choice when the entire group is acquainted with the patient. Bedside clinic and nursing care conference can be used to evaluate the students in clinical learning. Both should be planned earlier if it is to be made more effective. But the nurse instructor conducts it on the spot if she wishes to evaluate the students.

Nursing Rounds

Nursing round is a visit into patient's area or wards involving the students and discussion with head nurses. It provides rich learning experiences. In nursing rounds the patient history and the medical aspects of his/her care are included only as a background for understanding the nursing care. The head nurse is responsible for the patient should answer questions aroused in the group. Suggestions are made by the members of the group. Suggestions discussed in the rounds will be recorded. Rounds may extend only up to one hour

The nursing round is conducted with many purposes. They are information giving rounds, instructional rounds and problem solving rounds.

Advantages

- Nursing round increases the learning ability of student nurses
- Increases interest among students to share ideas and knowledge with others for the benefit of the patients
- During nursing rounds response of the patient is more natural
- Students can select patient with specific problem and plan for proper nursing care.

SUMMARY POINTS

- ✓ We are living in the era of consumerism and our health consumer (patient) has every right to have a safe, clean, noise free, spacious, fresh aired and restful environment for his speedy recovery from illness. Keeping these in mind many hospitals are constructed out skirts of the city.
- ✓ Earlier hospital wards were built with large open wards with high ceiling. A modern hospital today focuses to provide more privacy by constructing individual rooms or cubicles for 2–3 patients. While constructing every ward needs a good planning designed in such a way that it is constructed with minimum cost with maximum functioning capacity with quality.
- ✓ The ward should be located away from crowded, noisy, and parking area. It should be situated away from hospital mortuary. The pediatric ward, antenatal ward and causality ward should be preferably located in ground floor. Labor room, operation theater, and diagnostic services to be located adjacent to the wards
- ✓ The size of the ward varies from hospital to hospital.Normally it ranges from 20–80 beds. It should be kept to an optimum size because; the resources required are more or less same whether the ward size is 20, 30 or 40 beds.
- ✓ Nursing station occupies a very importance place in a ward. It should ensure adequate space, ventilation, light for nurses to work. There should be sufficient space or record cabinet for keeping records, stationeries, report forms charts, manuals and files. and a computer table with computer. The medication unit is very important aspect of nursing station.
- ✓ Good time planning is a managerial skill. The ward sister or head nurse has a responsibility to develop daily and weekly plan for nurses to utilize their precious time for patient care. The time planning refers to the plan of time in hours and days to be spend by nursing personnel for the activities for patient care. It helps in planning executing and evaluating the optimum use of time.
- ✓ Quality of patient care depends upon not only the availability of resources and infrastructure, but the ability of the head nurse in managing the ward also.She should be aware the factors involved in good ward management.
- ✓ One of the objectives of any health care facility is to ensure speedy recovery of patients from illness. This is achieved by facilitating patient safety, quality patient care, and maintaining a therapeutic environment. Therapeutic environment includes not only the physical structure of the unit, but also it envisages a psychosocially supported environment for patient, family and caregivers. In therapeutic environment the patient receives care that affects patient outcomes, patient satisfaction, patient safety, health workers efficiency, and satisfaction, and a positive organizational outcome.
- ✓ A good therapeutic environment can enhance patient care outcome, reduce or minimize stressors from environment, and promotes psycho social support for patients, family and health care providers.
- ✓ The head nurse plays an important role in clinical nursing education, helping to prepare nursing students for professional practice. A positive and enriched learning environment in the clinical setting has an impact on students perception of the ward unit as their future work is oriented to similar setting Facilitating a positive clinical learning experiences to students can motivate students to translate theory into practice on real patients.
- ✓ Nursing care conference is same like a bedside clinic but the patient is not usually present for the class. This may be a method of choice when the entire group is acquainted with the patient. Bedside clinic and nursing care conference can be used to evaluate the students. Both should be planned earlier if it is to be made more effective. But the nurse instructor conducts it on the spot if she wishes to evaluate the students. Nursing rounds also helps student nurses to improve their clinical learning.

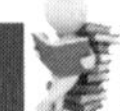

REVIEW QUESTIONS

1. Discuss the factors would you keep in mind while planning a ward.
2. Describe the functions and responsibilities of head nurse in time management for improving care of patients.
3. Explain in detail the factors influencing a good ward management.
4. Define therapeutic environment. As a head nurse how will you promote a therapeutic environment for your patients.
5. Describe the role of head nurse in enhancing student learning in a ward.
6. Write Short Notes on
   a. Objectives of ward planning
   b. Size of the ward
   c. Causes of time waste in a hospital ward
   d. Preventing interruptions in care
   e. Objectives of time planning
   f. Nursing care conference and nursing rounds.

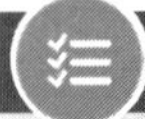

SELECTED READINGS

1. Gary W. Evans and Janetta M.M. Role of architecture in human health, *Environmental Psychology*, 18, 85-94, 1998.
2. Geri-Ann Galanti. Caring for Patients from Different Cultures, U.S. University of Pennsylvania Press, 2003
3. Jain Malkin Hospital Interior Architecture: Creating Healing Environments for Special Patient Populations. New York: John Wiley and Sons, Inc., 1992.
4. Jean Barret.Ward management and teaching, New Delhi: Konark publishers, 2004
5. Jean Barrette and G.H.Gessoner, The head nurse and her leadership role, 3rd edition, New York, Appleton century crofts, 1975
6. Kathryn H. Anthony and Nicholas Watkins Exploring Pathology: Relationships between Clinical and Environmental Psychology, Handbook of Environmental Psychology (pp. 129–146), R. Bechtel and A. Churchman (Eds.) New York: John Wiley and Sons, 2002.
7. Roger Ulrich "How Design Impacts Wellness". Healthcare Forum Journal, 1992.
8. Ron Smith Therapeutic Environments from the Therapeutic Environments Forum, AIA Academy of Architecture for Health, Design at the Intersection, LLC I Healthcare,
9. Stephen Kaplan, and Rachael Kaplan Human scape: Environments for People. Second edition. Ann Arbor, MI: Ulrich's Books, Inc. Inquiry by Design, 2006.

UNIT XIII
EDUCATIONAL ADMINISTRATION

23

Applications of Principles of Administration in Nursing Education

LEARNING OBJECTIVES

This chapter imparts learning about:

- Planning
- Organizing
- Staffing
- Directing
- Controlling
- Budgeting in nursing education

The principal is the head of college of nursing or school of nursing when a school/college of nursing to be started she has to plan ahead with the aim of getting the institution recognized by Indian nursing council. She /he should be knowledgeable, resourceful and exercise leadership while working with management and other concerned people responsible to start a college/school of nursing.

A good nursing school functions well when the management and controlling authority has interest in nursing education, supportive to nursing, cooperative, understand the objectives of nursing education, provides excellent infrastructure as recommended by national and state nursing statutory bodies, and facilitate adequate resources including faculty, materials and budget.

APPLICATIONS OF PRINCIPLES OF PLANNING IN NURSING SCHOOL ADMINISTRATION

Planning is the primary and key function of nursing school administration to fulfill the objectives for which the institution is established. The principal as an administrator requires managerial skills to establish a school of nursing. Good planning focuses on key fundamentals that enables to carry out the overall activities of the nursing school, envisions a futuristic needs of faculty and students for the development of the institution. It involves all levels of management in planning, stresses ongoing review for monitoring the progress and it is goal oriented. Further good planning gives direction to work, ensures control over administration and maintains cost-effectiveness.

Steps in Planning the School of Nursing

- Through a survey keeping curriculum determinants in mind, identify and ensure a need for a school of nursing in that area.

Planning for Obtaining Certificates from Statutory Bodies

- Establish a board of trustees or management for the establishment
- Develop vision, mission and philosophy for the nursing school
- Obtain permission to start the school from the State Government(NOC) **or essentiality certificate.**
- Send the proposal to Indian nursing council and being the national statutory body, the INC will conduct the first inspection to assess suitability with

regard to physical infrastructure, clinical facility and teaching faculty in order to give permission to start the programme. If the commission satisfied, **a suitability certificate** is issued by INC also advices the number of students could be admitted per year.

- After obtaining the suitability certificate from INC, the institution should move towards the state nursing council for approval of **registration.**
- Then the institution must obtain from examination board (for nursing school)/and university (for college of nursing) for affiliation.
- Both state council and university or state board nursing do inspection of the school/college simultaneously and give approval to start the college.
- Institution will admit the students only after taking approval of State Nursing Council and Examination Board.
- The Indian Nursing Council will conduct inspection every year till the first batch completes the programme. Permission will be given year by year till the first batch completes. The examination board and state nursing council conducts inspection every year before the next academic session starts.

Planning for Infrastructure Facilities

- The school should be built in 3 acres of land that is required to start nursing school/college subject to the conditions that they have minimum 54470 sq. ft. constructed area.
- It will be in a separate building or unitary building owned by the management.

Planning for Selection, Recruitment and Appointment of Faculty

The principal should know the staffing norms for each year as per INC recommendations. Before, the students are admitted, the required number of faculty to be recruited, selected and appointed as per norms. She needs to be updated with the staffing norms for school/college of nursing for the definite number of students.

Planning for Selection of Students

- Develops and finalize admission policies for students as per INC norms
- Develops college or school of nursing brochure for students
- Plans for sources for getting students (advertisement, media word of mouth, through friends, talk about nursing among students of twelfth standards nursing journal, film on nursing profession).
- Finalizing application form, admission policies, selection committee, criteria for selection.

Criteria for selection should be based on the recommendation of statutory bodies. Plan for starting program the members of the selection committee should include: the principal the senior tutor a representative of the local controlling authority (hospital) a representative from the nursing section of the state (if applicable), physician and an academician and a psychologist.

Planning for Student Hostel

- Develop hostel policies, hostel facilities-living room, toilet and bathing facilities, extracurricular activities (playground) and facilities for indoor games.
- Policies for visiting parents.
- Food and accommodation.
- Plan for student health and a sick room in hostel and facilities.
- Rest room for night shift student nurses.
- Plan for medical check-up examination on joining and every year.

Planning for Clinical Facilities

To start a college of nursing 300 bedded and for school of nursing a minimum 200 bedded parent/affiliated hospital is recommended. The staffing pattern 1:5 nurse patient ratio to be maintained by the affiliated hospital. The hospital having less than 500 beds 60 seats and more than 500 beds 100 seats can be admitted as per INC norms and as per sanction by statutory bodies by inspection and verification regarding other infrastructure norms.

Planning for adequate budget to run the school as well as budgetary policies to be finalized for the smooth running of the school/college.

Planning for Curriculum Implementation

The school/college should formulate its **philosophy, objectives.**

Selection of learning experiences including classrooms, library, preclinical labs, teachers offices, principal offices, toilet facilities for boys and girls separately, dining room for day scholars, selection instructional aids both projected and nonprojected aids to be planned.

Organization of learning experiences include teaching system, curriculum, syllabus, course outlines, unit plans, lesson plans, and all registers for clinical experiences master rotation plans, individual subject rotation plans, internal rotation plans to be developed.

Evaluation policies for both formative and summative evaluation, evaluation of knowledge attitude and skill, evaluation techniques for theory and practice, internal examination for theory and practice and clinical records to be developed.

Planning for students extracurricular activities and planning for student nurses association at unit level to be kept in mind.

Planning for various committees like curriculum appraisal committee, committees for student hostel and health, food, library, quality assurance, extracurricular activities, recruitment and selection, student grievances and evaluation to be taken care of.

APPLICATIONS OF PRINCIPLES OF ORGANIZATION IN NURSING SCHOOL ADMINISTRATION

Organization is defined as a group of people who work together in an organized way for a shared purpose.

In nursing education institutions, organization refers to the systematic, and orderly process of identifying teachers and staff, and grouping the work to be performed in their departments, specifying the work by ensuring job descriptions, defining and delegating the responsibility with authority to the teachers, and establishing inter personal relationships for the purpose of intra and interdepartmental coordination of work so as to get the work done together effectively in accomplishing the objectives of the nursing school/college of nursing.

- The head of the school/college should exercise transformational and transactional leadership in dealing with the faculty, staff and students. She should be a visionary and communicates the vision, mission and philosophy of school/college of nursing to all faculty and students as planned.
- Proper educational policies, procedures and standards are developed and implemented.
- Since, the authority flow from top to bottom, she prepares an organization chart of the college to communicate organizational relationship. (see Box 23.1). It is a design of the organizational structure specifying various departments with staff and line relationship.
- All the teachers and staff are accountable to one person in the organization that is the principal.
- A definite job description is given to all faculty members including the principal to know their functions and it is essential to avoid duplication of work and enhance organizational effectiveness.
- Delegation is one of the principles of organization. The principal delegates the tasks according to the competency and experience of the faculty and various departmental heads. Once the task is delegated the principal monitors the faculty by effective supervision to achieve the organizational objectives. Mentoring, coaching and counseling is facilitated to the needed faculty by the principal to maintain academic standard.
- The principal ensures prompt decision-making and good communication among faculty and students that influence organizational effectiveness.
- Maintains a conducive academic environment for faculty and students to enhance an academic environment.
- The principal organizes meeting with various committees of the college/school and maintains the minutes of the meetings.
- Departmental meetings are planned for the development and implementation of curriculum.
- Regular meetings with nursing staff of the affiliated hospital to maintain integration of theory and practice

Clinical supervisors are posted in the clinical area with 10 students each keeping in mind the span of supervision principle.

APPLICATIONS OF PRINCIPLES OF STAFFING IN NURSING SCHOOL ADMINISTRATION

The standard of nursing education is influenced by many factors and staffing is the most important factors. It is also interpreted as Human Resource Management (HRM).

Human resource management is the management process of combining various activities that are designed to enhance the effectiveness of the manpower in an organization in the achievement of organizational goals. Human resource management (HRM) may be defined as the function of planning for human resource needs, recruitment, selection, development, compensation and evaluation of performance to fill those needs.

Staffing ensures that the organization has the required number of people and the needed kind of people at the right places, at the desired time ,and that they are skilful to do the services. Importance of staffing helps in identifying and getting the right personnel who for higher performances, by putting their effort for various jobs. Staffing ensures the continuous survival helps in the growth of the establishment through the succession planning for managers.

The concept of staffing includes planning for, recruiting, selecting, and training and developing faculty members, as well as compensating them and providing for their health and safety.

Box 23.1: A sample organization chart of a college of nursing

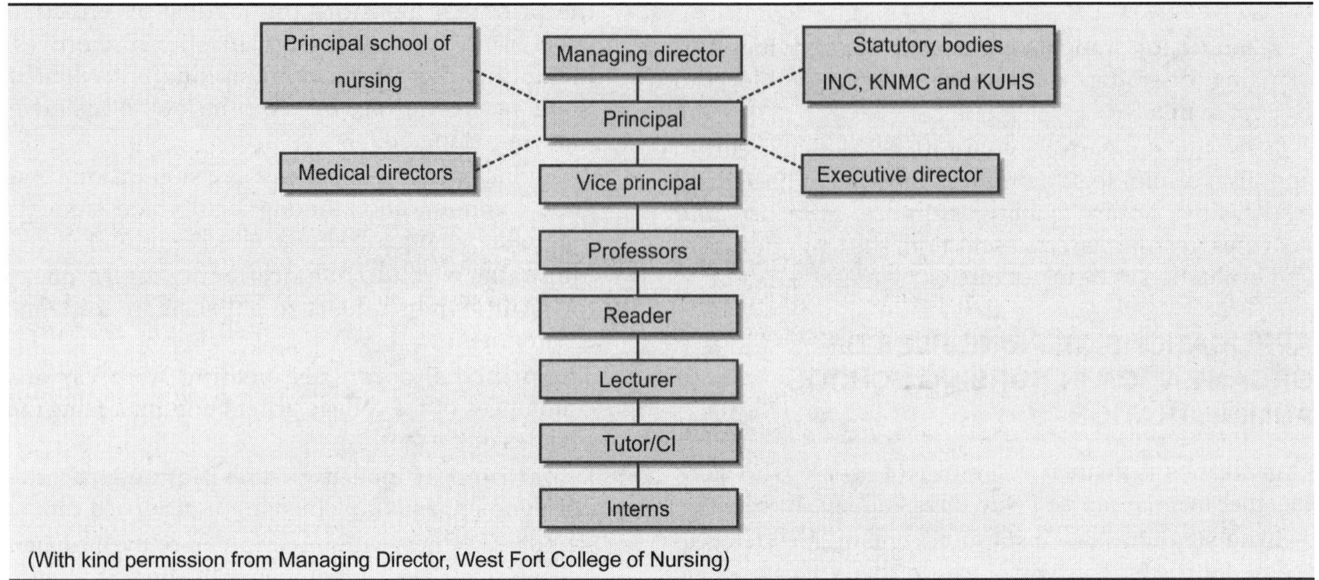

(With kind permission from Managing Director, West Fort College of Nursing)

RECRUITMENT

It refers to the process of inducing the candidates to apply for the job in the organization. After assessing the number and cadre of faculty member required, the Principal tries that more and more people should apply for the job so that the organization can get more choice and select better candidates.

Definition

Recruitment is a method of finding suitable candidates to fill various positions in an organization. According to Edwin B Flippo, 'Recruitment is a process of searching for prospective employees and stimulating them to apply for job in an organization.'

Purposes of Recruitment

- To attract and motivate more number of candidates
- To create a pool of candidates and select the suitable candidates as required
- To select the best candidate for the job as specified.

Recruitment of Faculty is One of the Staffing Functions

It is a continuous process. It is a systematic procedure and the principal ensures the following steps in recruiting faculty:

- Identifying vacancies for the post of clinical instructor, lecturer, reader, professor, etc.
- Developing criteria for selection of the particular cadre of faculty, his or her job and specification.
- Advertisement for filling vacancies in professional journals, media.
- Receiving responses from applicants.
- Short listing candidates based on criteria developed
- Arrange and inform candidates for interviews
- Conducting interviews by recruitment and selection committee comprising.
- After recruiting candidates from external or internal source, the selection process is the next step.

SELECTION OF FACULTY

- The principal receives the application forms.
- Scrutinizing committee scrutinizes applications. The committee ensures by checking age of the candidate, gender, educational qualification and experience, religion and community, references and medical fitness. It helps the employer to eliminate incomplete as well as ineligible application forms.
- Conducting preliminary interview.
- According to the job different tests are planned and conducted. Aptitude test, attitude tests, personality tests intelligent tests, etc. When a nurse teacher comes for preliminary interview usually a model teaching for actual students are asked to conduct on the candidates specialty area.
- The committee conducts final interview.
- The candidates who clear the tests successfully are called for final interview.
- Facilitate proper seating arrangement, drinking water facility for the candidate.
- Ensure adequate light and ventilation in interviewing venue.

- The panel members of interview to be informed about the interview well on time.
- Criterion sheet for evaluating the candidate with score to be given to each panel members.
- After interview all panel needs to sign and justify the cause for the selected and rejected candidates. Rank list is prepared by panel members.
  - The principal checks with persons (references) who were given in the application form for further verification of the candidates.
  - A complete medical examination is done by an authorized medical officer to ensure the candidate is medically fit to take up the job.
  - When all the selection procedures are conducted and satisfied the principal sends an appointment letter showing the title of the post, place of work, date of joining, testimonials to be submitted along. with joining report, salary and other benefits, probation and confirmation period, etc.

ORIENTATION AND PLACEMENT OF THE FACULTY

Once the selection process is over, the appointed faculty member is made familiar to the job settings (class rooms, library, preclinical labs, office, community centers, affiliated parent hospital and the management) and work environment through an orientation program to make the newly appointed teacher feel a sense of belongingness to the school/college of nursing.

PROMOTION OF THE FACULTY

- Promotion is the upward reassignment of a faculty member in the school administration's hierarchy. This is accompanied by increased responsibilities, enhanced status, and usually with increased monetary benefits Higher the position, the employee is promoted, that increases responsibilities and accountabilities more than the previous position. Further it brings changes in the designation, status and work facilities.
- All promotions are considered for a trial period, in case the promoted faculty is not found capable of handling the assigned task.
- The principal ensures the promotion policy is communicated to all faculty members.

RETENTION OF FACULTY MEMBER

The principal uses various employment strategies to retain faculty and prevent frequent turnover, such as:

- Cultivating e a positive work environment in school/college.
- Recognition of skill of the faculty and provides adequate supervision and support to novice teachers.
- Ensures benefits and compensation by discussing with faculty members.
- Recommends for increment, higher pay and benefits and promotion for eligible teachers who do a good teaching and supervisory job.
- Facilitates professional growth of the faculty by the following activities:
  1. Cultivating a learning culture in the hospital and nursing school/college environment.
  2. Encouraging and motivating faculty to create individual learning plans.
  3. Encouraging all faculty members to join professional associations.
  4. Organizing regular training and mentoring programme for faculty.
  5. Providing incentives for updating knowledge.
  6. Fostering faculty member's development through deputation, relieve from duty to attend seminar, conferences and guest lectures.
  7. Using contests and incentives to help nurses keep motivated for learning.
  8. Facilitating coaching, mentoring and guiding faculty for higher positions.
  9. Enhancing computer literacy.
  10. Motivating to conduct or participate in research
- Fosters a supportive culture in school of nursing/college.
- Facilitates for job flexibility by scheduling vacation, leave, shift time, and work load.
- Conducts regular staff meeting.
- Arranges for informal gathering time to time for open up feeling.
- The principal demonstrates organizational commitment as a role model.
- Proper dealing with low morale as and when the principal identifies them.

PERSONNEL POLICIES

As a principle of staffing the principal develops and communicates personnel policies for the faculty members

- Personnel policy is developed on the basis of school's objectives.
- A personnel policy is a written document that defines the expectations of management to faculty members and expectation of faculty to the management.

- A policy provides guidelines to the faculty in organization for choosing a course of action.
- All policies related to personnel decision is complied and is called personnel policy manual.
- The faculty can be terminated or retained as per personnel policies.

STAFF DEVELOPMENT PROGRAM

In nursing school/college administration there is a staff development department with a teacher as a coordinator with the main aim of enhancing the personal and professional growth of faculty members and other personnel while they are on the job.

The regulatory bodies of nursing at the national and state level recognize the need of staff development to renew the registration of nurses. To bring uniform standard the Indian nursing council has made it mandatory that nurses should obtain 150 nursing credit hours in five years or 30 nursing credit hours in a year by attending in-service education program otherwise nurses need to do re-registration to practice nursing in the country.

While organizing staff development program the principal keeps in mind the following objectives:

- Assist each faculty member to acquire and enhance personal and professional performance.
- To ensure safe and effective teaching and clinical supervision of student nurses by professional knowledge, attitude and professional competency.
- To help faculty to cope with newer trends in curriculum administration.
- To enhance job satisfaction among faculty members

The various types of staff development program for faculty members planned by the school are:

- Orientation
- Skill training
- Continuing education program
- Leadership and managerial skills

SUPERVISION

Supervision is a managerial tool envisages working together to achieve organizational goals the principal:

- Supervises and guides all teaching and non teaching faculty members
- Facilitates a good infrastructure facilities and learning environment for students.
- Procures and maintains instructional materials for teaching and learning.
- Ensures the safety and security of nursing students in the hospital.
- Supervises patient care in all units wherever nurses are posted by nursing rounds.
- Initiates and coordinate research program in nursing practices.
- Organizes and chairs Institution Review Board (IRB) and a member of Ethical committee.
- Promotes evidence based practices in clinical area.

DEVELOPING JOB DESCRIPTION FOR NURSING FACULTY

In order to maintain smooth running of the school/college, the principal. Develops and communicate their job responsibility in orientation program and providing personnel policy manual

APPLICATION OF PRINCIPLES OF DIRECTING IN NURSING SCHOOL ADMINISTRATION

- The principal of the nursing college/school exercises transformational and transactional **leadership** in realizing the vision and goals of the school As a leader she administers the institution observing all principles of directing the institution.
- Establishes effective **communication** between members of the faculty, students, staff and parents.
- The principal applies techniques, skills and knowledge of **motivational theory** to help teachers and students to achieve the goals of nursing school.
- Creates a **conducive working environment** that enhances job satisfaction among members of faculty and other staff.
- Facilitates a **motivational climate** where teachers work with autonomy and able to meet basic needs
- Provides counseling and guidance, coaching and training to increase individual teacher/students' performance and creates a productive climate.
- Applies positive and negative reinforcements, punishment and extinction approaches of motivation to enhance organizational behavior teachers and students.
- Ensures the knowledge **of group dynamics** that is needed for the head of the institution to improve leadership competencies and facilitates group discussions and communication. She is aware of groups that are a common platform of a majority of experiences of all nurses. As a principal she identifies problems, creating choices and providing alternatives courses of actions.

- The principal is aware of her success in leading her department depends on her ability to create a **health human relation climate.** Nursing leaders need to understand that nurses are human beings with social and emotional needs.
- Demonstrates **transformational leadership**, optimistic and positive outlook towards nursing personnel and ensures trust in teachers, students and staff members.
- Shows concerns about the satisfaction of nursing staff.
- Involve teachers in planning, implementing and **participatory decision-making**.
- The principal maintains a **good public relation** with community agencies, parents and patients She communicates to the public what nursing education is its scope and advantages to the public.
- As a **decision-maker** the principal makes-decisions and initiating new ideas to improve the performance of nursing school.
- Takes corrective decisions when there is a disturbance in the school to cope up with the situation.
- She decides for resource allocation such as man, money, materials and time for the smooth functioning of the school/college.
- **Delegates** the work effectively to the competent faculty.
- **Manages conflict** that occurs sometimes in school is handled effectively.
- Uses best possible **negotiation strategies** to overcome dispute or conflict occurs in school/college of nursing
- In order to direct the organization, she encourages all faculty and students to become member of the professional organization and participates in **collective bargaining** through professional organization (refer Chapters 14 and 15 for theory part of directing)

APPLICATION OF PRINCIPLES OF CONTROLLING IN NURSING SCHOOL ADMINISTRATION

- Nursing care excellence depends on **quality** education To prepare competent nurse practitioners, versed in the practice environment today, the principal and faculty of school/college of nursing have a great responsibility.
- In order to enhance and improve academic activities the nursing school administration strives to maintain **Quality Assurance** program. The principal chairs the quality assurance committee and conducts **educational audit** periodically to ensure the objectives of the school are achieved various **quality improvement** models are used to monitor academic excellence of the nursing school.
- **Performance appraisal** is a systematic and planned process to assess the performance capabilities of the faculty on his job based on criteria, and serves as an effective control mechanism in organization The principal prepares goal oriented performance standard for all staff of school of nursing. The performance appraisal include criteria for appraisal, who will appraise, when and how it will be assessed, how it will be communicated to the appraise and follow-up activity after appraisal. This also provides for counseling, coaching, training or mentoring for the teachers if needed after performance appraisal. As per the policy the performance appraisal is done. periodically and a follow-up interview and observation of the staff is done.

Box 23.2: A sample box format of performance appraisal (West Fort College of Nursing)

Performance appraisal for faculty member

A. To be filled by the faculty

Name of the institution______________________

Name of the faculty member______________________

Designation______________________

Date of joining the institution______________________

Date of confirmation______________________

Present address______________________

Permanent address______________________

I. Academics

1. **General education**__________Board/ University_______Year of passing _______Division/ Rank
2. **Professional education**______School/University________Year of Passing__________ Division/ Rank__________

II. Professional up-date.

1. **Continuing education** (seminar, workshop, conferences, academic meeting undergone/undergoing____(attach certificate of at-tend ance, certificate of presentation/ chairing session/ resource person if any)______________
2. **Research**____________ Departmental/ Institutional______________ Details of the study protocol, study report, (attach in a separate sheet)
3. **Details for publication** if any ___________ (Enclose the abstract of the study in a separate sheet)

III. Co-curricular activities

Areas of activities organized/ participated

1 ______________________

2 ______________________

3 ______________________

4 ______________________

IV. Counseling and guidance

1 ______________________

2 ______________________

3 ______________________

4 ______________________

V. Leadership activities

(Specify organization of workshop, conferences, field trip for students and your role as leader (as chairperson, secretary, treasurer, committee chairperson, etc.)

____

____

____

VI. Participation in college administration/ curriculum administration

Specify your participation as class coordinator, clinical coordinator, Laboratory In charge, student advisor, chairperson of college committee, inspection by statutory bodies, paper evaluator or any administrative work entrusted by the head of the institution

____

____

____

____

____

(Attach additional sheet if required)

B. Self-evaluation

(Write a paragraph on your own evaluation on what has been assigned during the academic year, how far you were able to achieve the objectives, what type of innovation you could bring in your teaching and student learning, what you could not achieve and why? Write your own suggestions to improve your teaching learning and research activities)

____

____

____

Signature of the faculty member **Date**

S.No.	Criteria	Always (AL)	Usually (US)	Sometimes (SM)	Never (NV)
A TEACHING (To be filled by the Principal)					
1	**Content preparation**				
	• In relation to the syllabi requirements appropriate • Content prepared according to the level of learner • Content is recent in discipline • Presentation of divergent view points • Lesson plan,assignments,instructional aids appropriate				
2	**Organization of the content** • Logical sequence of topics • Pace of the lecture, discussion topics • Provision of summary and re-enforcement • Appropriate use of class time				
3	**Clarity of presentation** • Definition of new term, concepts, principles • Relevance of examples • Co-relation of theory with lab, clinical practice • Questioning ability • Students participation				
4	**Style of presentation** • Stimulates students thinking • Professional and ethical behavior • Demonstrates mutual respect • Personal mannerism, voice and vocabulary				
B CLINICAL SUPERVISION (Applicable to nursing school/Nursing college only)					
	• Maintains punctuality, professional dignity, professional attitude • Maintain professional competency • Provides quality clinical supervision including maintaining appropriate documentation				
C ADMINISTRATIVE RESPONSIBILITIES					
	• Participates in college committees • Participates in organizing and conducting any college functions/ activities • Attends professional conferences/staff development programme and updates professional knowledge and participates in co- and extra curricular activities				
D RESEARCH					
	• Participates in conducting research, demonstrates interest in publishing scholarly articles, guides students in their research work				
	Total marks allotted _________100 **Marks obtained** ___________ **Grade:** • Excellent > 90 marks • Very good 75–89 marks • Good 61–74 marks • Need for improvement < 60 marks **Areas need to be improved**___________________				

Comments by the Principal
Eligible for promotion.........Yes/ No
Eligible for confirmation ... Yes/No
Eligible for higher education./sponsorship Yes/No
Eligible for increment Yes/No
Signature of the Principal ....
Date............

*My signature indicates that I have read this format and received a copy of it. If I disagree with it, I will be responding in writing within 10 working days and my comments will be attached to this observation form

Signature of the faculty ....
Date

Comments by the Managing Director

....

....

....

....

Signature..Date

(This evaluation covers the Planning skills, management skills, cognitive skills, human relation skills, and professionalism of the faculty being assessed)

(With the kind permission from the Managing Director, West fort college of nursing)

- When the performance of the teacher is not satisfactory, the principal facilitates **counseling, mentoring and coaching** to the faculty for improving her job.
- **Maintaining discipline** in school of nursing is one of the tools of principle of controlling the administration. The principal identifies disciplinary problem among faculty, staff and students and take effective disciplinary strategies to maintain discipline in nursing school/college
- **The grievance** committee (cell) of the school investigate the grievances among staff and report to the principal. Necessary grievance handling procedure is taken promptly to prevent adverse incidents (Refer Chapters 16 and 17 for principles of controlling.

APPLICATION OF PRINCIPLES OF BUDGET IN NURSING SCHOOL ADMINISTRATION

Budget is a managerial tool. It is very important function of principal. Planning, organizing implementing and evaluating the budget are important aspects of financial administration. The principal of school/college of nursing must understand fiscal terminology and aware of budgetary responsibility. She is accountable to the school of nursing for maintaining a cost — effective unit

- The principal **forecasts unit fiscal needs** and prepare unit needs to ensure sufficient funds or budget.
- Formulates **philosophy, objectives and goals** for effective financial administration of school.
- Involves herself and participates in **budgetary decisions and policies.**
- Prepares a **budgetary projection** to meet the institutional needs.
- The principal **monitors** aspects of budget control and involve the faculty members in fiscal planning.
- **Monitors revenues and expenditure** throughout the budget year and day to day expenses.
- Prepares a **budget calendar** for the school/ college
- She should be able to **include flexibility, creativity** and vision regarding future needs **anticipate budget constraints** and act proactively.
- She ensures that **cost containment** does not jeopardize patient safety.
- The budget prepares for the following areas like receipt, non-plan expenditure and plan for expenditure (see Boxes. 23.3, 23.4 and 23.5)

Box 23.3: Sample format for budget for BSc nursing college*

	SAMPLE FORMAT FOR BUDGET FOR BSc NURSING COLLEGE				
	RECIEPTS				
S. No	Particulars	Accounts 2014-15 (₹)	Budget estimates 2015-16	Budget estimates 2015-16	Budget estimates 2016-17
1	Registration fee				
2	Tuition fee				
3	Library fee				
4	Laboratory fee				
5	Hostel fee				
6	Student service and amenities fee				
7	Miscellaneous fee				
8	Caution deposit				
9	Other fee				
	Total				

* It is a sample only

Box 24.4: Budget format for nonplan expenditure*

SNo	NON-PLAN EXPENDITURE				
	Particulars	Accounts 2014-15 (₹)	Budget estimates 2015-16	Budget estimates 2015-16	Budget estimates 2016-17
1	Salaries and allowances				
2	Medical expenses				
3	TA and conveyance				
4	Rent, tax, insurance				
5	Vehicle maintenance				
6	Electricity and water charges				
7	Postage, telephone telegram				
8	Internet access				
9	Repair and maintenance				
10	Office expenses				
11	College function—lamp lighting annual day celebration				
12	College sports				
13	CNE program				
14	Deputation expenses				
15	Students scholarship				
16	Clinical affiliation expenses				
17	Bank charges, interest				
18	Student welfare				
19	Contingency expenses				
20	University exam expenses				
21	Awards for outstanding student and faculty				
22	Celebration of college day				
23	External teachers expenses				
24	Imprest (petty cash)				
	Total				

* It is a sample only

Box 24.5: Plan expenditure*

SNo	PLAN EXPENDITURE				
	Particulars	Accounts 2014-15 (₹)	Budget estimates 2015-16	Budget estimates 2015-16	Budget estimates 2016-17
1	Land				
2	Building				
3	Equipment—furniture and fixures				
4	Office equipment				
5	Laboratory equipment				
6	Library equipment				
7	Computers and soft wares				
8	Hostel building and equipment				
9	Total				

* It is a sample only

The items (Particulars) may vary as per the nursing school policy.

All the principles of administration such as planning, organization, staffing, directing, controlling and budget can be applied in nursing school/ college administration.

The sample format for performance appraisal, formats budget plans given in boxes are only ideas presented by the author. The principals of school/college of nursing can build up or delete some of the item presented.

The theoretical part of budget is presented in Chapter 19 for depth understanding.

SUMMARY POINTS

- ✓ Planning for nursing school include getting essentiality certificate from the government, and suitability certificate from Indian Nursing Council. Apart from this certificate for registration from state nursing council and permission from the university is required for affiliation if it is a degree program.
- ✓ Planning for infrastructure of college and hostel is very important, clinical facilities to be well planned before we start a college or school of nursing. The principal is responsible to plan for faculty and students.
- ✓ Budget planning is important function in nursing school administration.
- ✓ Organization principle is well applied in nursing school administration. Preparation of organization chart, job description of faculty to be developed Exercising effective leadership the principal implements academic policies, administrative decision and proper delegation to faculty to maintain organizational effectiveness.
- ✓ Application of staffing includes calculation faculty as per recommended norms, recruitment, selection, placement orientation and in-service education program for faculty members.
- ✓ Directing is another principle of administration. The principal as a leader translates the vision and philosophy to achieve the institutional goals. Group dynamics, human relations, public relation in context of nursing, decision making, delegation, conflict management, negotiation and collective bargaining are some of the principles applied in directing the smooth functioning of the nursing school.
- ✓ The nursing school is controlled by implanting quality assurance, quality control, educational auditing, and quality improvement program. Performance appraisal is used to monitor and develop the faculty and students competence. Grievance handling is done promptly to prevent organizational conflict The principal maintains discipline in nursing school and takes disciplinary action if adverse event occur.
- ✓ In order to maintain standard of the institution, the principal gives proposals of budget including all resources. She makes a budget plan and monitor every day the status of finance. She helps in quarterly and annual auditing of the budget.

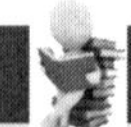

REVIEW QUESTIONS

1. Discuss the principle of planning applied in nursing school administration
2. What are organizational principles? How they are applied in nursing school administration?
3. Describe the responsibilities of a principal in staffing a college of nursing.
4. Describe academic leadership in directing the nursing school.
5. Define controlling. How this principle of controlling is applied in nursing school administration?
6. Write Short Notes on:
    a. Orientation to novice faculty
    b. Job description of a tutor in school of nursing
    c. Outline a performance appraisal performa to assess a faculty
    d. Role a principal in maintaining discipline in nursing students hostel
    e. Nursing school budget
    f. Providing an academic culture in nursing college.

SELECTED READINGS

1. Excite Education – Nursing Administration Degrees,...
   www.excite.com
2. http://nursinglink.monster.com/education/articles/6534-tips-for-a-nursing-school-budget
3. Indian nursing Council, Staffing http://www.indiannursingcouncil.org/pdf/
4. INC Land norms http://www.rajswasthya.nic.in/Inc.pd
5. Learning theories application in nursing education
   www.ncbi.nlm.nih.gov › ... › v.4; 2015
6. Mapping the literature of nursing administration
   www.ncbi.nlm.nih.gov ... v.94(2 Suppl); 2006 Apr...
7. Nursing Leadership and Management - Carter Center
   www.cartercenter.org/resources/pdfs/.../nursing_students
8. Nursing Leadership and Management ... effective in application. Nursing service administration is the ... regarding career planning. Application to Nursing
9. Principles of Management Lecture Notes for MBA -... www.scribd.com/doc/30457447Cached
10. Staffing Pattern Collegiate Programme www.indiannursingcouncil.org/pdf/ST

UNIT XIV
ISSUES AND CHALLENGES

24

Issues and Challenges in Nursing Administration

LEARNING OBJECTIVES

This chapter imparts learning about:

- Issues and Challenges in Nursing Service Administration
- Issues and Challenges in Educational Administration
- Research Highlights

INTRODUCTION

Nursing service administration is more exciting and as well as more challenging than ever before. Effective nursing administration offers wide range of opportunities to innovate, to grow personally, and to inspire patient care excellence. The task of managing, organizing, delivering and improving safe and effective nursing care in this changing health care environment requires sound managerial skills. The main challenge into nursing management faced by nurses today is how to facilitate safe, reliable, cost-effective high quality patient care in today's challenging environment.

Nursing service administration is a process of planning, organizing, leading and controlling the efforts of the members of the organization. It is the effective utilization of available resources to achieve the pre-established goals of the organization that is to bring better quality patient care outcomes.

Current Trends in Health Care Delivery System

- Emphasis on quality, patient safety, benchmark and accreditation.
- Patient average length of stay in the hospital need to be reduced.
- Growth of outpatient care is increasing.
- High rocketing health care cost that is not affordable to a common man.
- Shifting trends in demographics—born earlier and living longer, living with chronic illness.
- Long-term care and assisted living is very important for nurses.
- Emphasis on prevention and quality of life in health care industry.
- Global shortage of nurses.
- Health care consumerism and E-health, rapidly changing technology.
- Complementary and alternative therapy in nursing.
- Disparities in urban and rural health care.
- Globalization of health.
- Legal and ethical issues in nursing.
- Terrorism/bioterrorism, disaster nursing
- Web-based nursing degrees.
- Generational diversity—work force differences in attitude, work habits and expectation.

ISSUES AND CHALLENGES IN NURSING SERVICE ADMINISTRATION

Global Shortage of Nurses

Why There is a Shortage of Nurses?

Some of the major causes of shortage of nurses are steep rise in population growth, majority of nurses are retiring, job opportunities within the health care system is expanding and nurses report high level of job dissatisfaction.

In spite of opening of nursing schools and colleges in large scale, our country still need 6.8 lakhs nurses by the end of this year. 55% of nurses are expected to retire by 2015. In India, Nurse: Doctor ratio = 1:1.5 and in abroad it is 3:1 and nurse population ratio, 1:1248. According to 2006 World Health Report, India had 0.60 doctors, 0.80 nurses, 0.47 midwives, 0.06 dentists for 1000 population.

Therefore, supply of nursing workforce remains a real and evident problem in many countries/states in India:

As per Nursing Human Resource in India: Current scenario (INC 2011) the nursing workforce available is:

- Registered ANM: 576 810
- Registered Nurse Midwife: 128 116
- Lady Health Visitors: 52 490.

Shortage of nurses poses a great problem for nurse administrators and is challenging. The nurse administrators need to develop innovative strategies to recruit and retain nurses. The vacant posts need to be filled. There should be manpower planning at central, state, district and institutional level.

Shifting Trends in Demographics

Due to the advancement in public health and clinical care, the life span of individuals is increasing rapidly. India is in a phase of demographic transition, has already acquired the label of 'aging nation'.

The population of elderly people in India is 57 millions and it is projected that India will have 324 millions of elderly by 2050. 75% of these will occupy the rural community. They live with chronic illness that needs greater attention.

This is a challenge for both community and hospital nurse administrators. Greater the life expectancy, individuals with acute and chronic illness, psycho-social and other age related problems are increasing. Long-term care and assisted living are recent trends. Nurses have high scope to work in geriatric settings and chronic care clinics/setting. Nurse administrators need to plan and organize geriatric care settings, develop policies and facilities for elderly care. Further, they need to develop geriatric specialized nurses with nursing care competencies to care such population.

The strengthening of primary health care is essential in addressing the burden of chronic diseases as well as in reaching the most vulnerable population and nurses play a key role in this area. To make best use of nurses in the health system, they should be encouraged and supported to perform at their highest potential.

Health Informatics System

Health Information Technology (HIT) is using computers to store, protect, retrieve and transfer information electronically within the health care system. Though, INC has introduced this subject in nursing curriculum recently, many senior nursing personnel may not be exposed to these trends.

Nurse managers at various levels need to know the benefits of using computers and its application in nursing practice, and administration such as patient informatics system, nursing informatics system, electronic documentation diagnosis and treatment packages. It poses a great challenge to nurse mangers to get updated knowledge on telehealth, video conferencing, telenursing among themselves and among all nurses.

Today, nurse administrators use computers for financial administration to monitor the cost of nursing services and to compare the expenses between the past and the present. Computers help in the calculating of salary and benefits and tax calculation for all nurses and health workers. At the same time, it helps to assess the bills of the hospitals paid. It ensures the administrator that the health care given to patients are cost-effective and efficient. Computers evaluates the quality assurance program of the hospitals and the utilization of available resources appropriately. Computers help to justify new roles and job description of nursing personnel, and estimation of staff and scheduling.

Globalization

Nursing services need to address health issues such as emerging and remerging infection that results from globalization.

There is an epidemiological transition in the world. Apart from Non-Communicable Diseases (NCD) such as diabetes, hypertension Cerebro-Vascular Accidents (CVA) cancers, and accidents, reemerging infectious diseases like Swine flu, Leptospirosis, chicken guinea, malaria are highly prevalent. TB (tuberculosis) is back again due to drug resistance. HIV/AIDS is also posing issues.

Nurse managers of hospitals and community need to strengthen their primary role of a case manager, and they have varied case loads of individuals and families whom they assist with illness oriented concerns.

Consumerism

We are living in the era of consumerism. Our consumers expect safety and quality care in clinical settings. When nursing care is inadequate, there is a greater overall incident of adverse events which are commonly patients fall, pressure ulcers, urinary tract infections, developing ventilator associated pneumonia, etc. that needs a greater attention. Our consumers are more knowledgeable today.

This poses a great challenge for nurses and nursing administrators. Nurses need to have significant leadership role in designing patient care delivery system. Care environment element must be optimized alongside nursing staffing and education to achieve high quality care. Nurse administrators need to develop clinical pathways to support implementation of practice standards, clinical guidelines, patient care protocol and clinical audit. Clinical supervision, continuity of staffing, more effective nurse-patient ratios and educational preparation of nurses are to be strengthened. Nurses must do nursing functions.

Nurses need to exhibit exemplary professional nursing practices by providing safe and quality care, protecting patients and avoiding risk or legal liabilities, protecting reputation of the organization and preventing illegal and unlawful practice.

Lack of Empowerment and Autonomy

Within the clinical setting, nurses are not able to make decision that affects the design of facilities, process of management and delivery methods which in turn affects patient care. Even with higher education in nursing they are not empowered to make independent decision for patient care.

Nurse administrators must exercise and promote transformational leadership role at all levels of their work and continue to encourage multidisciplinary collaboration in care. At postgraduate level, advanced practice nurses (APN) are prepared. The role of APN is clinical expert, educator, researcher, consultants and manager. APNs have competency in making clinical judgments, leadership skills, are an agent of change, and help in collaboration and communication. They must be fully utilized.

Nurses are not Involved in Policy Making at Various Level

The nursing management structure is majorly managed by senior policy makers from the medical fraternity, and provides very little scope for nursing professionals to participate in policy decision-making and to bring about any reforms. Lack of coordination between the senior nursing positions under the Department of Family Welfare/Department of Medical Services (DMS) and Director Medical Education (DME) is seen as one of the issues.

The weak supervisory structure for nursing staff both in clinical and public health cadres may be partially explained by the absence of nursing leadership positions at the state directorates.

Nurses to be included in all level of policy making. Accountability, autonomy and empowerment are closely related. In shared governance model, the traditional controlling roles of management must be replaced by a system which recognizes the importance of supporting nurses and nurse administrator need to reflect on respect, justice and trust in work place.

In January 2010, under 11th Five Year Plan, ₹ 1 crore was released to each of the 15 states for upgradation/ strengthening of Nursing Councils.

Special task force committee of TNAI developed job description and suggested restructuring of nursing services at various level stressing involvement of nurses in policy making.

Cost of Health Care

It is a major issue. The high rocketing price in hospitals for outpatient as well as in-patient care is alarmingly increasing. A common man cannot afford the cost for health care today.

To make patient care cost-effective, nurse managers implement the best practices evidence informed in clinical setting. They need to bring innovation in patient care to reduce the number of days in hospital stay and promote early discharge. They must utilize the services of postgraduate nurses with advanced nursing practice preparation in the clinical nursing care.

The administrators should make aware of nurses regarding health Insurance schemes available for individuals and they can help patients to utilize such benefits through Health Insurance Agencies.

Role Conflict and Poor Interpersonal Relationship

Role conflict in nursing occurs when nurses are confronted with incompatible role expectations in nursing. When nurses disagree about what the expectations are for a particular role or when someone simply has difficulty in satisfying expectations because their duties are unclear, too difficult, or disagreeable. These roles are based on institutional expectation, expectation from top level administration, expectations from peer group/subordinates and patient's expectation.

Conflict occurs in members of any occupation including nursing. Personality clashes are highly common among nurses, as nurses are confronted with many physical and psychosocial stressful circumstances that affects not only for nurses themselves (example, burnout syndrome) but also for patients and their families.

Some of the causes of role conflicts are long working hours, inadequate information about job responsibilities, varied job expectation, unable to make prioritization in patients care, lack of autonomy and unable to make patient care decision for care. There is a generational diversity in work force working in a unit also cause role conflict among nurses.

When nursing conflicts are not resolved, they can trigger many pressing problems in the work environment. They can lead to dis-satisfaction, indiscipline, grievances, poor interpersonal relationship among nurses. Unresolved issues can make some nurses feel that they are not part of the nursing service department. This causes poor morale and decreased productivity in organization.

This creates a great challenge for nurse administrators. They should define the role and responsibilities to nurses, and practice effective communication to enhance clarity of role. Good appreciation and rewards booster the morale of nurses. The nurse administrator must have conflict resolution skills and develop collaborative relationship with the members of the health team.

Inadequate Budget

Budgeting is a planning function of financial administration. It is an essential managerial tool. Nurse administrator requires sufficient funds to support quality services. Budget is required for salary of nursing personnel, equipment and supplies for patient care, maintaining day-to-day electricity, water supply, telephones, health education program, organizing in-service education program for nurses. Inadequate allocation of budget, and lack of knowledge and skills among nurse administrator in preparation of budget are some of the barriers in budgeting and inadequate budget negatively affect quality care outcome. Preparation of adequate budget for nurses and nursing care is a great challenge for nurse administrators.

Other Issues

Lack of personnel policies, hospital policies, lack of motivation among employees, inadequate equipment and supplies, poor working condition and work schedule are some of the other issues.

- It is a great challenge for nurse administrators to redesign and restructure nursing care delivery system.
- The nurse administrator should consider to re-engineering nursing information technology in academic and clinical work settings and manage constant change.
- The nurse administrator makes evidence-based decisions in organizational, clinical and academic problems.
- She/he should prepare nurses and faculty for health system transition.
- She/he should practice servant leadership to transform nurses and work environment.

The role of nurse administrator has been discussed in previous respective chapters as per the theory.

ISSUES AND CHALLENGES IN EDUCATIONAL ADMINISTRATION

Educational leadership is a term applied to school administration that attempts to create a positive change in educational policy and academic processes. Educational leaders are trained to advance and improve educational system or institutions. They are utilized as school principals or administrative head or an academic dean.

Impact of educational trends in academic leadership:

- **Entry to nursing practice is BSc Nursing:** Many countries in the world has accepted a BSc Nursing, is required as entry level qualification to nursing practice. In India still we have diploma in nursing program.
- **Educational mobility**: The outcome of educational mobility is the educational advancement of nurses prepared at levels on the educational continuum lower than the Baccalaureate degree. Educational mobility enables an individual to move from one educational level to another with acknowledgment of acquired competencies and minimal repetition of previous learning. The development and implementation of efficient and creative methods for identifying and evaluating prior learning: experience is the responsibility of nurse educators.
- **Education in a university without wall**: Online nursing degree programs is common now, and students can advance their careers in best universities. Students should be prepared to spend two or three years for earning their master's degree in nursing online, and graduates can then be certified with an advanced license as a nurse. The best online nursing degree programs, include faculty credentials, and academic credit courses after graduation.

- **Computerization in nursing**: It necessitates the faculty to be literate in computer use. Today apart from Computer assisted teaching, university has started with online theoretical examination and evaluation of nursing students.
- **Globalization in nursing**: Globalization has created a world market mobility for nurses. There should be mechanism to compare nursing education and qualifications of nurses against global standards. Because all countries have specific requirements related to technology and disease prevalence, as well as cultural, social, and environmental differences. There is a possibility of non-uniformity in nursing education. The challenge is to develop appropriate procedures and systems to cover foreign university's program in order to maximize the benefits and limit the potential drawbacks of internationalization of higher education in nursing.
- **Increased community-based competencies:** Community-based competencies are required for nurses today as most of the patients are coming from different communities. The learner should be prepared with behavioral competencies relate to nursing performance and work setting, professional knowledge to improve work, integrated competencies and holistic competencies include professional attitude. Lifestyle modification to be taught to all patients along with discharge planning instruction.
- **Advance nursing practice** (Transition planning in hospital): In order to become more advanced in nursing practice, nurses need to self-monitor, evaluate, and create opportunities for improvement that are required in their future position as an advanced nurse. She must possess clinical nursing competencies, research competencies, leadership competencies and consultation and collaborative competencies.
- **Clinical teaching models:** Nursing is a practice discipline. Excellent nursing teachers focus on individual students' learning growth, and clinical teaching enables them to do this by:

  Assessing, monitoring and evaluating their impact on learning and adapting the subject to meet the needs of each student—rather than expecting the student to keep up regardless of their circumstances. Various clinical teaching method are used to improve and translate the theory into practice.
- **Faculty nurse practioners:** A newer concept where nursing teachers take over a patient unit or ward and take care of patients. They teach the students according to the curricular needs specific to their clinical posting. These faculty practice do interact with clients/patients, collaborate between the faculty member in academic setting, and clinical facility; transfer and integrate clinical role and evidence-based practice to nursing students; and conduct clinical research.
- **Community-based nursing**: It emphasizes client empowerment, health promotion and disease prevention services.
- **New pedagogy: Learner-centered curriculum.**
- **Increasing specialization.**
- **Flexible curriculum design, student-teacher partnership.**

ISSUES AND CHALLENGES

Research shows that the capacity of educational program to prepare safe competent nursing graduates is often hindered by:

- Insufficient emphasis on clinical learning hours
- Absence of clearly defined clinical educational outcome
- Use of ineffective clinical teaching methodology
- Unsuitable, poor quality, overcrowded clinical learning environment
- Lack of ideal clinical role model
- Many nursing schools run out of a single room establishment (TOI April 13, 2014)
- In order to meet the demands of nursing workforce in hospital, private nursing colleges had come up with no entrance exam. And some institution run on 'non attending program. (TOI , April 13, 2014)
- Faculty shortage
- Uneven distributions of nursing training institutions
- Actual hands-on experience limited, varies from institution to institution
- Numbers of teaching institutions not commensurate with the number of hospitals and improper attachment of multiple teaching institutions with a single hospital
- Physical facilities and teaching aids grossly inadequate in various government and private institutions
- Many colleges/schools of nursing do not have independent budget and the principal is not given financial powers
- Educational institutions should be in a separate building as per norms, and is violated by some of the institutions.

Challenges

Developing academic leadership: The educational administrator should:

- Identify who should be targeted for leadership development vs other types of development among faculty members
- Identify input from teaching staff
- Do not ignore the quieter teachers or give extra consideration to the more talkative faculty
- Be explicit in what leadership or other skills the school /college of nursing needs

An academic leader:

- Provides opportunities for growth, allowing mistakes and reward the success
- Clarifies and communicate her expectations for the department
- Holds regular retreats for planning, developing, and learning as well as feedback
- Plans for regular In-Service Education (ISE), skill training, conferences, journal clubs and other activities
- Facilitates autonomy and financial powers to the principals
- Enhances mentoring and supervisory role of the faculty
- Believes hands on training not to be compromised for students
- Provides compulsory attachment with the hospital for skill practice
- Implements INC syllabus both theory and practice
- Arranges regular in-service training for the faculty
- Establishes a healthy learning environment.

Leadership Framework for Today and Tomorrow

Nurses are dissatisfied with their practice setting with limited professional growth and oppressive organizational hierarchies that hinder autonomy in practice, lack of job status and power. The transformation of our society profoundly affected nursing organization and leadership strategies needed for the 21st century that demands leaders will need to be facilitators, organization must humanize by the work place and leaders to empower nurses.

A visionary nurse leader shares the power and recognition and she/he must be charismatic, inspirational, respectful, and stimulating, invigorative and creative when leading nurses looks for 'shining eyes' in others and makes others powerful and empowered.

NURSING LEADERSHIP IN EDUCATION

It is the process of influencing nurses to accomplish goals of the hospital or nursing school. They innovate nursing practice and focus on nurses empowerment. Nurse leaders do; influence fellow nurses to achieve long-term and short-term goals. Nurse leaders inspire nurses through personal trustworthiness and self-confidence Nurse. leaders communicate a vision that turns self-interest into commitment to nursing profession.

A Nurse Leader should be Visionary

What is nursing want to become?

It should be resonate with all members of nursing and help them to feel proud, excited, motivated and part of something much bigger than themselves.

for example: Our vision—nursing to be recognized and respected as one of the premier health care profession and service organization in the world.

Informs Mission Statement

Mission defines what you are doing and for the purpose the organization (nursing) exists currently. Each member of the organization should be able to express this mission. For example, our mission is to provide high quality education based on our strong commitments to practice nursing profession.

Inculcates Values in Nursing

Values are that shape Nurse's action. Nurses should participate in an organization with certain personal values.

For example: Competency, integrity, respect, commitment, dedication, dignity, collaborativeness, innovativeness, compassion, assertiveness, etc.

Values of nursing focus on preserving and improving human health. Nurses are committed to the highest standards of ethics and integrity. Nurses are dedicated to the highest level of scientific excellence and commitment. Nurse leaders and academicians:

- Empower nurses and faculty for exemplary services and recognize expertize
- Demonstrate risk taking behavior is a prerequisite for creating tomorrow's leaders
- Determine the priorities for care, based on need, acuity and optimum time for intervention, innovation and research
- Select and utilize resources efficiently
- Promote private public partnership and collaboration in nursing and education
- Encourage nurse led and nurse managed health care

- Develop and coach for preparation for tomorrow's work force in nursing education and service
- Participate in planning, at all levels of nursing system.

Understands and Work for Future Focus

Nursing leadership in education continue to view nursing as profession with systematic body of knowledge, formal college bound education, unique role, standards of practice, academic excellence, research climate and professional accountability.

Nursing Schools and Colleges each will have a Future Committee The future trends in nursing education would be:

The virtual classroom will become a reality due to their availability of broadband internet, through mobile data cards or mobile phones.

Faculty will teach in classroom over a web camera and phone from their offices which will provide global learning—a step forward opens a world of learning.

PhD faculty for MSc program may be mandatory.

Nurse educators and health care technology companies will be partners in designing and implementation of technology in nursing education.

Emergence of Nursing Universities

Other activities such as providing safety and security of nursing human power by:

- Strengthening nursing at the Central/State Nursing Directorate
- Promoting nurses' role in developing Nursing universities
- Promoting reforms in the educational institutions for strengthening the nursing workforce
- Solving nursing management issues arising from service and nursing education with the central and state level nursing councils/association (INC, SNC, TNAI)
- Networking, partnership and advocacy at the national and international levels
- It is very essential that nurses and leaders of every country focus on nursing workforce as a key priority for achieving better health for all by:

1. Developing workforce planning
2. Providing safe environment
3. Commitment to education and learning
4. Justifying human and financial resources
5. Efficient utilization of resources
6. Justifying allocation of resources
7. Trend analysis would be a routine activity in nursing schools.

The role of educational administration is a challenge for academicians. They need to have leadership skills, administrative skills and curriculum administration skill.

Box 24.1: Research highlights

Evidence in research shows that the role ambiguity and role conflict had low job satisfaction. Job ambiguity has a stronger negative correlation with job satisfaction compared to role conflict. The greater the role ambiguity and greater the role conflict, the lesser the job satisfaction.The nurse administrator should develop a clear cut job description to all levels of nursing personnel and discuss with them during their induction period.

Box 24.2: Research highlights

VOICES EMERGING FROM NORTH EASTERN STATES: KEY NURSING ISSUES REQUIRING REFORMS

Rajni Bagga, Ms Vaishali Jaiswal conducted a study on voices emerging from north eastern states: Key nursing issues requiring reforms with the aim to review the current nursing and midwifery organizational/Management structure and HR processes and to obtain a perspective to strengthen nursing management capacities to address to the RCH needs appropriately in the three North Eastern States, i.e. Assam, Manipur and Tripura. Three carefully planned Focus Group Discussion (FDG) were conducted with the groups comprising of homogenous mix of nursing, midwifery professionals including nursing administrators from state directorate, registrar of state nursing council, nursing faculty from teaching institutes, and practitioners from health facility to obtain their true feelings, attitude concerns, perception, and constrains and challenges faced by nursing professionals. Findings were-lack of decision making power, mushrooming of private nursing colleges, diluting of midwifery component in nursing course, supervisory role reduced over the years, gross pay and career graph disparity, needs of a separate nursing division at the state directorate, need for nursing leadership. Study concluded that nursing profession need autonomy in all sectors including education, services and community health and administration.

(Rajni Bagga and Vaishali Jaiswal, NRSI Con'14)

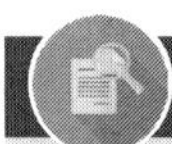

SUMMARY POINTS

- ✓ Nursing service administration is a process of planning, organizing, leading and controlling the efforts of the members of the organization. It is the effective utilization of available resources to achieve the pre-established goals of the organization that is to bring better quality patient care outcomes. One of the major causes of shortage of nurses are steep population growth, majority of nurses are retiring. Job opportunities within the health care system is expanding and nurses report high level of job dis-satisfaction.
- ✓ The population of elderly people in India is 57 millions and it is projected that India will have 324 millions of elderly by 2050. 75% of these will occupy the rural community. They live with chronic illness that needs greater attention. It has an implication for hospital and community health nursing practice.
- ✓ Today, nurse administrators use computers for financial administration to monitor the cost of nursing services and to compare the expenses between the past and the present. Computers help in the calculating of salary and benefits and tax calculation for all nurses and health workers. At the same time, it helps to assess the bills of the hospitals paid. It ensures the administrator that the health care given to patients are cost-effective and efficient. Computers evaluates the quality assurance program of the hospitals and the utilization of available resources appropriately.
- ✓ There is an epidemiological transition in the world. Apart from non-communicable diseases (NCD) diabetes, hypertension, CVA cancers, and accidents, re-emerging infectious diseases like swine flu, Leptospirosis, chicken guinea, malaria are highly prevalent. TB is back again due to drug resistance. HIV/AIDS is also posing issues.
- ✓ Within the clinical setting nurses are not able to make decision that affects the design of facilities, process of management and delivery methods which in turn affects patient care. Even with higher education in nursing they are not empowered to make independent decision for patient care.
- ✓ Nurses to be included in all level of policy making. Accountability, autonomy and empowerment are closely related. In shared governance model, the traditional controlling roles of management must be replaced by a system which recognizes the importance of supporting nurses and nurse administrator need to reflect on respect, justice and trust in workplace.
- ✓ Some of the causes of role conflicts are long working hours, inadequate information about job responsibilities, varied job expectation, unable to make prioritization in patients care, lack of autonomy and unable to make patient care decision for care. There is a generational diversity in work force working in a unit also cause role conflict among nurses.
- ✓ Lack of personnel policies, hospital policies, inadequate budget for nursing service department, lack of motivation among employees, inadequate equipment and supplies, poor working condition and work schedule are some of the other issues.
- ✓ Educational leadership is a term applied to school administration that attempts to create a positive change in educational policy and academic processes. Educational leaders are trained to advance and improve educational system or institutions.
- ✓ Nursing leadership is the process of influencing nurses to accomplish goals of the hospital or nursing school. They innovate nursing practice and focus on nurses empowerment. Nurse leaders do influence fellow nurses to achieve long-term and short-term goals. Nurse leaders inspire nurses through personal trustworthiness and self-confidence. Nurse leaders communicate a vision that turns self-interest into commitment to nursing profession.
- ✓ The role of educational administration is a challenge for academicians. They need to have leadership skills, administrative skills and curriculum administration skill.
- ✓ This chapter also discussed current trends in nursing administration. Global shortage of nurses, cost of health care consumerism, globalization of health, inadequate budgeting, shift in demography, lack of personal and hospital policies, role conflict among nurses, poor interpersonal relationships lack of empowerment and autonomy have negative impact on quality of nursing care. The nurse administrator needs to address these issues with effective leadership and administrative skills.

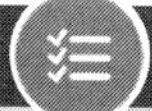

REVIEW QUESTIONS

1. Discuss the issues and challenges in nursing service administration.
2. What are the causes of shortage of nurses in hospital? As a nurse administrator, how will you solve this problem?
3. As a nursing administrator, how will you utilize postgraduate nurses in hospital setting?
4. What are the issues confronting academic administration in nursing in the country? What is your role in making personnel policies for nursing school?
5. Write a paragraph on impact of academic leadership in nursing school administration.
6. Write short notes on the following:
   a. Philosophy of nursing education
   b. Globalization in nursing
   c. Nursing empowerment and autonomy
   d. Student discipline
   e. Role conflict in nursing
   f. Implications of information technology in nursing education.

SELECTED READINGS

1. Charan, Drotter and Noel. The Leadership Pipeline. Jossey-Bass, 2001
2. Creating Leaders for the Future - Lippincott Williams & Wilkins journals.lww.com › Home › November 2009 - Volume 109 - Issue 11 by PA Thompson - 2009
3. Dolezalek. "Got High Potentials?" Training Magazine, January/February 2007.
4. George, Sims, McLean and Mayer. "Discovering Your Authentic Leadership." Harvard Business Review, February 2007
5. Grasberg, Boris and Michael Slind. "Leadership is a Conversation." Harvard Business Review, June 2012.
6. Growing Future Nurse leaders ...nursingworld.org/Main Menu Categories/.../Growing-Nurse-Leaders.html by R Sherman Jan 1, 2010 -
7. Heifetz, Grashow, Linsky. "Leadership in a (Permanent) Crisis." Harvard Business Review, July-August, 2009
8. Hill. "Becoming the Boss." Harvard Business Review, January 2007.
9. Jurow. Cultivating Your Career. The Business Officer, July 2006.
10. Katzenbach, Stefen and Kronley. "Culture Change that Sticks." Harvard Business Review, July – August 2012.
11. Leadership, whether I Nursing leadership: bringing caring back to the future www.ncbi.nlm.nih.gov › ... › Qual Health Care › v.10(Suppl 2); Dec 2001 by A Kitson - 2001
12. Various. "Global Executives Talk about the Challenges that Shaped them as Leaders." Harvard Business Review, January 2007.
13. Z enger and Folk man. The Extraordinary Leader. McGraw Hill, 2002

25

Emergencies and Disaster Management

LEARNING OBJECTIVES

This chapter imparts learning about:

- Epidemiology of Disasters
- Role of Nurses in Disaster Management
- Role of Nurses in Rehabilitation

INTRODUCTION

By using epidemiological triad of agent-host-environment disaster can be studied and analyzed and predict, prevent or control the outcomes of a disaster.

A disaster is described as an event that causes destruction damage, loss of human life and deterioration in health services on a large scale which affect a community or area.

Epidemiology of Disaster

- Disaster agents are the physical item that actually causes the injury or destruction, falling buildings, heat, wind and smoke. (Primary agents) bacteria or viruses that produce contamination or infection later. (Secondary agents)
- Host factors are the individual characteristics that has an impact on the severity of disaster effect such as age of the person, gender, immunization status, pre-existing health status and emotional stability of persons.
- Disaster Environment: This include physical factors such as the weather conditions, availability of food and water electricity. Chemical factors such as spread of stored chemicals into the air, soil, ground water. Biological factors such as contaminated water, improper food storage, lack of refrigeration can cause adverse effect on human health and social factors such as social support system, loss of family members, and changes in their roles.

Magnitude of the Problem

The coastal Tamil Nadu state was hit by **Cyclone Nilam** followed by heavy rains at Chennai. 282 schools were converted temporarily as relief camps by state Government. About 150,000 people were moved to shelters in Nellore. The cyclone with speed of 75 kph caused Pratibha Cauvery ship, an oil tanker to dip ashore and five sailors aboard the tanker lost their lives.

Uttarakashi flash flood killed 31 people and left thousands of pilgrims stranded on the Char Dham Yatra route to Gangotri, Yamunotri, Badrinath and Kedarnath. An estimated 20,000 people were affected due to this flood.

Assam floods took at least 33 people life and more than 17.60 lakh people affected. The flood in Brahmaputra caused the death of 595 wild animals. (Indian Express, 2016).

In September 2014, monsoon rains in **Jammu and Kashmir** and the neighboring region in Pakistan resulted in the worst flooding in 60 years. It resulted in 200,000 houses were destroyed.

The biggest storm of the Pacific and Indian Ocean season was **Cyclone Hudhud** made land fall near Visakhapatnam in Andhra Pradesh with winds blew to 200 km/124 miles per hour and a storm surge of up to three meters in some areas which left with heavy loss of lives.

In recent years, we have witnessed many disasters in Asia. There was catastrophic destruction by the **Indian ocean Tsunami, Kashmir earthquake, Sichuan earth quake and Nargis cyclone.**

Summer heat in India and Pakistan in the year 2015, caused the deaths of 3,600 people.

Chennai floods and heavy rains, destroyed Chennai city with initial estimates suggesting a loss of ₹ 15,000 crore losses (2015).

(http://indianexpress.com/article/india/india-news-india/after-the-chennai-floods-revisiting-the-natural-catastrophe-pool/#sthash.9AAQBGfP.dpuf)

In India, 60% of landmass prone to occur earthquakes. 8000 km long coastline affected with two cyclone seasons. Drought—low and medium rainfall region which constitute 68% of the total area. 40 million hectares (8%) of landmass prone to floods and vulnerable to drought. Hilly regions are vulnerable to avalanches/landslides/Hailstorms/cloudbursts. Different types of manmade hazards caused 1 million houses damaged annually including human, economic, social, other losses.

Classification of Disasters

Natural Disasters

- Tectonic
- Meteorological
- Topological.

Manmade Disasters

- Chemical contamination
- Mass intoxication
- Fire
- Mass accidents
- Victims of social violence
- Explosion.

Health Consequences of Disaster

- Unexpected number of deaths, injuries, illness in the community
- Affects psychological and social behavior of affected community.
- Shortage of food with severe nutritional consequences
- Large population to areas where health services cannot cope with the new situation
- Destruction of local health infrastructures such as hospitals adding to morbidity and mortality
- Risk for epidemics and environmental hazards premature deaths, and diminished quality of life.

Phases of Disaster Management

Nondisaster (Interdisaster Phase)

It is also termed as disaster preparedness. The role of nurse include:

- Participates in national or local predisaster planning
- Cooperates with international programs in case of disasters in other countries
- Works with community programs to reduce harmful pollutants
- Improves community nutrition
- Encourages family planning.

Predisaster (Warning) Phase

In this phase the following activities are taken:

- Mapping the potential locations for disasters and associated risks.
- Analysis of vulnerability
- Taking an inventory of existing resources
- Planning appropriate, preventive, preparedness and mitigation measures.
- Conducting education and training of health personnel and the community.

Impact Phase

The impact of these disasters on human health varies according to the nature of the disaster itself, population density, pre-disaster health, nutritional status, climate and organization of health services.

Emergency Phase

The activities included in this phase are search and rescue operation, first aid, emergency medical assistance, restoration of emergency communication and transportation network, public health surveillance and evacuation. Greatest emergency occurs in the first few hours and first responsibility is search, rescue and first aid and prioritize the most injured persons or dead people according to 'TRIAGE' (Triage is the method of determining the priority of patients' treatments based on the severity of their illness or condition). This phase also include establishing centers for inquiries from relatives of victims.

RECONSTRUCTION PHASE (RESTORATION OF PRE-DISASTER CONDITION)

In this phase, re-establishing normal health services and assessing repairing and reconstructing damaged facilities and buildings are concentrated and it is the time to improve current emergency preparedness plans. The phase begins when the assistance from outside starts to reach the disaster area. Do a rapid damage assessment to identify the needs and resources. Help the disaster managers in receiving donations. Help in the management of humanitarian supplies for acquisition, transportation, storage and distribution.

ROLE OF NURSES IN DISASTER MANAGEMENT

Role of Nurses in Providing Outreach Health Services During Emergencies

- The public health nurse/nurse is the first contact for the community to provide outreach services during emergencies
- Educate the community on vital health issues
- Serve as a vital link between the community and the health system
- Provider of 'holistic' care to the affected community.

The Following Basic Nursing Skills are Required for Managing Emergencies

- Assessing the needs of the community
- Identifying vulnerable groups (women, children, adolescents, elderly, etc.)
- Providing appropriate medical assistance and care
- Providing health education on vital health issues including feeding practices
- Prevention of epidemics and addressing environmental health issues
- Providing psychosocial support
- Use of emergency nursing kit.

Basic Steps in Nursing Management

- Assessment of the need of the affected community by collecting and analyzing all the available data
- Diagnosing the community disaster threats
- Planning for the management and do an ongoing monitoring and supervision of the plan
- Implementing the plan effectively
- Evaluating the result.

Step I Assessment of the Need of the Affected Community by Collecting and Analyzing all the Available Data such as

- Previous disaster experiences
- Local climate
- Local industries
- Personnel available for disaster interventions (nurses, doctors, etc.)
- Locally available disaster resources (e.g: food, clothing, shelter)
- Local agencies and organizations (hospital, schools, churches).

What are the Objectives of Assessment?

- To determine the number of individuals affected
- To identify the health needs of the population
- To establish priorities for action
- To identify existing and potential public health problems
- To identify local resources
- To setup the basis for a health information system.

Collection of Data

Panchayats or local authority officer gives the background data about the area. Data is also available from government or private health facilities. We can also get data maintained by ANM or Anganwadi workers or any local health volunteer. The nurse does the field visit to get first hand information. Some of the other methods like participatory mapping of the area by inviting a group of affected population and house survey using family health card which will help to collect data on age and sex distribution and details of health related matters.

Step II Diagnose the Community Disaster Threats

The nurse needs to diagnose both actual and potential threats of the disaster such as:

- Toxic waste spills
- Explosion
- Mass transit accidents
- Tornadoes
- Flood, earthquakes, etc.

Step III Plan for the Management and do an Ongoing Monitoring and Supervision of the Plan

The main aims of community planning are to prevent or deal with identified disaster threats, to identify community communication system to identify disaster management personnel, including private and professional voluntary agencies and resources and find out specific responsibilities of various personnel involved.

Monitoring and Supervision

While monitoring and supervising, the nurse should see that only useful information is to be collected, and avoid collecting too much data and over burden the staff engaged in management. She should provide accurate feedback on time through the use of reporting format which can be interpreted easily. These documents are vital.

Step IV Implement the Plan Effectively

The nurse acts as a principal investigator and should focus on primary prevention activities to prevent the occurrence of manmade disasters and practice the plan with all personnel carrying out their previously identified responsibilities (triage, providing supplies, grief counseling) She must make sure that the available resources are well-utilized to implement the plan effectively. She must assess the environmental hazards if any. The nurse educates the general public about environmental and other health hazards, participates in research providing data for early warning, prevention of environmental hazards, and to discover ways, and means of improving living and working conditions.

Step V Evaluate the Results

The nurse evaluates the following for the effectiveness of management:

- Critically evaluates all the aspects of the plan
- Evaluates the practice drills for speed, effectiveness, gaps and revision
- Evaluates the impact of disaster on community and surrounding regions
- Evaluates the response of personnel involved in disaster relief efforts.

Epidemiological Surveillance and Role of the Nurses

- Implement as soon as possible of all public health measures to reduce disease transmission
- Organize a reliable reporting system to identify outbreaks and promptly initiate control measures
- With the other team members investigate all reports of disease outbreaks rapidly
- Begin mass vaccination program
- Ensure supply of safe drinking water and proper disposal of excreta
- Ensure adequate nutrition as during a disaster the components of food chain are affected
- Ensure good food hygiene
- Emergency latrines should be made available where toilet facilities are destroyed
- Take vector control measures
- Educate the community regarding early warning signs for prevention of health hazards Improving living and working condition, monitoring the environmental pollutants and preparing to face disasters
- Have a nursing kit ready to use at the time of emergency that include dressing materials, first aid medications, ORS packets, IFA tablets, DD kits, assessment articles (scale, tape, thermometer etc), Handwashing articles, urine testing kit, hemoglobin estimation kit, chlorine tablets, medicines for treating minor ailments, and Family health cards.

ROLE OF NURSE IN REHABILITATION

Rehabilitation is the process of assisting someone to improve and recover lost function after an event, illness or injury that has caused functional limitations.

Disasters impose a huge burden on the community in terms of physical as well as psychological trauma they suffer.

For disaster victims, rehabilitation does not simply mean physical care but the psychosocial care and counseling are much important.

Physical Rehabilitation

The nurse provides physical health care as a part of relief work and refer them to centers for further care.

Psychological Rehabilitation

Disasters cause psychological impact on each and every person in the population and hence, the magnitude of the problem is as large as the population affected by the disaster. Immediately after a disaster there is an out pouring of concern, sympathy and desire to assist the victims as much as possible. Psychosocial interventions are interrelated and interdependent. These can be carried out effectively by community level relief workers, if they are trained and supervized to do so. Psychological responses of affected population varies from transient reactions to lifelong emotional problems.The need for emotional support is crucial in order to enable people to begin recovery.

Immediate reaction within 24 hours observed in people are:

- Tension, anxiety or panic
- Stunned, dazed, shocked, disbelief

- Elation or euphoria among survivors or people suffering lesser losses
- Restlessness or confusion
- Agitation crying or withdrawal
- Survivors' guilt.

These reactions are seen in nearly everybody in the affected region and are called as 'NORMAL REACTIONS TO ABNORMAL SITUATIONS'.

Reaction within days to weeks observed are:

- Being fearful or vigilant
- Become hyper alert (irritable, angry and unable to sleep)
- Worried or despondent
- Repeated flashbacks
- Weeping, guilt feeling
- Sadness
- Some positive reactions including hoping, thinking of future, getting engaged in helping other victims.
- Acceptance of disaster as 'natures doing'. These are normal responses and they usually adapt positively to the situations. But some go to maladaptations such as substance abuse.

After 3 weeks, the people demonstrate the earlier reactions may persist and manifest as:

- Restlessness
- Feeling panicky
- Continued intense sadness, unrealistic pessimistic thoughts
- Outward inactivity, isolated and withdrawn behavior,
- Anxiety manifested as physical symptoms.

These reactions also may not necessarily indicate mental disorder. They can be helped by trained relief workers. But some disaster survivors may go into full blown mental disorders such as acute stress reactions—bereavement and grief. Diagnosable mental disorders which causes significant impairment in social, occupational and other important areas of functioning (anxiety disorders, somatoform disorders and depressive disorders).

Psychological Interventions During Acute Emergency Phase

Allow the person to perform the last rites of the dead. Avoid undue burdening by relief operations, but provide basic necessities to survive. Rehabilitation workers can help people to cope with the disaster situation more effectively during this phase.

POST DISASTER PHASE—AFTER 3 WEEKS

The nurse provides psychosocial care along with general relief work continues general measures such as counseling to help them to adjust. Specific psychological interventions like emotional first aid, grief counseling, etc. to be given. When the situation found worst identification and referral to mental health professionals prove better results.

There should be commitment to being involved in community planning activities, participating in exercises and actual disaster work and ongoing updating of knowledge by all those involved in disaster preparedness.

ROLE OF NURSE ADMINISTRATOR IN DISASTER MANAGEMENT

The nurse administrator as a proactive leader should have plan of disaster preparedness in hospital and a team of nurses should be prepared by preserving open lines of communication, ensuring quality patient care providing continuing education, influencing policy and financial decisions providing security for staff, patients, and families.

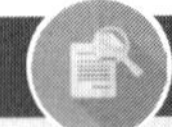

SUMMARY POINTS

- ✓ A disaster is an occurrence of a severity and magnitude that normally results in death, injuries and property damage that cannot be managed through the routine procedure and resources of government. It can be explained as an occurrence either by nature or manmade that causes human suffering and creates human needs that victims cannot alleviate without assistance.
- ✓ In India, 60% of landmass prone to occur earthquakes. 8000 km long coastline affected with two cyclone seasons. Drought—low and medium rainfall region which constitute 68% of the total area. 40 million hectares (8%) of landmass prone to floods and vulnerable to drought. Hilly regions are vulnerable to avalanches/landslides/hailstorms/cloudbursts. Different types of manmade hazards caused 1 million houses damaged annually along with human, economic, social, other losses.
- ✓ The disasters are classified as natural and manmade.

- ✓ The epidemiological aspect of disaster is caused by agent, host and environment which are preventable.
- ✓ Phases of disaster management include inter disaster (non-disaster) phase, pre-disaster (warning)phase, impact phase, emergency (Relief) phase and reconstruction (Rehabilitation).
- ✓ Role of nurses in providing outreach health services during emergencies include being the first contact of the community with the health care provider educate the community on vital health issues serve as a vital link between the community and the health system and provider of 'holistic' care.
- ✓ The basic steps in managing emergency and disasters are assessment of the need of the affected community by collecting and analyzing all the available data, diagnose the community disaster threats, plan for the management and do an ongoing monitoring and supervision of the plan, implement the plan effectively and evaluate the results.
- ✓ Rehabilitation is the process of assisting someone to improve and recover lost function after an event, illness or injury that has caused functional limitations.
- ✓ Disasters impose a huge burden on the community in terms of physical as well as psychological trauma they suffer and nurses have great responsibility in providing psychosocial rehabilitation for affected disaster victims.

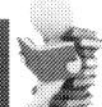

REVIEW QUESTIONS

1. Define disaster. Discuss the incidence and classification.
2. Describe the various phases of disaster management.
3. Discuss the role of nurses in providing outreach services during emergencies.
4. Explain the various steps in nursing management of disaster.
5. Describe the role of nurses in physical and psychosocial rehabilitation for the disaster affected victims.
6. Write Short Notes:
   a. Health related consequences of disaster
   b. Epidemiological surveillance and the role of nurses in disaster
   c. Diagnosis of community disasters threats
   d. Mental health and disaster
   e. Epidemiology of disaster
   f. Disaster nursing kit.

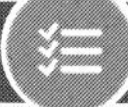

SELECTED REFERENCES

1. A national strategic plan for public health preparedness and response. http://www.cdc.gov/phpr/publications/A_Natl_Strategic_Plan_for_Preparedness.htm CDC. March 2011.
2. American Nurses Association (ANA). 2008. Adapting standards of care under extreme conditions: Guidance for professionals during disasters, pandemics, and other extreme emergencies. http://www.wsna.org/Topics/Emergencypreparedness/documents/ASCEC_WhitePaper031008FINAL.pdf
3. Association for Community Health Nursing Educators (ACHNE) Task Force on Disaster Preparedness. 2008. Disaster preparedness white paper for community/public health nursing educators. http://www.achne.org/files/public/DisasterPreparednessWhitePaper.pdf
4. Association of Schools of Public Health (ASPH). 2010. Public health preparedness and response core competency model. http://www.asph.org/userfiles/PreparednessCompetencyModelWorkforce-Version1.0.pdf
5. Centers for Disease Control and Prevention (CDC). 2012. Public health preparedness: 2012 state-by-state report on laboratory, emergency operations coordination, and emergency public information and warning capabilities. http://www.cdc.gov/phpr/pubs-links/2012/documents/2012%20State-ByState_Preparedness_Report.pdf CDC. 2011.

6. http://indianexpress.com/article/india/india-news-india/after-the-chennai-floods
7. http://www.business-standard.com/article/current-affairs/india-among-the-top-10-most-natural-disaste...
8. http://www.hindustantimes.com/india/top-10-natural-disasters-of-2012/story-Oadfb0IscYHZSiTkgcIWvJ.ht...
9. ICN framework of disaster nursing competencies. http://www.icn.ch/images/stories/documents/networks/DisasterPreparednessNetwork/Disaster _Nursing_Competencies_lite.pdf Institute of Medicine (IOM). 2012
10. Independent study program (ISP). http://training.fema.gov/IS/NIMS.aspx International Council of Nurses (ICN) and World Health Organization (WHO). 2009.
11. Presidential Policy Directive (PPD) 8 components: http://www.fema.gov/preparedness-1/learn-about-presidential-policydirective-8#NPF FEMA Emergency Management Institute (EMI). 2013.
12. Public health preparedness capabilities: National standards for state and local planning. http://www.cdc.gov/phpr/capabilities/dslr_capabilities_july.pdf Federal Emergency Management Agency (FEMA). 2013.

26

Nursing Standards

LEARNING OBJECTIVES

This chapter imparts learning about:

- Concept and Definition of Standards
- Importance of Standards
- Characteristics and Sources of Standards
- Levels and Types of Standards
- Framework of Standards
- Steps in Developing Standards

INTRODUCTION

Nursing is a science and art. The aim of professional nursing is to render excellent patient care by compassion, commitment and competent quality care that is determined by criterion or standard that are verifiable, observable and measurable to achieve quality care outcome. Standards ensures safety, and reliable care. The mission of nursing profession is to render quality nursing care to the population served as health is the patient's right. The vision of nursing is to render exemplary nursing care to those who need care irrespective to caste, creed, religion or ethnicity in the country.

The quality of nursing care can be assessed by monitoring degree of outcome results of patient care rendered by nurses. This will enable the nurse to improve her performance for the future. The standards are important managerial tool to assess quality patient care to enhance quality management.

STANDARDS: CONCEPT AND DEFINITION

- According to Webster's Learners' dictionary, standard means a level of quality, achievement, that is considered acceptable or desirable.
- Standards are ideas about morally correct and acceptable behavior.
- Standard is also something that is very good and that is used to make judgments about the quality of other things.
- Standard is measured quantitatively and qualitatively as against set criteria. Based on the criteria, the activities or things are measured and compared.
- Standards are professionally agreed levels of performance, which are observable achievable, and measurable.

According to Oxford Dictionary, the definition of standards explained in many ways, they are:

- Standards represent a degree of excellence
- Standards serve as a basis of comparison
- Standards are acceptable behavior.

A nursing care standard is a statement of various nursing activities rendered by nurses with a desired quality against which one can evaluate nursing care and care outcome. It is a protocol/guidelines to carry out delivery of professional nursing performance with safety and reliability.

IMPORTANCE OF STANDARD

Standards of nursing profession is based on the definition of nursing practice that explains nursing is a science and art which concentrates on prevention of illnesses, promotion and maintenance of optimum health of the individual, family and community, diagnosing nursing care problems and provide care according to the patients' reaction to illness. Nursing practices advocacy in the care of individuals, families, and communities. One of the criteria of any profession is that the members of its profession accept and adopt standards of practice of their profession. Today in almost all health care facilities nursing care standards are developed and enforced to enhance job satisfaction of nurses and improve quality of patient care. It is the responsibility of nurse administrator to see that standards are maintained in nursing service department.

Nursing standards provides criteria for meeting clinical, education, administration and research areas of practice.

The major aim of the Professional Standards is to enhance, guide and direct professional nursing practice.

Nurses, the health care consumers, employers of health, statutory bodies and other stakeholders are well benefited by professional nursing standards.

- It helps the registered nurses better understand their professional responsibilities and obligations
- It helps nurses to encourage and support their own continuing skill and competence and professional development
- It makes nurses aware of the concept of nursing and nursing practice
- It guides for making changes in health care policies and practices for enhancing status
- It is ongoing and dynamic in nature
- It guides nurses to solve problems arising from nursing care practice and nursing education
- It is useful for patients and families to understand the expectations for nursing practice
- It can be utilized by the management or stakeholders to develop an ideal systems that support nursing profession to meet the day today challenges
- In nursing practice such as to develop job descriptions, to develop in-service education, and formulating performance appraisal tools, etc. standards are referred
- Statutory bodies like Indian Nursing Council (INC), State Nursing Council and universities use the Professional Standards to justify its legal responsibility to protect safety of patients. This also helps regulatory bodies to prescribe regulation for nurses' practice such as to develop norms for entry-level and re-entry education programs for registered nurses and nurse practitioners in India or state, to justify the health care consumers and other members of health care profession what the profession expects from nurses. Nursing standards also facilitate guidance to nurses regarding their professional obligations and it provides a base for the development of performance appraisal tool.

CHARACTERISTICS AND SOURCES OF STANDARD

Characteristics

- Standards should be developed by nurses for nursing profession
- It must reflect value of the profession
- It must reflect changes and advancements in nursing profession
- The language used should be simple and explicit
- It should be unbiased, acceptable, and achievable
- It is not static but flexible
- It should be phrased in both qualitative and quantitative form.
- Must prescribe the level of competence in each phase of nursing care
- Must be recent and scientific
- Must be dynamic, ongoing, reviewed and revised periodically.

Sources of Standard

Standards are developed by professional nursing association, like TNAI, ANA, statutory bodies like INC, State Nursing Council, board of nursing studies in university and are reviewed or enforced. Department of institutions like Nursing Department Critical care unit, ICU, NICU or PICU Medical ICU, etc. also make their own standards for caring patients admitted in their units.

LEVELS AND TYPES OF STANDARD

Levels of Standards

- **Minimum standards** are generally described to represent a level of acceptability below which they are unacceptable.
- **The desirable standards:** It is an optimal standard represent a level of high degree of excellence.

TYPES OF STANDARDS

- **Ideal standard:** These standards are considered ideal by authority to provide highest quality of nursing care practices.
- **Empirical standard:** These are developed by regulatory or legal authorities which are achievable practice standards.
- **End standard:** These are standards which are patient oriented, based on patient care outcome.
- **Nursing standard:** These are standards which are nursing oriented; that defines the tasks and behavior expected in nursing practice.
- **Means standard:** These standards are process standards define how to reach the goals and that supports the care outcome or end standards.

FRAMEWORK OF STANDARDS

This is described under structure, process and outcome standards.

Structure standards

These include availability of the standards for patient care like:

- Vision, mission and philosophy and objectives of the hospital.
- Infrastructure facilities for various types of patients in the hospital.
- Resources like manpower both professional and technical, in quality and quantity with adequate in-service program and job description.
- Budget for running the health facility.
- Equipment and supplies.
- Policies, protocols and standards for patient care
- Technology and innovation, for improving patient care.
- Organization of administration, channel of communication, hospital committees, meetings and minutes.
- Recording and reporting system.

Process Standard

These are means to carry out to achieve the outcome of care. Nursing oriented actions are important in process standards such as:

- Standards and procedures for planning, implementation, and evaluation of care
- Nurses interpersonal and human relationship
- Nurse patient interaction and communication
- Patients and families involvement in care
- Communication process
- Inter- and intra-departmental coordination
- Records and reporting system
- Nursing care plans and nurses notes
- Performance appraisal of nurses
- Nursing audit
- Clinical nursing research
- Periodical nursing conference with nurse administrator
- Patient care conferences.

Outcome Standard

These standards are meant to assess patient care outcome. These are the description statement of result of care for the patient and can be both positive and negative outcome.

Positive outcome like early discharge, patient empowerment, quality of life provision of nutritional screening and care planning. Patients' experience of the provision of educational information and patient satisfaction.

- **Negative outcome** like mortality
- Morbidity like occurrence of bed sore
- Incidence of health care associated pressure ulcers
- Incidence of health care associated infection (HAI)
- Incidence of Catheter Associated Urinary Tract Infection (CAUTI)
- Patients' experience of pain management
- Healthcare Associated Infection (HAI) rate—the number of individuals who develop any infection while in an inpatient setting and hospital infection
- Disability.

Outcome standards are assessed periodically and necessary action is planned to prevent further complication.

STEPS IN DEVELOPING STANDARDS

Standards are developed at various levels such as National and state level, Community level, Institution level, Department level. Nurses use standards mainly in health care facilities. The nurse administrator has an important role to play in standard setting for nursing service department. The following steps can be used to develop standards. The nurse administrator:

- Organizes small groups of nurses who work in the same type of departments and nursing experts are invited to guide
- Organizes meeting periodically to develop standards
- Identifies the area of practice needs to review and revise
- The members review philosophy, purposes and objectives of institution

- The members assess existing nursing care practices, nursing process and identify the role of patients and strategies for nursing care services
- Formulates the relevant statement with accepted criteria which are achievable, observable and measurable
- Before finalizing the statement many meetings are conducted to assess its practicability
- The statements are sent for approval with other nurse administrators, clinical supervisors and unit in charge nurses
- Develops a format to assess the standard like observation checklist, assessing nursing records, self-evaluation report by nurses, opinionnaire from patients
- Send the standard developed for content validity from nursing experts
- The standards need to be tried out for its reliability and feasibility to use
- When it is found viable and feasible the nursing service department implement standards of nursing practice
- Documents the date and year of its development
- The quality of the standard proforma to be audited periodically and renew if necessary.

The role of nurse administrator is dynamic and functions according to the trends in change in health care delivery system. Nursing standards are important in terms of quality patient care as well for legal purposes and professional accountability.

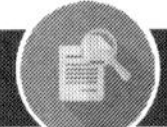

SUMMARY POINTS

- ✓ Standards ensure safety, and reliable care. Our mission is to render quality nursing care to the population we serve as health is their right. The quality of nursing care can be assessed by monitoring degree of outcome results of rendered patient care by nurses. This will enable the nurse to improve her performance for the future.
- ✓ The standards are important managerial tool to assess quality patient care to enhance quality management.
- ✓ Standard is measured quantitatively and qualitatively as against set criteria. Based on the criteria the activities or things are measured and compared. Standards are professionally agreed levels of performance, which are observable achievable, and measurable.
- ✓ The major aim of the Professional Standards is to enhance, guide and direct professional nursing practice. Nurses, the health care consumers, employers of health, statutory bodies and other stakeholders. are well-benefited by professional standards.
- ✓ Standards are developed by professional nursing association, like TNAI, ANA , statutory bodies like INC, State Nursing Council, board of nursing studies in university and and various nursing service departments.
- ✓ Types of standards include ideal standard, empirical standards, end standards nursing standard, and means standard.
- ✓ The framework of standards comprises structure, process and outcome standards.
- ✓ The role of nurse administrator is dynamic and according to the trends in change in health care delivery system standards are reviewed and modified. Nursing standards are important in terms of quality patient care as well for legal purposes and professional accountability.

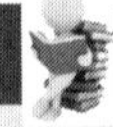

REVIEW QUESTIONS

1. Define nursing standards. Explain the importance of standards in nursing practice.
2. Describe the characteristics and sources of nursing standards.
3. What are various types of standards? Explain with examples.
4. Describe the framework for nursing standards.
5. Discuss the steps involved in developing nursing standards.
6. Write short notes on:
   a. Nursing care standards
   b. Regulatory bodies and nursing
   c. Structure standards
   d. Process standards
   e. Outcome standards
   f. Criteria and standards.

SELECTED READINGS

1. American Nurses Association (ANA) Scope and Standards of Nursing Practice, 2010
2. Clinical governance website http://www.clinicalgovernance.scot.nhs.uk
3. Donabedian A (1986) Criteria and standards for quality monitoring. Quality Review Bulletin 12 (3): 99-100
4. Higher Education Academy (2006) The UK Professional Standards Framework for teaching and supporting learning in higher education, London, HE Academy
6. Kitson A, Hyndman S, Harvey G and Yerrell P (1990) Quality Patient Care: The Dynamic Standard Setting System London: Scutari Press
7. Mllby R (1995) Clinical audit for nurses and therapists. London: Scutari Press
8. NHS e-library http://www.elib.scot.nhs.uk/portal/elib/pages/index
9. Nursing scope and standard www.worldcat.org/title/nursing-scope-and-standards-American nursing association
10. Nursing: Scope and Standards of Practice -..www.nursesbooks.org/ebooks/.../NursingScopeStandards.pdfNursing: Scope and Standards of Practice, 2nd Edition
11. Nursing: Scope and Standards of Practice:... www.amazon.com, › ...
12. The Nursing and Midwifery Council (Midwives) Rules Order of Council 2004 (SI 2004 No 1764), Norwich, Office of Public Sector Information (OPSI)

UNIT XV
NURSING AS A PROFESSION

27

Nursing as a Profession

LEARNING OBJECTIVES

This chapter imparts learning about:

- Introduction to Nursing as a Profession
- Philosophy of Nursing Practice
- Aims and Objectives
- Characteristics of Professional Nurse
- Regulatory Bodies: INC, SNC Acts and Functions

INTRODUCTION TO NURSING AS PROFESSION

A profession is different from an occupation or job. Profession is a calling that requires a specific body of knowledge, skill and training for a period of time in order to meet the societal needs for special services. Thus the profession builds upon advanced knowledge, renders a needed service to the society and protects its members and facilitates for practice.

Nursing is a practice discipline that renders the best possible health care to its community with the aim of maintaining health and well-being of the population it serves. Nursing is a science and art. Nursing profession is characterized by:

- It has a body of knowledge leading defined professional knowledge, professional attitude and professional skills to practice
- It requires a planned and sound education including skill of its members
- Its members provides specific services to society
- Its members have autonomy in decision-making while rendering care
- It has defined well-developed code of ethics.

Criteria for a Profession

When we describe a profession, it must have certain criteria. Various experts had defined nursing as a profession:

- First of all, it must have a body of knowledge
- It is dynamic and ongoing
- The members of the profession have the ability to solve professional problem
- It is built on nursing theories on which the the professional nursing practice is carried out
- It is different from job or vocation
- Nursing practice has its own code of ethics and professional nursing standards
- The profession is accepted by the society and members can exercise autonomy in caring their patients
- The main aim of the profession is service to society
- There is an accreditation body that give license to practice nursing.
- Nurse who violates ethics are liable to be penalized.

Philosophy of Nursing Practice

Nursing is a profession that concentrates patient centered, care that gives importance of interpersonal relationship with patient, family and community.

Nursing believes that each individual patient is unique in knowledge attitude and personality makeup. Nursing respects each individual and imparts selfless care without any difference to caste, creed or gender, cultural and ethnic diversity. The professional nurse serves as care manager for the patient aiming at prevention of diseases, promotion of health, restoration of health and rehabilitation health care services with excellence to attain quality care outcome.

Nursing also believes that nursing practice is based on standards of professional excellence, and the framework to achieve positive patient outcomes.

Nursing accepts that each nurse is a professional who functions independently, interdependently and collaboratively with members of the health team and makes informed and independent decision for care. She is an authority of nursing by the virtue of her education and position in nursing and exercises autonomy in her practice.

Nursing profession recognizes that the nurse is responsible and accountable for the nursing services rendered by her. She is responsible for empowering herself with professional knowledge, attitude and practice and also empower her patients for self-care and enhance quality of life through teaching, demonstration and counseling and guidance. Nursing further recognizes the best practices evidence informed in nursing that warrants nurses should carry out research for professional advancement.

Nursing recognizes that it is flourished when professional nurses have opportunity of professional growth and exemplary practice environment to perform their nursing functions. Nursing practice recognizes that excellent nursing care depends upon each nurse's professional responsibility to maintain continual self-learning and enrichment, and to pursue professional growth opportunities, including education, and professional competency and community involvement.

Aims and Objectives of Nursing Profession

- To prepare professional nurses who will provide comprehensive health care to the population with commitment and compassion utilizing critical thinking to apply knowledge derived from nursing, natural and behavioral sciences, humanitics and arts in the practice of professional nursing.
- To develop professional nurses who will render service in different levels of health care delivery system.
- To prepare nurses to render competent professional nursing care in variety of settings, utilizing competency in caring.
- To enable nurses to perform preventive, promotive, restorative and rehabilitative nursing interventions with individuals at various stages in the life span by using nursing process application.
- To help professional nurses to utilize the professional knowledge and professional competency to practice independently and collaboratively with other members of health care team.
- To enhance the professional growth of nursing through continued research Process. Integration of research findings and nursing theory that helps in decision-making in professional nursing practice.
- To prepare for professional leadership competency according to the level of educational preparation and maintain autonomy in clinical nursing management including decision-making for professional patient care practice.
- To empower the professional nurse as an individual, citizen and as a perspective member of the profession in order to uphold the dignity of the profession and able to integrate professional caring into practice decisions that integrate values, ethical, moral and legal aspects of care.
- To empower nursing personnel to maintain the dignity and standard of the nursing profession. Prepare nurses to accept authority, responsibility and accountability for the excellence of care of patient, family and community.

Characteristics of a Nurse

A nurse

- maintains professionalism and ethics that are qualities to nurses' practice each day. It is comforting for the patients to work with professionals.
- demonstrates diligence in making decisions for matters affecting patient care.
- always exhibits compassion towards the individuals, family and community to whom the nursing services are rendered.
- demonstrates sensitivity to human suffering is one of the important characteristics of a nurse.
- Exhibits a sense of pride being a nurse.
- Shows awareness of collaboration and interpersonal, and interprofessional relationship to enhance nursing care.
- Believes nursing is caring profession and strives to enrich a body of knowledge through nursing research.
- Accepts that nursing is committed to excellence in practice, and contributes to achieve better care outcome that in turn contribute to achievenational health goals.

- Accepts that nursing is committed to care to all patients irrespective to caste, creed, religion, gender, age or socioeconomic status.
- Works within the framework of professional and ethical standards developed by the statutory bodies of the country.

REGULATORY BODIES: INC, SNC ACTS

Indian Nursing Council (INC)

Under the Ministry of Health and Family Welfare, the Government of India constituted an autonomous body called INC under section 3(1) of the INC Act, 1947 of parliament in order to establish a uniform standard of education and training for nurses, midwives and health visitors.

It has 17 sections and each section describes the specific legislative role of the INC (INC Act 1947).

Aims and Objectives of INC

The purpose of INC is to formulate a national policy for training and practice of nursing in India.

Organizational set up of INC

The office bearers of INC are:

- The President
- Vice-president
- Secretary
- Joint secretary
- Deputy secretary
- Assistant secretary and office staff.

Functions of INC

- To establish and maintain a uniform standard of nursing education for nurses midwife, auxiliary nurse-midwives and health visitors in India
- To recognize the qualifications of nurses to practice in the country.
- To give approval for registration of Indian and foreign nurses who obtain required qualification.
- To prescribe syllabus and regulations for all nursing programs conducted in the country.
- INC has the power to withdraw the recognition of an institution in case the institution fails to maintain the prescribed standards.
- To counsel and guide the various statutory bodies like the State Nursing Councils (SNC), Examining Boards, State Governments and Central Government in various important aspects pertaining to nursing education.
- To monitor the standards of nursing education in the country.
- To recognize nurses as a separate branch in health service.
- To regulate nursing practice.
- To permit title, badges, uniforms for registered nurses.
- To inspect schools and colleges of nursing power to make regulations.
- To initiate prescribe, advise and monitor the various nursing program.
- To prescribe the qualification for the admission, registration and employment of nurses in the country.

State Nursing Council (SNC)

Established in the year 1948, the State Nurses and Midwives Council under the provisions of Nurses and Midwives Act functions in each state with the aims of training of nurses, midwives and health visitors. It is an autonomous body under the respective government, Department of Health and Family Welfare.

Salient Features of SNC

- It is an independent autonomous body.
- It is composed of majority of members of nursing profession.
- It has the power for making decision in terms of nurses and nursing problem of the state.
- It advocates compulsory registration for all nurses, midwives to practice in the state.
- SNC has the power to regulate nursing education, implementation of curriculum and monitor examination policies without violating INC norms.
- All SNCs have the provision to have a nurse registrar to implement the functions of the SNC.
- Provision for recognition of educational institutions of nursing and withdrawal of such recognition, as and when they violate norms if observed.

Functions of SNC

As per the act

This council is an autonomous statutory registration body for registering qualified nurses, midwives, auxiliary-nurse-midwives/multipurpose health workers/health visitors as per the provisions of the Act. It extends its registration to union territories.

Nurses and Midwives Act VII of 1934 and Act XXVI(26) of 1960, till today we follow the same.

- Recognition of nursing institutions as per the Act.
- Registration of qualified nursing professionals

mentioned above and maintenance of state register for the purpose.

- Development of inter linkages and reciprocities with corresponding councils in other States of India.
- Monitoring of professional ethics.
- Regulation and surveillance of professional conduct and take action against practice of their professional by quacks and check malpractice.

Example: **Functions of Tamil Nadu Nurse Midwife Council Act**, registration of nurses within the state, other state (reciprocal verification) and foreign verification.

- Regulation of training programs for nursing and granting recognition to the nursing institutions who satisfy the prescribed norms.
- Monitoring professional ethics, regulation and surveillance of professional conduct and take action against practice by quacks and check malpractice.
- Compilation, maintenance and publication of State Nurse Register.
- Developing and conducting model continuing nursing education program with emphasis on periodical refresher course for updating nurses knowledge, bridging courses for advanced professional education, in-service education in various specialties and dissemination of new knowledge and exchange of views.
- Conducting periodical conference for nursing personnel [With kind permission from Prof Dr S. Ani Grace Kalaimathi MSc (N), PhD, Registrar (FAC), Tamil Nadu Nurses and Midwives Council]

Nursing Boards

Nursing boards are state government institutions that are functions for the regulation of nursing practice.

Role of Nursing Boards

- To establish and maintain a uniform standard of nursing education as per INC norms with affiliated schools of nursing
- To verify the eligibility requirements before each examination of the students
- To arrange and conduct examination
- To issue certificates to successful candidates
- To appoint the examiners before each examination.

Role and Function of University in Nursing

- A university is an institution of higher education and research which grants academic degrees in a variety of courses and provides both undergraduate education and postgraduate education in nursing apart from other disciplines. It maintains regulation of its own affiliated colleges and institutions.
- To conduct inspection and granting permission for admission and continuing affiliation.
- To conduct examination and announcing the results.
- To conduct the graduation, postgraduation and doctoral programs
- To facilitate faculty and student welfare and development.
- To conduct research program.
- To organize various programs such as book exhibition, job fair, seminars, conferences, inter-college competitions, sport meets, etc.
- The Board of Nursing Studies (BNS) in the university helps the university in implementing INC syllabus for its affiliated colleges. Nursing representatives in Senate and University Governing Council has a great role in maintaining standards of nursing education in the state by interacting with academic council and standing academic board with regards to nursing problems (academic) and policies.

SUMMARY POINTS

- ✓ A profession builds upon advanced knowledge, renders a needed service to the society and protects its members and facilitates for practice. Thus a profession is different from occupation.
- ✓ The main aim of nursing profession is to prepare professional nurses who will provide comprehensive health care to the people/public with commitment and compassion utilizing critical thinking to apply knowledge derived from nursing, natural and behavioral sciences, humanities and arts in the practice of professional nursing.
- ✓ The important characteristics of nurse is that she maintains professionalism. It is comforting for the patients to work with professional nurses. She demonstrates diligence in making decisions for matters affecting patient care.

- ✓ Indian Nursing Council, State Nursing Councils, State Nursing Boards, University Board of Nursing study are regulatory bodies in nursing.
- ✓ INC maintains a uniform standard of nursing education in the country.
- ✓ The State Nursing Council is an autonomous statutory registration body for registering qualified nurses, midwives, auxiliary-nurse-midwives/multipurpose health workers/health visitors as per the provisions of the Act. It extends its registration to Union Territories.
- ✓ State Boards of Nursing are state governmental agencies that are responsible for the regulation of nursing practice.
- ✓ A university is an institution of higher education and research which grants academic degrees in a variety of subjects and provides both undergraduate education and postgraduate education.

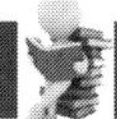

REVIEW QUESTIONS

1. Differentiate profession and occupation or job. Is nursing a profession? Justify.
2. Write philosophy of nursing in your own words.
3. Discuss the objectives and functions of nursing profession.
4. Describe the structure and functions of Indian Nursing Council.
5. Describe the function of State Nursing Council in maintaining quality of nursing in the state.
6. Write Short Notes on:
   a. Criteria for a profession
   b. Characteristics of nurse
   c. State Nursing Boards
   d. Board of Nursing studies.

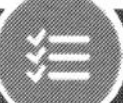

SELECTED READINGS

1. Draper Elaine; LaDou Joseph; Tennenhouse Dan J (2011). 'Occupational Health Nursing and the Quest for Professional Authority'. New Solutions 21 (1): 57–88.doi:10.2190/ns.21.1.i.
2. http://www.nursingworld.org/EspeciallyForYou/What-is-Nursing
3. http://www.slideshare.net/Sujatamoh...
4. Indian Nursing Council Act 1947 Act No. of Year: ...
5. Prof. Dr.S .Ani Grace Kalaimathi M.Sc (N), PhD., Registrar (FAC), Tamilnadu Nurses and Midwives Council)
6. Indian Nursing Council Act 1947 Act No. of Year: www.indiannursingcouncil.org/pdf/inc-act-1947.pdf
7. Schneider, John. "Healthcare advocacy experts aid workers." Miami Herald 31 August 2010
8. Taylor, C. R., Lillis, C., LeMone, P., Lynn, P. (2011) Fundamentals of nursing: The art and science of nursing care. Philadelphia: Lippincott Williams and Wilkins, page 735-736.
9. Taylor, C. R., Lillis, C., LeMone, P., Lynn, P. (2011) Fundamentals of nursing: The art and science of nursing care. Philadelphia: Lippincott Williams and Wilkins, page 468.
10. www.indiannursingcouncil.org/pdf/inc-act-1947.pdf)

28

Professional Advancement

LEARNING OBJECTIVES

This chapter imparts learning about:

- Introduction to Professional Advancement
- Continuing Education
- Career Opportunities
- Membership in Professional Organization
- Participation in Research Activities
- Publication of Research Report

INTRODUCTION TO PROFESSIONAL ADVANCEMENT

Advancing nursing education helps nurses to update their knowledge and skills in order to meet the day to day challenges in health care delivery system.

There are various opportunities available now in nursing to move upward in professional career to provide the best possible patient care. Advancing nursing education is useful for nurses' status, patient care outcome and achieving goals of the administration and appropriate recognition.

Advancement in nursing serves as a viable means of improving professional competence with improved patient care outcome.

Evidence suggests that Internationally Educated Nurses (IENs) progress relatively slowly through the career ladder and participate less in professional development compared with nurses educated in the United States (UENs). Mentorship and self-efficacy are considered major determinants of career advancement.

Recognition of professional nursing practice is achieved as a nurse student progress to first level position in nursing and with advanced professional preparation becomes expert nurses from novice to expert.

CONTINUING NURSING EDUCATION (CNE)

Introduction

Florence Nightingale had said, that nurses should not think that they have completed their learning but should continuously learn in life. Today, the concept of lifelong learning is very important for nurses so as to keep them updated with the changes that occur in health care delivery system. The nurse administrators have great responsibility to facilitate continuing education for their nurses to bring excellence in nursing care practice

Definition of Continuing Education

- According to American Heritage Dictionary of the English Language, (Fifth Edition) it is an instructional program that brings participants up to date in particular area of knowledge and skills. It is the Instructional courses designed especially for part-time adult students.

- **It is a program of courses** for adults offered by a university extension or other institution (Random House Kernerman Webster's College Dictionary).
- Continuing education is planned for a short duration after the basic qualifying examination to practice. Sometimes the term is interchangeably used with adult education.
- Continuing Nursing Education in nursing is a planned educational program organized by the administration of any health care facility or educational institution to keep their professional nurses updated with the current trends in nursing or nursing education.

Need for CNE

Following factors warrants nurses to undergo continuing education in nursing:

- Medical and technological advancement
- Specialization and super specialization in medicine and nursing
- Consumerism
- Knowledge explosion and its influence in nursing practice
- Theory practice gap in nursing
- Emerging and re emerging diseases
- Best practices in nursing
- Quality and patient safety are the benchmark of nursing
- Organ transplants, ART, etc. brings ethical dilemmas for nurses
- Clinical nursing research poses a major challenge to prepare themselves updated and enable to provide evidence based patient care.

Philosophy of Continuing Nursing Education

Nurses as unique individuals and their learning needs are diversified. Therefore, the educational institutions or health care facility has a responsibility to recognize and respond to nurses working under them as unique persons, as individual learners, and as citizens.

Nursing profession accepts that Nurses have individual responsibility to update themselves in professional knowledge and competency by attending seminar, conferences and short courses. The hospital and educational administration should provide a forum for all nurses working under them to provide facility to advance their knowledge by providing additional days off or study leave as well as deputation.

Nursing profession recognizes that continuing nursing education should be carried out in a well-planned, organized educational setting and the providers giving education should exhibit strong support and leadership. Continuing nursing education should help the nurse practitioners in the advanced Professional knowledge, professional commitments, the development of human relation, interprofessional relationship, and the enhancing skills in problem solving to excel in professional nursing practice. That in turn will bring quality health care outcome CNE should bring the innate potentials of the nurses, quality of life and current trends, issues and challenges in nursing.

Types of Continuing Professional Development

- **Orientation** develops a sense of belongingness of the new staff to the hospital/education institution and also to explain the job responsibilities to perform nursing care effectively.
- **Continuing education** enhances knowledge, skills and attitudes for better patient care.
- **Skill training** is another way of updating nurses with competency in nursing care procedures.
- **Management skills and leadership training** helps to manage patient care effectively.

Steps in Conducting Continuing Education Program

Planning Phase

- Need analysis
- Establish goals
- Set priorities
- Identify resources (man, money and materials)
- Explore constraints to conduct the program and find alternative solutions
- Determine scope and sequence of training program (by task and job analysis).

Designing Phase

- Determine the content to be taught
- Determine training approach
- Select teaching learning objectives
- Decide performance measures with training program specifications.

Development Phase

- Prepare course outline, lesson plans
- Select supportive instructional aids
- Revise material if needed.

Implementation Phase

- Conduct training as per the schedule developed
- Document training results.

Evaluation Phase

- Conduct summative evaluation
- Analyze collected information
- Initiate corrective action.

Follow-up Phase

- The participants are to be followed-up regarding their improvement in knowledge and change in behavior by mailing letters of questionnaire, observation and reports from the employer.

Benefits of Continuing Nursing Education

- Update nurses knowledge
- Facilitate lifelong learning
- Improve patient care outcome
- Develops self confidence
- Develop resourcefulness and public relations
- Promotes broader career opportunities
- Earn more credit points to maintain registration to practice
- Job satisfaction for nurse, satisfaction for patients and status for employer.

CAREER OPPORTUNITIES

Introduction to Career Guidance and Career Opportunities in Nursing

Nurses play an important role in health care delivery system. Their role as nurse in promotion of health, prevention of diseases, care of the sick as well as well people in the family and community, restoration of health and rehabilitation of patients and families are commendable. Nurses practice independently, inter dependently and collaboratively with all members of the health care team to provide quality patient care and achieve excellence in care outcome. The nursing profession has a wide range of job opportunities, ranging from first level staff nurse practitioner position to nurse scientist with doctoral degree. Nurses also serve as advocates, counselors, managers, educators and practitioner of nursing to individuals, family and community to achieve health related goals.

There are many opportunities for a person who wants to be a nurse.

- If the candidate is 10+2 or equivalent examination passed can opt **for Auxiliary Nurse and Midwife** training for 2 year duration.
- If a candidate is passed 10+2 or equivalent examination with minimum 40% of marks obtained can opt for **General Nursing and Midwifery Diploma** training for 3 years and six months duration
- If a candidate 10+2 Class passed with 45% aggregate marks in PCB group can opt for **Basic BSc nursing** with 4 years duration
- If a candidate is 10+2 + GNM can opt for **BSc (Post Basic**) program for a period of 2 years training
- If a candidate wants to opt for **MSc nursing** the minimum education requirements shall be the passing of: BSc Nursing/BSc (Hons). Nursing/Post Basic BSc Nursing with minimum of 55% aggregate marks. It is conducted for a period of 2 years
- If a nurse wants to do **M Phil nursing** should be MSc nurse. It is a program for 1 year as a full time candidate and 2 years duration for part-time candidate
- If a nurse wants to do **PhD in nursing** it is a program for 3-8 years after MSc or M Phil nursing as per the ordinances of a the particular university where she or he is registering.
- **Postbasic specialty courses** for one year as prescribed Indian Nursing council. Many colleges of nursing are conducting such program. The nurse can choose the course according to his or her interest and the institution. After getting RN, RM the candidates can pursue the following courses:
  - Diploma in neurosciences in nursing
  - Postbasic diploma in neonatal nursing
  - Diploma in cardio thoracic nursing
  - Diploma in operation room nursing
  - Postbasic diploma in emergency and disaster nursing
  - Postbasic diploma in nurse practitioner in midwifery
  - Diploma in nursing education and administration.
- A nurse with BSc nursing degree having obtained 55% marks aggregate in BSc nursing examination with minimum one year of experience can apply for Nurse Practitioner in Critical Care Postgraduate Residency program (NPCC). This program is for two years. The selection is based on entrance examination and interview by authorized experts in nursing. (This program is expected to start by 2016–17.) The course is already developed by Indian Nursing Council.

Other Scope, Designation and Role of Nursing:

- Clinical nurse
- Clinical instructor
- Clinical specialist nurse
- College/university professor
- Midwifery practitioner

- Staff development specialist
- Nurse midwife
- Patient education specialist
- Occupational health nurse
- Manager/administrator
- Educator
- Clinical Nurse researcher.

The Nurse can Function in the Following Hospital Settings

- Critical Care unit
- Emergency/Casualty Block
- Maternal/Child Care units
- Medical: Cardiology, Diabetes, Gastroenterology, Gerontology, Nephrology, Neurology,wards
- Oncology, Pulmonary, Rehabilitation, Renal, Rheumatology, Urology department/ OPD
- Operating Room/Recovery Room
- Pediatrics Wards
- Psychiatric/Mental Health
- Surgical: Burn, Cardiovascular, Ear/Nose/Throat, Gastroenterology, Orthopedics, Plastic Reconstructive, Transplant units
- The nurse can also function in the following non-hospital settings
- Public/Community Health centres
- Mental Health Agencies
- Home Health Care setting
- Health Maintenance Organizations
- Managed Care Companies
- Geriatric homes
- Occupational Health in factories, industrial plants
- Research Centers
- Special Clinics
- Outpatient Surgery Centers
- Hospices
- Community Schools, Day Care Centers
- Military Branches
- Independent Practice
- Schools/Colleges of Nursing.

(With kind permission from Prof DrS Ani Grace Kalaimathi MSc (N), PhD, Registrar (FAC), Tamilnadu Nurses and Midwives Council)

MEMBERSHIP IN PROFESSIONAL ORGANIZATION

The Trained Nurses' Association of India (TNAI)

In 1905, at Lucknow Association of Nursing Superintendents was established by few European nurses who were holding administrative position in hospitals.During the Annual Conference held in Bombay in 1908, it was decided to establish Trained Nurses' Association and it was inaugurated in 1909.

Both the Associations of Nursing Superintendents and Trained Nurses' Association were united in 1910 during the first annual conference of TNAI held at Banaras and named as The Trained Nurses' Association of India (TNAI) and the TNA members elected their own office bearers simultaneously the following became part of TNAI. They were: Health Visitors' League (1922) Midwives and Auxiliary Nurse-Midwives Association (1925) and Student Nurses Association (1929-30). In 1912 the TNAI got affiliated with the International Council of Nurses (ICN). The TNAI along with various responsibilities as a member had participated in the ICN Nursing Abroad Programme since 1950. Due to unavailability of funds TNAI felt difficult to pay the heavy subscription and was disaffiliated from the ICN since May 1995. From 2011 India has become a member of ICN again through Indian Nursing Council. In 1974 the TNAI became a member of the Commonwealth Nurses Federation (CNF). From 2014, the name of Commonwealth Nursing Federation (CNF) changed into Commonwealth Nurses and Midwives Federation (CNMF).

The Main Objectives of TNAI

- Upholding the dignity and honour of the Nursing profession
- Promoting a sense of *esprit de corps* among all Nurses; and
- Enabling members to take counsel together on matters relating to their profession.

Functions of TNAI

- Rapport with government of India
  - Government Recognition as Service Association:
  - Issue of Railway Concessions:
- Affiliation with Government Committees and Councils (The Indian Nursing Council (INC)
- Affiliation with Other health related Organizations'
- TNAI takes part in the activities of important social organizations
- Affiliation with International Council of Nurses (ICN)
- Affiliation with Commonwealth Nurses Federation
- Affiliation with Scholarship Funds

Membership in TNAI

As per 2013 statistics, TNAI has 2,13,565 life mebers, 1858 TNAI members and 10515 SNA to TNAI members

Life Membership fees in rupees (India)

Trained Nurses..3600
Retired Nurses (Provide Certificate)..................1200
Religious Sisters (drawing no salary)...............1100
HVL/ANM/MPHW...1800
SNA to TNAI (for student)..................................2200

Life membership Foreign nurses

Life membership... $303(USD)
Add postal charges (subject to change)...... $55 (USD)
Air mail charge.. 55 (USD)

Student Nurses Association (SNA)

The Student Nurses Association (SNA) is a part of TNAI which was established in 1929 at the time of the Annual Conference of the Trained Nurses' Association of India (TNAI). It is a great achievement of the growth of SNA units from its establishment from 1929. At present there are over 1000 SNA units with more than 1 lakh Student Nurses as members all over the country (2012).

The SNA and TNAI used to have combined Annual Conference, but due to the increase in number of delegates it was felt in 1960 to hold separate Conferences for the student Nurses. Since, 1961 the students Nurses are having separate Biennial Conferences. These are held alternately with TNAI Conferences.

The students are being given more and more responsibility to manage their affairs both at the State and national levels. In 1975 it was agreed by the TNAI Council that one student representative be included in the State Branch Executive Committee on trail basis before the students are included in the TNAI Council as representatives of SNA.

Organization of SNA

At the unit level, the unit executive committee has the power to manage SNA affairs.Its composition is as follows:

- SNA Advisor,
- President (TNAI member),
- Vice President who presides over the unit meetings,
- Secretary,
- Treasurer and the conveners of various committees.

At the State level

- The State TNAI President as ex-officio member,
- SNA Advisor,
- Student Vice President
- Secretary,
- Treasurer,
- Programme chairperson and the representatives of Units/Zones.

At the National level

- TNAI President,
- Honorary Treasurer,
- Secretary-General, SNA Advisor,
- State SNA Advisors and
- State SNA Vice President and Secretaries.

Membership of SNA to TNAI

- When a student nurse/ graduate nurse wants to become a member of TNAI should down load the application form from TNAI website.
- Read the current journal to know the current membership fees.
- Fill the application form and give it to the principal/ nursing director of hospital who is a TNAI member to recommend for membership.
- True attested copies of registration certificates along with the application form can be sent when there are authorized persons for recommending your application is unavailable
- A nurse who is already a TNAI member is interested to become a life member, need not to send a fresh application form. She is required to send Life membership fees along with application form with current TNAI membership number to TNAI.
- Complete filled application should be sent to the Secretary, TNAI, L-17, Green Park, New Delhi-11 0016, along with the membership fee.
- Any change in present/mailing address, should be intimated immediately quoting TNAI number, and pin code to ensure regular supply of nursing journal of India.
- The membership card given by TNAI to be kept carefully because some time it is needed for attending conferences presentation of papers and in election of office bearers.

ROLE OF A NURSE IN PARTICIPATING RESEARCH ACTIVITIES

Introduction

One of the criteria of a profession is it must have its own body of knowledge. If we say nursing is a profession, the body of knowledge comes from nursing research findings.

The main purposes of conducting nursing research are:

- Research generates theory and tests theories in nursing where nurses demonstrates a crucial role in clinical settings.

- When nurses demonstrate the best practices evidence informed, that enable them to function with Professional accountability and independent and informed clinical decision making skill for effective patient care.
- Research based practice is cost effective and reduces the hospital stay of patients.

Importance of nursing research

- Research develops academic curiosity among nurses to earn status of professional nursing.
- Research develops new information which helps to define the functions of a nurse as a professional.
- Evidence based practice or the best practices evidence informed promotes professional accountability of nurses to their patients by incorporating taking informed clinical decisions in caring.
- Another reason for nurses to engage in research involves the reduction days of hospital stay of patients because of evidence based practice. It brings cost effective care for patients, reduction of cost in health care facility that enhances good public relation.
- Research also enable nurses to understand about which a little is known
- It helps to assess the need for intervention
- Helps to identify factors that must be considered in planning nursing care.
- Helps to predict probable outcome of certain nursing decisions.
- Helps to control the occurrence of undesired outcomes.
- Helps to initiate activities to promote appropriate client behavior.

Thus, it has been seen that clinical nursing research is necessary for developing nursing's body of knowledge and improving the quality of nursing care. The support and participation of nursing staff are crucial to conducting interventional research and determinant research in their work settings that facilitate new knowledge to nursing.

Nurses play a major role in their contact with patients as well as in collecting data and giving treatment for the study group. It is extremely important that the nurses to understand the treatment and its indications. They must also be attentive to what effects they have and how to ensure patient safety.

The Institutional Review Board (IRB) is another essential group within each research institution. The objective of the IRB is to ensure the protection of human subjects while selecting a problem for nursing research. The IRB consists of doctors, advanced practice nurses, nurse scientists, and nonmedical persons, often from the community, who must review and approve all clinical research.

Ethical Committee (EC) is a forum where nurses participate with other members. There are three main principles to be observed when dealing with ethical concerns with human subjects. Is described as the obligation of the investigator to respect each study subject as a person capable of taking an informed decision whether or not participate in the research study. The nature study to be explained to the subjects by the investigator and ensure that the subjects understands the nature of the study, the risks, benefits and alternatives, with an extended opportunity to clarify any doubts Principle is beneficence, is another ethical aspect of research which means the obligation of the investigator to give maximize benefits for the individual participant and/ or society, and to decrease risk of harm to the individual. The researcher to be honest in risk-benefit calculation.

The last principle of ethics in research is Principle of justice that warrants fair selection of participants, with voluntarily participation.

Nurses are involved in research both clinically and scientifically.

Clinically, nurses have contact with the research subjects, observe them, provide care, and collect research data. Clinical research nurses are on the cutting edge of improvements in health care. Nurses should have and continue to build upon their knowledge and skills which are required to enable them to become competent in identifying, assessing and acting upon all aspects that may affect the integrity and data of research protocols.

Commitment for the well-being of patients to whom they serve, is to become more knowledgeable about what they can do to contribute for the improvement in independent research studies. Working with patients help nurses to appreciate and develop an understanding of the research process and health care setting.

Scientifically, nurses conduct independent research studies. Because of the they want to build up a body of professional knowledge to nursing.

The outcomes associated with new treatments that enable to improve the quality of life, functionally, psychologically and socially, of an individual and family.

PUBLICATION OF RESEARCH REPORT

What is a Research Report?

Reports are documents which presents specific, focused content- often the result of an experiment, investigation, enquiry or otherwise research.

Purposes of Writing Report

- The purpose writing research report is to document the research findings, to share the results with other interested groups, and apply the results in practice
- Exchange knowledge with expertise with colleague, scientists, locally and internationally.
- Used as a tool for evaluation of personnel.
- Career making (impact factors of journal)
- Personal satisfaction
- Dissemination of results is a general requirement by research funder.

Where to Publish Your Report?

- Match your manuscript with the most appropriate journal
- Assess what is the impact on the quality status of the journal
- Assess what is the impact factor of the journal.

What is Impact Factor?

The decision of where to publish research results is one that every investigator takes into account when preparing a manuscript for publication. The topic of the investigation, the quality of the research, and the opportunity to publish in the most highly regarded journal all play a part in the researcher's final decision.

But how does a journal get a reputation as being better than other journals? Many researchers generally accept that a journal's reputation is based on the following factors: history of publication, breadth of readership, quality of individually published articles, and selectivity in deciding which articles to publish, and impact on the practice of nursing are the most popular attempt to quantify the impact, or importance, of a particular journal.

Structure of the Report Includes

- Title
- Authors
- Abstract
- IMRAD format
  - Introduction
  - Methods
  - Results
  - Discussion.

Title of the study

Write the title of the study first. The title of the paper can be given in different ways from being very short to very elaborate and descriptive, depending on personal preferences. Ideally, the title should be as short as possible, preferably less than ten words, but exhibiting the full nature of the subject presented. It should be able to attract the attention of the reader. The title should express the subject of the paper in a simple manner so that people might read or cite it.

Authors

The person who actually conducted the study would be the first author and the person can rectify if any problems comes would be corresponding author do not make it too specific, or people might not read or cite it.

Abstract

Abstract is the major element of the research. It is far more important part of the research. Abstract is very concise statement of the major elements of the research project. It states the purpose, methods, and finding of the project. It is condensed version of full scientific paper—means a short summary of 200–250 words, to be presented in the beginning of the main text of the report. The components of the abstract should include seven elements such as: Short theme of the study in one sentence. A justification to conduct the study, nursing relevance of academic and clinical practice, of the study, a detailed methodology and results. Include probabilistic magnitudes of effects in the results (main findings).

Report Format: Follow IMRAD Format

1. **Introduction**
   - Pose the problem in one or two sentences.
   - Write the purposes clearly
   - Review the literature briefly in a manner that leads to the importance/justification of your study.
   - State variables under the study with brief description.
   - State or test hypotheses.
   - Explain theoretical/conceptual framework used in the study.
   - Justify the need and significance of the study
   - Conclude with the outcome expected from the study.
2. **Methods**
   - In methods use subheading like study design, variables settings, population, sample, sample size estimation, inclusive and exclusive criteria data collection instruments.
   - The technique for sample selection.
   - Data collection instruments.

- Content validity index, reliability.
- Method of data collection.
- In data analysis present clinical or mechanistic inference, rather statistical significance.
- Instead of standard errors of the mean it is better to present standard deviations.

3. **Results**
   - Explain the characteristics of the sample. If the study is interventional research, do not forget to mention pre-test means and SDs.
   - Present difference in mean - score and SDs to highlight any individual responses; with confidence limits.
   - Present the outcome in the form of figure or table to give the reader the magnitude of the important effects.
   - Repetition of outcomes presented in figures, tables, or text are to be avoided.
   - If the study adopted a quantitative approach report the findings it in numerical form.
4. **Discussion**
   - Discuss the main finding as per objectives laid down, interpret as per theoretical frame work.
   - Bring supportive studies and mention the hypotheses are accepted or rejected.
   - Bring clinical relevance to the main findings. Introduce the recent findings.
   - Study should explain major limitation in generalizing that may help to overcome those limitation by the future researchers.
   - Explain implication for the present study for nursing clinical practice, administration, education and research are the vital component of research report.
   - The report should end with conclusion in concise manner with recommendations for future research.
   - Acknowledge all the people who helped in contributed research with data collection, laboratory work and library materials.
   - Give credit to original author references and all sources of literature included in bibliography. Bibliography is a list of all materials that have consulted while give credit to original author.

Conclusions/Recommendations/Applications

- If the journal has such a section—state the main findings and/or applications in plain language, without being too repetitious.
- It must stand alone; therefore references, tables or figures.to be avoided.
- Avoid substantial or new points of discussion.
- Indicate useful future research, if it is not mentioned in discussion.
- **Acknowledgements**
  - Acknowledge the funding body.
  - Name the people who have provided help with equipment or testing.

Factors to be Considered while Writing the Report.

- Correct information to be presented
- Complete information to be included
- Concise descriptions will be more appealing
- Explicit explanations prevents ambiguity
- Convincing conclusions is more important in writing reports.

Submission of Report

- Take impact factors into account while choosing a journal to publish the study.
- Take the copyright policy into account, too.
- Follow the instructions for authors written in the journal!
- Check the report is the most recent version.
- If the paper gets rejected outright for bad reasons, ask the editor to send the manuscript out for further reviewing.

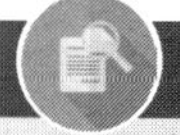

SUMMARY POINTS

✓ Advancement in nursing serves as a viable means of improving professional competence with improved patient care outcome.

✓ Recognition of professional nursing practice is achieved as nurse progresses from novice to expert. Novice nurses have minimal or no professional experience, whereas expert nurses demonstrate the most complex critical thinking skills and professional nursing practice, frequently are sought as resources by all members of the healthcare team, and serve as role models and clinical leaders.

- ✓ Continuing nursing education in nursing is a planned educational program organized by the administration of any health care facility or educational institution to keep their professional nurses updated with the current trends in nursing or nursing education.
- ✓ Continuing professional development includes orientation, skill training, continuing education and developing leadership and managerial skill.
- ✓ Steps in any continuing education program includes planning, designing, developing, implementing and evaluating phase.
- ✓ Nurses are hands-on health professionals who provide focused and highly personalized care. The field has a wide range of career opportunities, ranging from entry-level practitioner to doctoral-level researcher. Nurses also serve as advocates for patients, families and communities. They develop and manage nursing care plans, instruct patients and their families in proper care and help individuals and groups take steps to improve or maintain their health.
- ✓ The Trained Nurses Association of India is the important professional nursing organization in the country aimed at upholding in every way the dignity and honour of the nursing profession; promoting a sense of *esprit de corps* among all nurses; and enabling members to take counsel together on matters relating to their profession.
- ✓ Student nurses need to follow certain procedures to become member of TNAI from SNA. Becoming a member of TNAI has many benefits in professional career.
- ✓ Nurses have various opportunities in participating research as clinical nurse researcher, conducting scientific research, member of institutional review board and member of ethical committee in an institution .She/he can guide students to carry out research and teach research.
- ✓ The purpose writing research report is to document the research findings, to share the results with other interested groups, and apply the results in nursing practice.
- ✓ While publishing research report take impact factors into account while choosing a journal and take the copyright policy into account, the nurse researcher to follow the instructions for authors. Usually the model used is IMRAD and Check you have the most recent version.

REVIEW QUESTIONS

1. Define Continuing Nursing Education (CNE). Why CNE is important for nurses?
2. Describe the responsibilities of a nurse administrator in conducting CNE program.
3. Discuss the career opportunities in nursing for nurses in India.
4. Discuss the procedure for enrolling membership in TNAI from SNA.
5. Describe the role of nurses in nursing research
6. Write short notes on the following:
   a. Philosophy of CNE program
   b. Objectives and functions of TNAI
   c. Administration of SNA at various level
   d. Importance of nursing research
   e. Writing report of research for publication in a journal
   f. Orientation .

SELECTED READINGS

1. American Journal of Nursing. (2009). About the Journal. Retrieved from http://journals.lww.com/ajnonline/Pages/AbouttheJournal.aspx.American Medical Association (AMA). (2007). AMA manual of style: A guide for authors and editors (10 th ed.). New York: Oxford University Pres
2. Carlson, D. S., Masters, C., and Pfadt, E. (2008). Guiding the clinical nurse through research publication development. Journal of Nurses in Staff Development, 24, 222–225. 1097/01.NND.0000320679.73448.bf
3. Elcigil, A and Sari, H. (2006). Student's Opinions About and Expectations of effective Nursing Clinical Mentors. NYU Medical Center. (2004).

4. Glen Ellyn, IL: College of DuPage. Rickard, C., McGrail, M., Jones, R., O'Meara, P., Robinson, A., Burley, M., et al. (2009). Supporting academic publication: Evaluation of a writing course combined with writers' support group. Nurse Education Today 29, 516–521.
5. Heinrich, K. T. (2008). A nurse's guide to presenting and publishing: Dare to share. Boston: Jones and Bartlett Publishers
6. Hermann, M. H. (2010). Writing for publication in nursing: What every nurse educator needs to know Teaching nursing. The art and science. 146–166).
7. Hermann, M. H., Nordstrom, C., Wilmes, N. A., Denison, D., Webb, S. A., Featherston, D. E., . . . Striz, P. (2008). Dissemination of research in clinical nursing journals. Journal of Clinical Nursing 17, 149–156.
8. http://www.tamilnadunursingcouncil.com/career_guidance.phpCAREER GUIDANCE
9. http://www.tnaionline.org/membership.htm
10. International Committee of Medical Journal Editors. (2009). Ethical Considerations in the Conduct and Reporting of Research: Peer Review. Retrieved from http://www.icmje.org/ethical_3peer.html.
11. Megaghie, W. C., and Webster, A. (2009). Scholarship, publication, and career advancement in health professions education: AMEE Guide No. 43. Medical Teacher, 31, 574–590.
12. Policy guidance. Retrieved July 8, 2008, from http://www.hhs.gov/ohrp/ policy/index.html
13. Research ethics. Retrieved July 8, 2008, from http://depts. washington.edu/bioethx/topics/resrch. html # ques 1 U.S Department of Health and Human Services. (2008).
14. Shah, J., Shah, A., and Pietrobon, R. (2009). Scientific writing of novice researchers: What difficulties and encouragements do they encounter? Academic Medicine, 84, 511–516.
15. The TNAI http://www.tnaionline.org/membership.htm
16. What is clinical research and who is involved? Retrieved June 23, 2008, from http://gcrcwww.med.nyu.edu/public/rsso/clinical. html University of Washington School of Medicine. (1998).

Glossary

A

- **Abscond:** When an individual depart in a sudden and secret manner to avoid capture and legal prosecution. For example, a medicolegal case absconds from the ward.
- **Absenteeism:** It is an occurrence of habitual failure to appear at a work place or duty. It is an unauthorized absence reflects the morale of a person.
- **Abuse:** Mistreatment or neglect of vulnerable person(s) through the intentional or unintentional behavior of another person(s). This abuse may be physical, psychological, sexual, and financial in nature. For example, child abuse is common these days.
- **Access:** The ability of an individual or a defined population to obtain or receive the desired health care facilities without any barrier.
- **Accessible:** It is a term used to describe provision of health care facilities easily available to all people in a community.
- **Accounting:** Refers to financial reports related to budgeting transactions like assets, revenue, expenses and liabilities.
- **Accountability:** Accountability means being responsible for the task assigned as per the expectation set.
- **Accreditation:** It is referred as a process of recognizing an organization or institution by authorized agency officially to qualify or granting approval to perform a particular function for a specified period of time, e.g. hospital accreditation.
- **Accreditation standard:** A standard against which facilities or programs are assessed to decide if they will be accredited.
- **Administrative costs:** It refers to the costs which are not attributable to the direct delivery of health services and is not direct clinical care or service costs.
- **Administrative record:** A record concerned with administrative matters.
- **Administration:** It is an enabling process. The act of administering or managing an organization.
- **Administrator:** A person who manages to get the work done in order to achieve the goals of the organization.
- **Administration of nursing services:** It is the planning, organizing, directing, coordinating and controlling the members of the nursing service department to achieve the objectives of nursing services.

- **Advance directive:** A mechanism by which a competent individual expresses his or her wishes should circumstances arise in which he or she no longer is able to make rationale and sound decisions regarding his or her medical treatment. Usually 'advance directive' refers to orders for withholding and/or withdrawing life support treatments at the end of life, made by writing living wills and/or granting power of attorney to another individual.
- **Advocacy for health:** A combination of individual and social actions designed to gain political commitment, policy support, social acceptance and systems support for a particular health goal or program.
- **Affect:** It is a state of emotional condition of an individual which can be observed.
- **Agent of disease:** A factor, such as a microorganism, chemical substance, form of radiation, or excessive cold or heat, which is essential for the occurrence of a disease. A disease may be caused by more than one agent acting together or, in the case of deficiency diseases, by the absence of an agent.
- **Allied health personnel:** Specially trained and licensed people in occupations that support and supplement the functions of health professionals, e.g. health assistant.
- **Alternative and complementary health care/medicine/therapies:** Health care practices that are currently an integral part of conventional medicine. Such as AYUSH (Ayurveda, Unani, Siddha and Homeopathy).
- **Allocation:** It is the process of distributing by allotting according to the plan. For example, budget allocation for nursing service department, allocation of nurses for intensive care unit.
- **Ambulatory care:** Health services provided in an outpatient department. Patients can come from home, get the required health care services and does not require to stay in hospital as inpatient.
- **Ancillary service:** It refers to the supportive services provided in combination with medical or hospital care. For example, laboratory, radiology, CSSD, dietary services, etc.
- **Appropriate health technology:** It is described as methods, procedures, techniques and equipment that are scientifically valid, adapted to local needs and acceptable to those who use them and to those for whom they are used, and that can be maintained and utilized with resources the community can afford. For example, Disposable Delivery Kits (DDK).
- **Appraisal interview:** It is a face to face interview conducted between an employee and employer, to discuss job expectations, work performance and possible areas of growth for the employee. The appraisal interview is also gives a chance for an employee to air out any concerns.
- **Assault:** It is an unlawful sudden physical attack to another person in a threatening manner.
- **Assertiveness:** A person is being able to stand up for his own or other's rights in a calm and positive way without aggression.
- **Assessment:** It is referred as the process of collecting health care related data or information about a person's condition to identify individual needs and problem in order to develop a comprehensive care management plan as per the health needs and health problems identified.
- **Attitude:** It is a way of perceiving, thinking, feeling, or behaving that reflects a state of mind or disposition. For example, the nurse has a positive attitude towards geriatric patient care.
- **Auditing:** It refers to a thorough and sequential way of examination of ledgers, accounts, documents and vouchers related to money or budget of an establishment to ensure the accuracy of the financial statements presented, are properly maintained according to the legal requirements.
- **Authority:** A person in an organization, by the virtue of her/his power to give orders, make decisions, enforce discipline and control over its members.
- **Autonomy:** It is empowerment, to make personal decisions, according to one's own rules and preferences. For example, many a times Nurse lack autonomy in nursing practice.
- **Auxiliary worker:** A worker who has less than full professional qualifications in a particular field and is supervised by a professional worker. For example, Nursing assistant.

B

- **Basic health service:** It include all health care services such as communicable disease control, environmental sanitation, nutrition, health education, maintenance of records, vital statistics, nursing care and medical care facilities given to a definite population.

- **Battery:** It is a criminal offence involving the unlawful and deliberate physical touching without consent of that person.
- **Benchmark:** A level of care set as a goal to be attained.
- **Bench marking:** It is a standard or set of standards used as a reference point or yard stick to measure or evaluate quality of something.
- **Beneficiary:** A person eligible for benefits under a particular plan or policy. For example, Janani Suraksha Yojana scheme is planned for women and they are the beneficiaries.
- **Beneficence:** Doing well to other person. For example, researchers follow the principle of beneficence to do good for their subjects rather harming them. It is a principle of Ethics.
- **Budget:** The budget in simple words refers to financial statement or the documents which contains estimates of the revenue and expenditure for a year.
- **Budget plan:** It is planned according to the duration. It can be divided into (1) Short-range budget is planned month-to-month for 12 months and (2) Long-range plan which is planned for a period of three to five years.
- **Budget cycle:** It describes the activities and time frame that a budget covers. This is used in establishments who prepare monthly, quarterly and/or annual budget cycles to control costs and bring regularity in administrative duties.
- **Budgeting:** It is a process that includes various steps and activites to prepare a budget for a year.
- **Bureaucracy:** It is the division of power under different office position in hierarchical order to administer a large organization in a better way.

C

- **Capital:** It refers to fixed inputs or factors used in the production of goods and services. The value of such factors, or the money specifically allocated for their acquisition. For example of capital costs: the buildings, beds and equipment used in the provision of hospital services, etc.
- **Capital expenditure:** It refers to payment in cash to acquire asset. For example, money or funds to establish an auditorium in nursing college.
- **Care:** The application of professional knowledge and competency in caring individual or community in health and wellness condition. It include acute care/intensive care, intermediary care, long-term care, ambulatory care and day care.
- **Care package:** A series of health services provided to meet a person's assessed needs.
- **Care pathway/clinical pathway:** It is referred as a multidisciplinary set of daily prescriptions and outcome targets for managing the overall care of a specific type of patient, e.g. from pre-admission to post-discharge for patients receiving inpatient care. Clinical pathways are often intended to maintain or improve quality of care and decrease costs for patients in particular diagnosis-related groups. It is an agreed and explicit route an individual takes through health and social care services.
- **Career ladder:** It is a term used in HR management. It refers to the progression or upward mobility of an employee from entry level position to higher level position with increased salary benefits, responsibility and authority. For example, from the position of staff nurse to the nursing superintendent of the hospital.
- **Case conference:** A meeting of all professionals interested including doctors and nurses in an individual's care. for example, the head nurse conduct patient care conference.
- **Case manager:** A health care professional who is responsible for coordinating the care delivered to an assigned group of patients based on diagnosis that also include patient/family education, advocacy, and outcomes monitoring and management.
- **Case load:** The total number of patients taken care of by a case manager.
- **Case management:** A continuous process of planning, arranging and coordinating multiple health care services across time, place and discipline for persons with high-risk conditions or complex needs in order to ensure appropriate care and optimum quality, as well as to contain costs.
- **Centralization:** It refers to the administrative practice in which most of the decisions are taken by an officer from one central office.

- **Change agent:** An individual who encourages and motivates the people to change their behavior or opinion. For example, as a change agent the community health nurse motivate the people to make latrine for their family and use them.
- **Classification of disease:** Arrangement of diseases into groups having common characteristics.
- **Client:** A person who seeks or receives services or advice.
- **Client care:** In health care system client is referred as patient and is meant by interacting and managing patients or clients by providing good quality care within the framework of protocols and standards.
- **Clinical governance:** Refers to frameworks through which health organizations are accountable for continuously improving the quality services and protecting the population with high standards of care.
- **Clinical information system:** An information system that collects, stores and transmits information that is used to support clinical applications (e.g. transmission of laboratory test results, radiology results, prescription drug orders). Electronic medical records is one of the methods of clinical information system.
- **Clinical pathway:** *See* care pathway.
- **Clinical practice guideline:** A systematically developed document to assist practitioner and patient decisions about appropriate health care for one or more specific clinical circumstances.
- **Clinical trial:** A controlled research study of the safety and effectiveness of drugs, devices or techniques that occurs in four phases, starting with the enrolment of a small number of people, to the later stages in which thousands of people are involved prior to approval by the licensing authorities (for example, the Food and Drug Administration).
- **Closure:** Putting an end of the project/program/discussion over meeting.
- **Coding:** A mechanism of identifying and defining patient care services/activities as primary and secondary diagnoses and procedures.
- **Code of conduct:** A formal statement of desirable behavior that research workers or practitioners are expected to honour. There may be penalties for violation.
- **Coercive:** It refers to the practice of forcing a person to act in threatening or intimidation. For example, forcing a subject to participate in research without his voluntary consent.
- **Collective bargaining:** It is a discussion and negotiation between an employer and members of employees union about the welfare of the workers.
- **Communication skills:** Refers to the ways and means of transferring idea or thought from one person to another through the commonly used media of speech, written words, or bodily gestures.
- **Community empowerment:** Involves individuals acting collectively to gain greater influence and control over the quality of life in their communities. Community empowerment is an important factor for the success of goal achievement on health program.
- **Comprehensive health care:** Provision of a complete range of health services, from diagnosis to rehabilitation.
- **Computer-assisted diagnosis:** The use of information technology to assist health care professionals in diagnosis. This usually involves a dialogue between a computer system and a clinician. The systems are generally regarded as support systems for clinicians; the final responsibility for decision-making resides with the clinician.
- **Confidence:** A sense of assurance, faith or trust in a person, thing or oneself.
- **Confidentiality:** Privacy in the context of privileged communication (such as patient, doctor consultations) and medical records is safeguarded.
- **Conflict management:** It refers to an action of being able to identify and handle conflicts sensibly, fairly, and efficiently in an organization.
- **Consensus:** Agreement in opinion of experts. Consensus building is an important aspect of developing case management plans.
- **Consensus development:** Various forms of group judgment in which a group of experts interacts in assessing an intervention and formulating findings by vote or other informal or formal means, involving such techniques as the nominal group and Delphi techniques.
- **Consent form:** A document used during the consent process which is the basis for explaining to people the risks and potential benefits of a study or care intervention and the rights and responsibilities of the parties involved.

- **Consultation:** A technique of interaction where the opinions of several stakeholders are sought before a decision is made.
- **Consumer:** One who may receive or is receiving services. Any individual who avails services for which he has paid termed as consumer.
- **Consumer protection Act (CPA):** It refers to the act aiming to redress consumer grievances in a simple, speedy and inexpensive manner and the grievance caused by detective goods, deficient services and unfair trade practices.
- **Constitution:** The Indian Republic is controlled by her Constitution headed by the President of India. India became Republic on 26th of January in 1950, though the constitution was officially adopted on 26th November 1949.
- **Continuing education:** After formal basic education obtained by a health professional undergoes further education while on the job to advance their competency level.
- **Continuity of care:** The provision of barrier-free access to the necessary range of health care services over any given period of time, with the level of care varying according to individual needs.
- **Continuous Quality Improvement (CQI):** It is an important component of total quality management that uses systematic, organization-wide processes to achieve continuous improvement in the quality of health care services. It focuses on both outcomes and processes of care.
- **Continuum of care:** The continuum of care matches ongoing needs of the individuals being served by the case management process with the appropriate level and type of health, medical, financial, legal and psychosocial care for services within a setting or across multiple settings.
- **Coordinated care:** A collaborative process that promotes quality care, continuity of care and cost-effective outcomes which enhance the physical, psychosocial and vocational health of individuals. It includes assessing, planning, implementing, coordinating, monitoring and evaluating health-related service options. It may also include advocacy.
- **Coping:** An adaptive or otherwise successful method of dealing with individual or environmental situations that involve psychological and physiological stress or threat.
- **Cost:** It is referred as a price paid to acquire or maintain any objective or work.
- **Cost accounting:** It is referred as an accounting process with the objectives of assessing input costs incurred in each step of production and fixed cost such as depreciation cost of capital fixed equipment.
- **Cost containment:** It is referred as the process of controlling the expenses required to operate an organization within the framework of existing budgetary constraints.
- **Cost analysis:** It is a procedure of breaking down the costs of each activity and reporting on each factor separately to the administration.
- **Cost-benefit:** The relationship between the cost of an activity and the benefit that accrues from it.
- **Cost-benefit analysis:** It refers to the systematic comparison, in monetary terms, of all the costs and benefits of proposed alternative schemes with a view to determining: Which scheme or combination of schemes will contribute most to the achievement of predetermined objectives at a fixed level of investment; or the magnitude of the benefit that can result from schemes requiring the minimum investment.
- **Counseling:** Interaction offering an opportunity for a person to explore, discover and clarify ways of living with greater well-being, usually in a one-to-one discussion with a trained counselor.
- **Critical Path Method (CPM**): It is the sequential activities from start to the end of a project with time frame for each activity.
- **Cultural competence:** A practitioner's or institution's understanding of, and sensitivity to, the cultural background and primary language of people in any component of service delivery, including patient education materials, questionnaires, office or health care organization setting, direct care and public health campaigns.

D

- **Decentralization:** It refers to the delegation of decision-making power to middle level managers and lower level employees by the organization
- **Deception:** refers to the act of deceiving or the act of propagating false things as true.
- **Decision making skill:** It is an ability of the person (administrator) to select a good choice from various alternatives choices available in order to achieve organizational goals.

- **Declaration of Helsinki:** A set of rules that govern biomedical ethics to be observed while conducting research on human subjects.
- **Decoding:** In communication it is one of the elements. The sender encodes the message and the receiver decodes the message means interprets the message.
- **Defendant:** The person who gets sued or accused is called a defendant — they have to defend or answer their innocence the in court.
- **Delegation:** It is referred as the assignment of any responsibility or authority to another person. For example, the head nurse delegates the responsibility of inventory to the staff nurse.
- **Discipline:** It is a systematic training to control undesirable behavior.
- **Demography:** The scientific study of human populations. It include to size and density of population, fertility, mortality, growth, age distribution, migration and vital statistics.
- **Dependency:** It refers to persons who depend on others to provide physical, mental and/or social support.
- **Dependency ratio:** An indicator used in population studies to measure the portion of the population which is economically dependent on productive age groups (Adults). It is calculated as the sum of the 0-14-year-old (Children) and the over 60 or 65 years old (Elderly), depending on the working age limit considered, divided by the number of people aged between 15 and 59 or 64, respectively.
- **Dignity:** The right of individuals to be treated with respect as persons in their own right.
- **Discharge planning:** A process by which an admitted inpatient's needs on discharge are anticipated, planned and arranged.
- **Direct costs:** It refers to the cost incurred in a particular program or project.
- **Dissemination:** Any process by which information is transmitted (made available or accessible) to intended audiences.
- **DRG:** DRG stands for Diagnosis Related Group. A system of classification of patients on the basis of their diagnosis.
- **Duty:** It refers to moral obligation of a person to follow particular course of action. Example the nurse on duty resuscitated the newborn.

E

- **Efficacy:** The effect of a specific intervention, procedure, or service produces a beneficial result under normal conditions.
- **Efficient/efficiency:** The effect the specific resources used to provide a specific intervention, procedure, or service.
- **Effectiveness of care:** The effect of care that is provided to patients to achieve desired outcome.
- **E-health:** An emerging field in the intersection of medical informatics, public health and business, referring to health services and information delivered or enhanced through the Internet and related technologies.
- **Empowerment for health:** A process through which people gain greater control over decisions and actions affecting their lives. It is the process by which individuals or groups acquire the knowledge and skills needed to acquire desired health.
- **Enabling:** Taking action in partnership with individuals or groups to empower them, through the mobilization of human and material resources, to promote and protect their health.
- **Encounter:** A contact between an individual and a care provider.
- **Epidemiology:** The study of the various factors influencing the occurrence, distribution, prevention and control of disease, injury and other health-related events in a defined population.
- **Equity of care:** Fair treatment of needs, regarding both the distribution of services and allocation of resources.
- **Essential drugs:** Any of the therapeutic substances considered indispensable for the rational care of the vast majority of diseases in a given population.
- **Ethics of care:** The basic evaluative principles which (should) guide 'good' care. Principles typically refer to respect for, and the dignity of, human beings. Basic dimensions are autonomy (respect for self-determination), well-being (respect for happiness, health and mental integrity) and social justice (justifiable distribution of scarce goods and services). More specifically, ethics of care refer to ethical standards developed for the care professions which are designed to implement ethical principles in the practice of care provision.

- **Ethics committee:** A committee that can have a number of roles in relation to ethics. For example, it may develop policy related to the use and limitation of treatment; serve as a resource for individuals and their families regarding options for terminal illness; or assess research projects with respect to the consideration of ethical principles.
- **Ethnicity:** A social group within a cultural and social system that shares complex traits of religious, linguistic, ancestral and/or physical characteristics.
- **Euthanasia:** A deliberate act undertaken by one person with the intention of either painlessly putting to death or failing to prevent death from natural causes in cases of terminal illness or irreversible coma of another person.
- **Evidence-based care:** The care given to patients as well as care decision taken based on research findings by health care providers
- **Evidence-based decision-making:** It refers to decision applied in care, based on evidence available from research findings.

F

- **Factual database:** An indexed computer or printed source that provides information, in the form of guidelines for diagnosis, treatment and care indications, about older persons, or other authoritative information (For example, a computer database on drug indications, contraindications and interactions).
- **Finance:** It refers to various types of activities revolving around money and other valuable assets.
- **Financial administration:** It refers to financial activities such as planning, organizing, directing and controlling finance for the achievement of organizational objectives.
- **Financial control:** This refers to financial activities aimed at achieving desired return on investment.
- **First level position:** It is the first, entry position of an employee at the lower hierarchy after completing studies in an organization. For example, the staff nurse work in first level position in a hospital.
- **Fixed costs:** It refers to a cost that does not change irrespective of increasing or decreasing value of goods produces or sold.
- **Flexible scheduling:** It is the assigning of employees duty hours (Shift) to accommodate the employee's preference. For example, in nursing the flexible schedule include 7-11 am—break for one hour then 12-4 pm (Morning shift); 7-12 noon break for 4 hours 12-4 pm 4-7 pm (Evening shift) 7 pm to 7 am is the night shift.
- **Functional assignment:** This method refers to getting the greatest amount of tasks in the least time. In this method, the nursing care is divided into tasks and each staff member is assigning to perform one or two tasks for all patients in the unit according to the level of skill required for performance.
- **Functional organizational structure:** It refers to the activies of an organization structured around areas of specialization. For example, central sterile supply department, hospital laundry, maintenance department.
- **Functional status:** The extent to which an individual is able to perform activities that are associated with the routines of daily living.

G

- **General hospital:** A hospital providing a variety of services, including medicine and surgery, to meet the general medical needs of the community it serves.
- **Generation effect:** Variations in health status that arise from the different causal factors to which each birth cohort in the population is exposed as the environment and society change. Each consecutive birth cohort is exposed to a unique environment that coincides with its life span.
- **Goal:** A general or specific objective towards which to strive. An ultimate desired state towards which actions and resources are directed.
- **Gantt chart:** It is used in project management. It depicts project schedule including activities, tasks and events with starting and finishing dates.
- **Grapevine communication:** It is an informal and unofficial channel of business communication it stretches throughout the organization in all directions irrespective of the authority levels though there is an official channel of communication exists in an organization. The informal channels tend to develop when the employees interacts with other people in organization. It exists more at lower levels of organization.
- **Group dynamics:** It describes the manner in which the people in a group interact with each other.

- **Group process:** It is referred as the understanding of the behavior of people in the group such as task group and the process used to solve problem and make decisions. For example, establishing task force committee to make bye-laws of an association.
- **Guideline:** A direction or principle representing current or future rules of policy and clinical practice. Guidelines are more specific and more detailed than guiding principles, on which they are based.
- **Guiding principle:** A general rule that can be used as a guide. For example, to develop and implement policies, to set up a managerial process or to organize primary health care in communities.

H

- **Hazard (health):** A factor or exposure that may adversely affect health.
- **Health care institution/facility:** Any establishment that is engaged in direct patient care on site.
- **Health care technology assessment (HCTA):** The systematic evaluation of properties, effects and/or impacts of health care technology. It may address the direct, intended consequences of technologies as well as their indirect, unintended consequences.
- **Health centre:** A centre that may carry out promotive, protective, preventive, diagnostic, curative and rehabilitative health care activities for ambulant people.
- **Health goal:** An ultimate desired state of health towards which actions and resources are directed.
- **Health indicator/index:** A characteristic of an individual, population or environment which is subjected to measurement and can be used to describe one or more aspects of the health of an individual or population (quality, quantity and time). A health index comprises a number of indicators.
- **Health Information System (HIS):** The generation and the use of appropriate health information to enhance decision-making for health care implementation and management of health services at various level.
- **Health outcome:** Changes in health status which result from the provision of health (or other) services.
- **Health personnel:** All persons employed or contracted to provide health services.
- **Health planning:** It refers planning for the improvement of the health of a population or community, for a particular population, type of health service, institution or health program.
- **Health policy:** A formal statement or procedure within an institution (notably government) which defines goals, priorities and the parameters for action in response to health needs, within the context of available resources.
- **Health program:** An organized series of activities directed towards the attainment of defined health objectives and targets.
- **Health resources:** All the means available for the operation of the health system, including manpower, buildings, equipment, supplies, funds, knowledge and technology.
- **Health sector:** The sector consisting of organized public and private health services comprising of all activities like health promotion, disease prevention, curative treatment and care, the policies and activities of health departments, Non-governmental organizations (NGOs), community groups, and professional associations.
- **Health system infrastructure:** Services, facilities, institutions, personnel or establishments, organizations and those operating them for the delivery of a variety of health programmes.
- **Health technology:** The application of scientific knowledge to solving health problems. Health technologies include pharmaceuticals, medical devices, procedures or surgical techniques and management, communication and information systems innovations.
- **Health technology assessment (HTA):** The systematic evaluation of the effects or other impacts of health care technology on patient's health. It is aimed to inform decision-makers about health technologies and may measure the direct or indirect consequences of a given technology or treatment.
- **Hierarchy:** It refers to a system or organization in which people or groups are ranked one above the other according to status or authority.
- **Homeopathy:** A system of medicine based on the theory that a disease should be combated by giving drugs which would produce symptoms of the disease in an otherwise healthy individual.
- **Host:** A person or other living animal that affords subsistence or lodgement to an infectious agent under natural conditions; in an epidemiologic context, the host may be the population or group, or biological, social and behavioral characteristics of the group.

- **Human relation:** Human relation is a study of human behavior. It utilizes the philosophy and knowledge from various interdisciplinary sciences like sociology, psychology, anthropology and other sciences. Human relations are an action oriented process to build human cooperation towards achieving organizational goals.

I

- **Impact:** It refers to the total, direct and indirect, effects of a programme, service or institution on health status and overall health and socioeconomic development. For example, the impact of health services on morbidity pattern.
- **Indirect cost:** Indirect costs include costs which are frequently referred to as overhead expenses (For example, rent and utilities) and general administrative cost.
- **Input:** It refers to the resources, experts guidance and structural factors basic to planning.
- **In-service education:** It refers to planned education program for enhancing professional knowledge and professional competency of employees when they are on the job such as workshops, seminar.
- **Interview:** It refers to planned purposeful conversation between employer and employee to collect pertinent data for the benefit of the employer and employee.
- **Inventory control:** Inventory control is the process of overseeing and controlling of the ordering, storage and use of materials in an establishment (Hospital).
- **Incidence monitoring and reporting:** The reporting and tracking of adverse incidents by care providers.
- **Information and referral service:** A designated site or contact for locating needed services or care.
- **Informed consent:** A patient's/client's explicit agreement to the care and treatment to be provided, based on full information on his or her condition/diagnosis, the existing choices for treatment and the possible beneficial and adverse effects of those choices.
- **Intensive care:** It refers to highly skilled and specialized care provided to medical or surgical patients whose conditions are life-threatening and require comprehensive care and continuous observation. These type of patients are admitted in specially equipped unit having an adequate and specialized medical and nursing staff.
- **Intervention/intervention strategy:** An activity or set of activities aimed at modifying a process, course of action or sequence of events in order to change one or several of their characteristics, such as performance or expected outcome. For example, it is used in public health to describe a programme or policy designed to have an impact on an illness or disease.

J

- **Job:** It refers to assignment of work consisting of a set of tasks, duties and responsibilities that differs from other jobs.
- **Job analysis:** It is the process of collecting and analyzing information about jobs to write job description.
- **Job context:** It refers to the purposes of job, work environment and its place in the organization.
- **Job content:** It describes the duties and responsibilities of an employee who holds the job.
- **Job description:** It refers to the document that identifies the tasks and duties performed by an example.
- **Job specification:** It is a document that identifies the qualifications and attributes required to perform a job.
- **Job satisfaction:** It refers to the employee's cognitive and affective evaluation or evaluation of his or her job.
- **Job withdrawal:** It denotes the employee's intention to leave the job and organization.
- **Justice:** It is an ethical principle refers to the moral obligation to act to fairness, entitlement and equality. In health care ethics, this can described as fair distribution of scarce resources (distributive justice), respect for people's rights (rights based justice) and respect for morally acceptable laws (legal justice).

K

- **Key person:** A person who is very important, holding responsibilities, supervising and monitoring towards care given in a context. For example, the head nurse is a key person in her unit.
- **Knowledge explosion:** It refers to the sudden exposure of information or data to people.

L

- **Law:** It refers to rules, regulation and conduct that guides individual's action. It is established by a competent authority which each one of us needs to follow as a citizen of India.
- **Leadership:** Leadership is described as the activity of leading a group of people or an organization which involves establishing clear vision, sharing that vision with others so that they will follow willingly.
- **Legal document:** A document that depicts some contractual relationship or grants of some rights which are legal in nature. For example, Records of Medicolegal cases are legal document.
- **Legal liability:** It is described as legal responsibility for one's own action.
- **Legitimate**: It is referred as lawful or according to the law.
- **Legislation:** It refers to the act making or enacting law.
- **Liability:** It is an obligation that legally binds an individual or establishment.
- **License:** To give permission to act or practice.
- **Line and staff structure:** In line structure managers direct the tasks to subordinates and make decision. In staff structure the managers advise those with line of authority.
- **Line of authority:** It refers to the chain of commands within an establishment that gives power to order the subordinates to perform the job within the framework of job description.

M

- **Maldistribution:** It refers to either a surplus or a shortage of the type of health providers needed to maintain the health services to a given population at an optimum level. For example, there is regional (Urban and rural) imbalance in distribution of health care services in India.
- **Malpractice:** Professional misconduct or failure to apply ordinary skill in the performance of a professional act. For example, in nursing—it is the failure of a nurse with professional education and skills to act in a reasonable and prudent manner.
- **Management:** Management is referred as the art of getting the work done through the members of the health team by directing and controlling their efforts to achieve the organizational goals.
- **Managed care:** It refers to the care approach to health care with the objective to streamline medical and nursing services and render healthcare that is quality and cost effective.
- **Managerial planning:** Managerial planning refers to the process to identification of goal, and developing a realistic plan of action, for achieving organizational goals. The basic steps in the managerial planning is defining each task to meet the objectives of the establishment.
- **Management by objectives:** Management by objectives (MBO) is an orderly and systematic approach that helps the management to utilize available resources to achieve desirable goals in an effective manner.
- **Management information system:** A system of databases designed to process and exchange information to support decision-making as well as implementation, monitoring and evaluation of programmes, activities and projects.
- **Medical error:** An error or omission in the medical care provided to an individual.
- **Medical record:** A file kept for each patient, maintained by the hospital (medical practitioners also maintain medical records in their own practices), which documents the patient's problems, diagnostic procedures, treatment and outcome.
- **Mentoring:** It refers to an activity in which an experienced and professional person guiding, and supporting a junior employee for enhancing his professional practice and development.
- **Minimum standard:** A level of quality that all health plans and providers are required to meet in order to offer services to clients/consumers.
- **Modular nursing:** In modular nursing assignment, technical and nurse aides, as well as professional nurses are involved. In each module, two or three persons are assigned and the professional nurse becomes responsible for the care of assigned patients. The non-professional nurses are guided and trained by the professional nurse.
- **Monitoring:** A process of continuous observing and checking.

- **Motivation:** It refers to all the internal energizing forces or conditions that stir up activity and sustain activity of an individual.

N

- **National health policy:** It refers to decisions, plans and actions that are undertaken to achieve specific health care goals of a country. These policies are developed by a team of competent experts in health industry as well as officials recommended by the Government of the country.
- **Neglect:** This refers to not give enough care or attention to people or things that are your responsibility:, either consciously or unintentionally.
- **Nursing negligence:** It is described as when a professional nurse who is fully qualified and capable to care does not use such capability as a skilled care nurse would use, and as a result the patient suffers from complication or harm.
- **Negotiation:** It is the art of reaching an agreement by resolving differences through creativity.
- **Nongovernmental organization (NGO):** An independent, national or international organization. These organizations may be run either for profit or not for profit.
- **Norms:** These are informal guideline about what is considered correct or incorrect social behavior in a particular group or society.
- **Nursing record:** Data recorded by nurses concerning the nursing care given to the patient, including nursing care implementation and evaluation of care given.
- **Nursing audit:** It is a detailed review and evaluation of selected clinical records by qualified professional nursing personnel for evaluating quality of nursing care. It is a part of the cycle of quality assurance. It incorporates the systematic and critical analysis of care given by nurses.
- **Nursing rounds:** Nursing rounds is a visit into patient's area or wards involving the students and discussion with head nurses. It provides a rich learning experiences to nursing students and clinical nurses.
- **Nursing ethics:** It concerns clinical nursing issues. Issues regarding: Allocation of care and Resources, Confidentiality, Unethical or Incompetent conduct of colleagues.

O

- **Objective:** A measurable state that is expected to exist as a result of the application of procedures and resources.
- **Operational Planning:** It is the process of planning and objectives to tactical goals and objectives. It describes the development expected activities to be completed within a period of time specifically during the financial year.
- **Optimizing:** It refers to making a portfolio in such a way that the outcome is maximized for a given risk level, or risk is minimized for a given risk level.
- **Organization:** It is defined as a group of individuals who work together in an organized way for achieving organizational goals.
- **Organization chart:** It is visual communication of information which is more effective to understand by each employee in an organization.
- **Organizational culture:** It is referred as the values and attitudes of the employees of an organization that has an impact on the development of an unique social and psychological work setting of an organization.
- **Organization process:** It refers to various steps and synchronization of various activities to achieve organizational goal.
- **Organizational climate:** It is described as how members of an organization experience the culture of an organization. The climate of an organization is subject to change frequently and can be shaped by the upper management of an organization.
- **Organizational change:** It refers to the strategies adopted by the administration to improve the performance of employees and outcome of organization.
- **Organizational Effectiveness:** It refers to the functions and competency of the employees of the organization who are able to achieve the organizational objectives. Or in other words the organization that brings positive outcome or an organization that is productive to achieve its goals.

- **Orientation:** It is an induction training program to help novice nurses to acquit with organizational structure, functions, policies, etc.
- **Outcome:** Outcome is a change in a situation resulting from an action. An outcome can also be viewed as the end result obtained from utilizing the structure and processes of health care delivery.
- **Outcome measurement:** The methods for measuring health care responses from patients and providers.
- **Outcome standard:** The quality of care set by an authority which the service providers should strive to achieve for all patients/individuals in care settings.
- **Output:** It is the end product or service derived from care process.

P

- **Participatory management:** It is an open system of management where employees are actively involved in decision-making process.
- **Patient-centered care:** It is one of the methods of assigning patient care for nurses. It is also called case method of assignment. In this method one or more patients to a particular nurse for a specific period of time is assigned by the head nurse. She is responsible for the complete care including assessing vital signs, general nursing measures, treatment, medication administration nourishments and imparting health education, etc. Nurses assume total responsibility for meeting all the needs of assigned patients.
- **Patient classification system:** It is system of categorizing patients according to nursing hours needed for their care as per complexity of their illness. This is required to estimate staffing and scheduling nurses.
- **Patients' rights:** It refers to a set of rights, privileges, responsibilities and duties under which individuals seek and receive health care services.
- **Peer review:** It refers to review by individuals from the same discipline and with essentially equal qualifications.
- **Performance:** It is an activity—the level of attainment of a goal in comparison to a given effort.
- **Performance criteria:** It refers to criteria to be used to measure/assess performance.
- **Performance measure or indicator:** It is an evaluation tool to assess the extent to which the performance of an individual practitioner conform to practice standards of quality or allow comparisons between services.
- **Performance appraisal:** It describes the systematic evaluation of the performance of employees and to understand the abilities of that employee for further growth and development.
- **PERT:** Program (Project) Evaluation and Review Technique (PERT) is a managerial tool. It is used with the aims of scheduling, organizing, and coordinating work related activities in an establishment. It systematically analyses the data related to the tasks and the time required to complete each task in a given project.
- **Philosophy:** It refers to statements of beliefs and values of a person, agency, professionet.
- **Placement:** The act of placing a newly appointed employee on job in an appropriate setting.
- **Policy**: It refers to written document comprising of wide range of statements of institutional goals or prescribed course of actions to achieve organizations goals.
- **Policy formulation:** The development of a policy.
- **Politics:** It is the manner in which people use their power in order to overcome the deficiencies and inadequacies of employees to cope up with changing trends.
- **Population dynamics:** It refers to branch of life sciences that studies the size and age composition of populations as dynamic systems). The study of changes in the number and composition of individuals in a population and the factors that influence those changes. Population dynamics involves five basic components of interest, to which all changes in populations can be related: birth, death, sex ratio, age structure and dispersal.
- **Poverty level/line:** A minimum income level below which a person is officially considered to lack adequate subsistence and to be living in poverty.
- **Power:** When an individual uses his ability to achieve his goal in a manner in which he desires from other individuals or his subordinates is referred as power.
- **Power of attorney:** It is described as a written document in which one person A appoints another person to act as an agent B on his or her behalf, thus conforms authority to perform certain functions on behalf of the person A.

- **Practice guideline:** It is a descriptive document containing the standardized specification for care patients in a particular condition developed through a formal process that are based on the best scientific evidence of effectiveness with expert opinion.
- **Prioritization:** Arranging or dealing with in order of importance.
- **Primary nursing:** In primary nursing the patient is the central focus not the task rendered. It is a well-planned, comprehensive, collaborative and coordinated nursing process that maintains continuity of care facilitated to meet the total needs of each patient.
- **Process:** A continuous and regular action or succession of actions taking place or being carried out in a definite manner and leading to the accomplishment of some results.
- **Professional accountability:** It refers to ensuring professionals in a sound and sustainable manner, maintain accountability for their practices and are held accountable for any deficiencies in their professional activities.
- **Professional self-regulation:** The enforcement of certain rules of conduct among its members by a professional community. For example, nursing ethics.
- **Project:** A unique endeavor with a beginning and an end to be completed by one or more people within the constraints of time, budget and quality; a problem scheduled for solution.
- **Prompt attention:** The principle that those needing care are able to access it speedily.
- **Protocol for nursing:** The standards or practices developed to assist nurses to make and effect decisions about particular steps in the nursing management process.
- **Planning:** The process of determining specific objectives, goals, and actions designed to meet the organizational goals through the assessment process.
- **Practice guidelines for nurses:** Systematically developed statements on nursing practice that guides the nurse practitioner in making decisions about appropriate diagnostic and nursing care services for specific clinical conditions. Practice guidelines are usually developed by authoritative professional societies and organizations such as the Nursing Council, Trained Nurses Association of the country.
- **Primary care:** The first point when the patient first seeks assistance from the health care system.
- **Provider:** A person or entity that provides health care services.

Q

- **Quality:** It refers to a specific feature or attributes of a person or a thing.
- **Quality Assurance:** Quality Assurance is a broad practice used for assuring the quality of services. In quality assurance, there is an administrative effort to enhance the quality practices in the organization.
- **Quality control:** It is set of procedures focus to ensure that performed service adheres to a defined set of quality criteria or meets the requirements of the patients.
- **Quality improvement:** It refers to techniques and methods used for the collection and analysis of data gathered during provision of health care practices in a clinical setting and to identify and resolve problems in the system and improve the processes and outcomes of care.
- **Quality indicator:** A predetermined measure for assessing quality.
- **Quality management:** A formal and planned, systematic, organization approach to the monitoring, analysis, and improvement of organization performance, thereby continually improving the performance to which providers conform to defined standards, the quality of patient care and services provided, and the likelihood of achieving desired patient outcomes.
- **Quality monitoring:** A process used to ensure that care is being delivered at acceptable quality standards prescribed by the organization or national guidelines.

R

- **Recruitment:** Recruitment is a method of finding suitable candidates to fill various positions in an organization.
- **Reinforcement:** It is a psychological factor. It is a state that forces the behavior to strengthen. For example, the teacher summarizes the lesson to reinforce or strengthen the learning.

- **Referral:** The direction of people to an appropriate facility, institution or specialist in a health system, such as a health center or a hospital, when health workers at a given level cannot diagnose or treat certain individuals by themselves, or face health or social problems they cannot solve by themselves.
- **Reform:** A purposeful, dynamic process that involves systematic policy, structural and process changes and is aimed at achieving desired goals.
- **Re-orienting health services:** Health services re-orientation is characterized by a more explicit concern for the achievement of population health outcomes in the ways in which the health system is organized and funded.
- **Responsibility:** It refers to the state or fact of having a duty to deal with something. For example, the nurse is responsible for the care of the assigned patients.
- **Retention:** Employee retention refers to the ability of the organization to retain its employees using retention strategies.
- **Reward:** It is a token of appreciation for the excellent performance exhibited by the employee.
- **Right:** It refers to legal and ethical principles of freedom and are fundamentals rules about what is allowed to people such as child's right, women's right.
- **Role:** A part played by a performer.
- **Role ambiguity:** It refers to lacking of clear information regarding role expected.
- **Role conflict:** Role conflicts occur when an individual is forced to take on separate and incompatible roles.
- **Role expectation:** A role expectation is what you are expected to do depending on what role you obtain.

S

- **Safety:** It is condition of being protected from harm For example the patient's safety in ward refers to protection, from cross infections, prevention of fall.
- **Scheduling of nurses:** It is an activity of the nurse administrator to assign an appropriate number nursing personnel to the each service unit/ward for 24 × 7 days of care.
- **Self-reliance/self-sufficiency/self-management:** The capacity of individuals, communities or national authorities to take the initiative in assuming responsibility for their own health in other words empowering them for their own health.
- **Service:** A result of a provider's actions focusing at meeting the needs and problems of a consumer.
- **Skilled care:** It refers to advanced level of care provided by trained health professionals, including nurses, doctors.
- **Social security benefits:** Benefits that include income for eligible persons from social security, old age, disability, and survivors' pension schemes.
- **Specialized nursing care needs:** Nursing care needs that require the advanced and specialized clinical skills and knowledge of a registered nurse.
- **Specialist:** A health professional who is specially trained in a certain branch of his/her profession related to specific services or procedures. For example, ICU nurse.
- **Staff counseling:** It is a therapeutic and planned process which is designed to help and support the staff or employee at the time of difficulties encountered in work place.
- **Staffing:** The term includes planning for recruiting, selecting, and training and developing employees, as well as compensating them and providing for their health and safety.
- **Staff development:** It refers to a process that includes both formal and informal activities which are related to the employees to develop their performance.
- **Standard:** A quality, measure or reference point established as a rule or model by authorities, custom or general consent, against which things can be evaluated or should conform. For example, nursing standards.
- **Strategy:** A planning and managing an operation to achieve the organizational objectives.
- **Strategic planning:** It is a systematic and planned process developed to support an organization to identify and maintain a maximal alignment with the most important components of the organizational environment. It is a complex and ongoing process of organizational change.
- **Supervision:** It refers to monitoring and regulating of delegated tasks, activities and responsibilities by a supervisor of employees working under her/him.

- **Sustainable development:** A process of development that meets the needs of the present generation without compromising the ability of future generations to meet their own needs.
- **System:** A network of interdependent components that work together to attain the goals of the complex whole.
- **Systems approach:** A school of thought evolving from earlier systems analysis theory and propounding that virtually all outcomes are the result of systems rather than individuals.
- **System analysis:** It refers to the techniques to assess the adequacy of the functions, need for change if any and the quality of outcome of a system.

T

- **Tangible cost:** Objective elements in the production of care, i.e. number of personnel, beds, consumables, technologies, staff qualifications.
- **Target population/target group:** The group of persons for whom an intervention is planned. For example, the targeting of services to particular user like antenatal mothers.
- **Task:** A definite work assigned or done as a part of duties.
- **Team nursing:** It is a method of nursing assignment that comprises all personnel involvement in care of patients. This method utilizes all professionals, technical and nursing aids into small teams efficiently and effectively for patient care. The unit incharge becomes head of all teams who through the direct supervision, guidance, and teaching of professional nurses enhances patient care outcome.
- **Termination:** It is a managerial act of making an employee leaves a job. Sometimes it is referred as the act of dismissing an employee.
- **Technology:** The application of science to health care.
- **Telemedicine/telehealth:** The employment of communication technology to provide assistance in the diagnosis, treatment, care and management of health conditions in remote areas.
- **Throughput:** This is a process or means or activities to achieve the outcome.
- **Time management:** Utilization of time effectively by preventing interruptions.
- **Tort:** It is a legal system refers to a violation is made against a person or property causes damage, injury or harm to another person.
- **Total cost:** The sum of all costs incurred in producing a set quantity of service.
- **Total Quality Management:** Total Quality Management include quality assurance and quality improvement. That is QA + QI = TQM.
- **Transactional leadership:** Transactional leaders are of traditional type of leaders who are mostly focus their attention on day-to-day activities.
- **Transformational leadership:** Transformational leaders are visionaries, committed to work and the people and empower subordinates to achieve the vision of the organization.
- **Trend analysis:** It refers to a method of collecting information and studying the pattern or trend in the information.
- **Turnover of employees:** It is a measurement in percentage of how long employees stay in an organization and how often the employer have to replace the employees.

U

- **Underutilization:** The use of a service or facility below its potential.
- **Universal access:** The right and ability to receive comprehensive, affordable, care.

V

- **Values:** It is a person's principles or standards of behavior; one's judgment of what is important in life.
- **Veracity:** When the truthfulness or honesty is consistent or habitual.

W

- **Wages:** It is a fixed regular payment, typically paid on a daily or weekly basis, made by an employer to an employee, especially to a manual or unskilled worker.

- **Withdrawal:** Detachment, social isolation.
- **Working capital:** The sum of the institution's short-term or current assets, including cash, marketable (short-term) securities, accounts receivable and inventories. Net working capital is defined as the excess of total current assets over total current liabilities.

X

- **X Theory:** In 1960, Douglas McGregor, an American psychologist authored a book *The Human Side of Enterprise* described the characteristics of people in the work place. Based on the belief of Theory X and theory Y. In X theory a manager is strong authoritarian leader shows poor outcome in administration, exercises coercive power, uses punishment and disciplinary action when the work is not done and the manager concentrates on monetary gain.

Y

- **Y Theory:** The manager and employees are innovative and enjoy their work, demonstrate rewarding leadership, work with employees to bring better outcome uses participative power and motivates and supports the employees to get good results.

Z

- **Z Theory:** William Ouchi developed Z theory and introduced into Japanese industries. Z Theory is an extension of motivation and assumes that bigger establishments are human systems and their effectiveness depends on the quality of humanism used. Z theory focuses on trust and strong bonding between the employer and employees.
- **Zero budgeting:** It is the fundamental technique of finance and accounting. In this method, all expenses are justified for each new year period of budget cycle. It starts from zero based with scratch with no preauthorized funds. In this method each function and its needs are analyzed and the cost is calculated in relation to the performance to be achieved. Then budget is prepared for the next year whether the budget amount is higher or lower than the previous year.

PREVIOUS YEARS' QUESTION PAPERS

As per the requests from students and teachers of nursing, the book includes previous years' question papers on Management of Nursing Services and Education from Rajasthan University of Health Sciences, Rajasthan and Rajiv Gandhi University of Health Sciences, Karnataka.

The question papers of Rajasthan University of Health Sciences include from May 2011 to March 2016 and the old syllabus from 2008 to 2010. The answers of the questions are indicated in chapter and page number in brackets for each questions.

However the question papers from Rajiv Gandhi University of Health Sciences from 2011 to 2016 are not indicated the answers in brackets. The students are required to solve such questions at their end using this book or from other sources if needed.

Rajasthan University of Health Sciences, Rajasthan
BSc (Nursing) Part IV Examination
March 2016
Management of Nursing Services and Education

Q.1. A. Describe nursing as a profession. Enlist the characteristics of professional nurse. (*Chapter 27, pp 341, 342*)
B. Explain current trends and issues in nursing. (*Chapter 24, p 318*)

Q.2. A. Explain the principles of good ward management. (*Chapter 22, p 290*)
B. Describe various factors involved in good ward management. (*Chapter 22, p 293*)

Q.3. A. Define curriculum.
B. Describe the purpose of curriculum.
C. Briefly explain curriculum planning.

Q.4. A. Explain the purpose of job-description. (*Chapter 13, p 136*)
B. Write the job-description of nursing superintendent, ward-in-charge and community healthy nurse. (*Chapter 13, p 137*)

Q.5. Write short answers (any 4):
A. Cost benefit analysis. (*Chapter 19, p 234*)
B. Bench marking. (*see Glossary, p 359*)
C. Techniques of IPR. (*Chapter 15, p 163*)
D. Human resource management (HRM). (*Chapter 12, p 111*)
E. Performance appraisal. (*Chapter 17, p 198*)

Q.6. Write short notes on (any four):
A. Program evaluation review technique (PERT). (*Chapter 6, p 64*)
B. Disaster management. (*Chapter 25, pp 326–330*)
C. Affiliation and accreditation. (*Chapter 29, p 254*)
D. Principles of adult learning.
E. Anecdotal record.

Rajasthan University of Health Sciences, Rajasthan
BSc (Nursing) Part IV Examination
February 2015
Management of Nursing Services and Education

Q.1. A. Define leadership. (*Chapter 14, p 143*)
B. What do you mean by leadership style?
C. Explain in detail about the various types of leadership styles. (*Chapter 14, p 146*)
D. Which is the favorite leadership style? Explain.

Q.2. A. Describe the nature of theories of management. (*Chapter 3, p 36*)
B. Explain the principles of management applied in nursing services. (*Chapter 3, pp 40–41*)

OR

A. Define evaluation.
B. List out the steps of evaluation.
C. Explain the methods of evaluation used in nursing.

Q.3. A. Briefly explain about in-service education. (*Chapter 13, p 132*)
B. Write about regulatory bodies nursing. (*Chapter 27, p 343*)

OR

Short answers (any four):
A. Group dynamics. (*Chapter 15, p 159*)
B. Code of ethics in nursing. (*Chapter 20, p 246*)
C. Guidance and counseling.
D. Principles of nursing supervision. (*Chapter 13, p 136*)
E. Nursing audit (quality assurance). (*Chapter 16, p 191*)

Q.4. A. Define material management. (*Chapter 18, pp 213–224*)
B. Discuss about material management in hospital. (*Chapter 18, pp 213–224*)
C. Explain about patient classification system. (*Chapter 10, pp 92–94*)

Q.5. Write short notes on:
A. Collective bargaining. (*Chapter 15, p 178*)
B. Clinical facilities for BSc (N) 1st year.
C. Functions of INC. (*Chapter 27, p 343*)
D. Supervision. (*Chapter 13, p 134*)

Rajasthan University of Health Sciences, Rajasthan
BSc (Nursing) Part IV Examination
June 2014
Management of Nursing Services and Education

Q.1. A. Define performance appraisal. (*Chapter 17, p 198*)
B. Describe the factors influencing effective performance appraisal. (*Chapter 17, p 198*)
C. Enlist and discuss about performance appraisal tools. (*Chapter 17, p 200*)
D. 'Performance appraisal motivates the employee'. Explain. (*Chapter 17, p 199*)

Q.2. Explain the principles of management which are applied in nursing services. (*Chapter 3, pp 40–41*)

Q.3. Explain human resources management. Discuss process of recruitment for nursing personnel in any agency which is familiar to you. (*Chapter 12, p 112*)

Q.4. A. Describe objectives of GNM programme.
B. Describe physical facilities for GNM programme.
C. Explain affiliation for such institution.

Q.5. A. Describe the components of the learning experiences with help of a diagram.
B. Discuss the criteria as a nurse will use in selection of learning experiences for the nursing student (support your answer with examples from the clinical field).

Q.6. Define leadership. Discuss leadership style in nursing. (*Chapter 14, pp 143, 146*)

OR

Define profession. Describe characteristics of professional nurse. (*Chapter 27, p 342*)

Q.7. Write short note on any five:
A. Principles of adult learning
B. Group dynamics (*Chapter 15, p 160*)
C. Guidance and counseling
D. Budgeting. (*Chapter 19, p 229*)
E. Career opportunities for graduate nurses. (*Chapter 28, p 348*)
F. Negligence and malpractice in nursing. (*Chapter 20, pp 248–49*)

Rajasthan University of Health Sciences, Rajasthan
BSc (Nursing) Part IV Examination
July 2013
Management of Nursing Services and Education

Q.1. A. Define nursing. (*Chapter 27, p 341*)
B. Enlist characteristics of professional nurse. (*Chapter 27, p 342*)
C. Discuss nursing as a profession. (*Chapter 27, p 341*)

Q.2. A. What is job description? (*Chapter 13, p 135*)
B. Describe job description of nursing superintendent of any hospital. (*Chapter 13, p 137*)

Q.3. A. Define in-service education program. (*Chapter 13, p 132*)
B. Enlist aims of in-service education program. (*Chapter 13, p 132*)
C. Describe orientation method as component of in-service education. (*Chapter 13, p 130*)

Q.4. A. Define evaluation.
B. Enlist features of evaluation.
C. Discuss principles of evaluation.

Q.5. A. Define management. (*Chapter 3, p 35*)
B. Enlist functions of management. (*Chapter 3, p 40*)
C. Discuss principles of management. (*Chapter 3, p 40*)

Q.6. Explain in brief:
A. Current trends and issues in nursing. (*Chapter 24, p 318*)
B. Budgeting. (*Chapter 19, p 229*)

Q.7. Write short notes on any four:
A. Delegation. (*Chapter 15, p 167*)
B. Recruitment. (*Chapter 13, p 120*)
C. Code of ethics. (*Chapter 20, p 246*)
D. Records and reports. (*Chapter 21, pp 270–274*)
E. Indian nursing council. (*Chapter 27, p 343*)
F. Communication. (*Chapter 14, p 154*)

Rajasthan University of Health Sciences, Rajasthan
BSc (Nursing) Part IV Examination
Held in July 2012
Management of Nursing Services and Education

Q.1. Define leadership. Discuss the skills of a good leader. Enlist the various leadership styles (theories) and explain the situational theory of leadership in detail. (*Chapter 14, pp 143–157*)

Q.2. A. Define the material management. (*Chapter 18, p 215*)
B. Discus the various elements of material management system. (*Chapter 18, pp 217–220*)
C. Explain the procedures for material management in an organization. (*Chapter 18, pp 217–220*)

Q.3. Short notes on any THREE:
A. Performance appraisal. (*Chapter 17, p 198*)
B. Cost benefit analysis. (*Chapter 19, p 234*)
C. Nursing audit. (*Chapter 16, p 191*)
D. Team nursing. (*Chapter 10, p 96*)

Q.4. Discipline is important part of an organization:
A. Define the discipline. (*Chapter 17, p 204*)
B. What should be the criteria to treat an employee for misconduct? (*Chapter 17, p 206*)
C. Write down the procedure to take disciplinary action against an employee. (*Chapter 17, p 205*)

Q.5. Discuss the guidelines to open a GNM training in India.

Rajasthan University of Health Sciences, Rajasthan
BSc (Nursing) Part IV Examination
May 2011
Management of Nursing Services and Education

Q.1. Define management. Discuss the principles of management. Write in detail management theory. (*Chapter 3, pp 35–36, 40*)

Q.2. A. Describe types of budgeting. Explain. (*Chapter 19, p 229*)
B. Role of nurses manager in budgeting. (*Chapter 19, p 237*)

Q.3. Discus the process of recruitment, selection, and placement of nurses in 500 bedded general hospital. (*Chapter 13, pp 120–138*)

Q.4. A. Enumerate the principles of organization. (*Chapter 7, p 73*)
B. Explain the role of nurses administrator in programme (staff development). (*Chapter 7, p 129*)

Q.5. Write short notes on any three:
A. Ethical issues in nursing. (*Chapter 20, p 252*)
B. Effective records and reports. (*Chapter 21, p 270*)
C. Public relations. (*Chapter 15, p 163*)
D. Consumer protection act. (*Chapter 20, p 256*)
E. Accreditation. (*Chapter 20, p 254*)

Rajasthan University of Health Sciences, Rajasthan
BSc (Nursing) Part IV Examination 2010
Old Scheme
Introduction to Principles of Administration and Nursing Services

Q.1. Define administration. List out the principles of nursing administration and explain how the nursing administration will apply these in day-to-day activities. (*Chapter 3, pp 38, 39*)

Q.2. Discuss in detail the functions, organization and line of authority of a hospital. (*Chapter 7, p 75; Chapter 8, p 80*)

Q.3. 'Head of nursing is a combination of administrator, supervisor and teacher.' Comment. (*Chapter 22, p 287; Chapter 4, p 45*)

Q.4. What are the duties of a supervisor when posted in public health field?

Q.5. Write short notes on any four:
   A. Principles of supervision. (*Chapter 13, p 134*)
   B. In-services education. (*Chapter 13, p 132*)
   C. Evaluation of students.
   D. Maintenance of records and reports in hospital. (*Chapter 21, pp 271–275*)
   E. Counseling of staff. (Chapter 17 see mentoring and coaching page 201)

Q.6. Describe the method of selection and counseling of students in school of nursing.

Q.7. Explain with suitable examples the process of decision making and problem solving. (*Chapter 15, p 165*)

Rajasthan University of Health Sciences, Rajasthan
BSc (Nursing) Part IV Examination
Held in June 2009
Introduction to Principles of Administration and Nursing Services

Q.1. A. How will you differentiate the term administration and management. (*Chapter 3, p 35*)
B. Discuss the functions of management. (*Chapter 3, p 40*)
C. Focus on the various techniques of management which are used by nursing manager. (*Chapter 3, p 40*)

Q.2. A. What do you mean by personnel management?
B. How staff development program help in personnel management. (*Chapter 13, p 129*)
C. Explain objectives and elements of health man power of effective personnel management. (*Chapter 13, pp 120–138*)

Q.3. A. Define a term evaluation in view of administration. (*Chapter 17, pp 198–200*)
B. Explain evaluation process and its components.

Q.4. A. Define budget. (*Chapter 19, p 225*)
B. Explain various types of budget used in nursing school. (*Chapter 19, p 229*)
C. Prepare a budget and plan for a school of nursing with yearly intake of 20 students. (*Chapter 28, pp 310, 311*)

Q.5. What are all administrative responsibilities of a nursing superintendent of 'A Grade' hospital. Discuss in detail. (*Chapter 4, pp 43–44*)

Q.6. A. What are the modern concept of hospitals. (*Chapter 10, pp 99–100*)
B. Explain its various department in details.
C. Prepare a diagrammatic structure of 10-bedded ICU set-up. Discuss the complete requirement of ICU. (*Chapter 10, pp 100–102*)

Q.7. Write short notes on any four of the following:
A. MBO (*Chapter 6, p 66*)
B. Nursing audit (*Chapter 16, p 191*).
C. Administrative and supervisory function of public health nurse in district level.
D. Steps to be followed in community health planning.
E. Guidanfe and counseling.
F. Role of SNA in view of leadership quality. (*Chapter 28, p 350*)

Rajasthan University of Health Sciences, Rajasthan
BSc (Nursing) Part IV Examination 2010
October 2008
Old Scheme
Introduction to Principles of Administration and Nursing Services

Q.1. A. List down the objectives of public health administration. (*Chapter 1, pp 7–8*)
B. Explain the factors which contribute to effective ward administration. (*Chapter 22, pp 293–295*)

Q.2. A. Discuss the role of public relation in hospital administration. (*Chapter 15, pp 163–165*)
B. Importance of relationship of nursing service department with other departments of hospital. (*Chapter 8, pp 80, 82*).

Q.3. A. Define organization. (*Chapter 7, p 73*)
B. Describe various characteristics of an organization. (*Chapter 7, p 75*)
C. Describe in brief about the various responsibilities of a ward incharge working in ICU. (*Chapter 13, pp 135, 137*). (modify for ICU head nurse).

Q.4. Write short notes on any four of the following:
A. Supplies and equipment in nursing unit. (*Chapter 18, p 220*)
B. Authority of responsibility. (*Chapter 15, p 168*)
C. Quality patient care. (*Chapter 3, p 35*)
D. Patient's clinical record. (*Chapter 21, pp 270–272*)
E. Classification of hospital. (*Chapter 10, pp 92–98*)

Q.5. Write about the following:
A. POSDCORB, (*Chapter 3, p 39*)
B. Nature and scope of supervision. (*Chapter 13, p 134*)

Q.6. Explain about following:
A. Decentralization of authority. (*Chapter 7, p 79*)
B. Importance of separate budget for nursing educational institutions. (*Chapter 23, p 310*)

Q.7. Write about two of the following:
A. Nursing audit. (*Chapter 16, p 191*)
B. Advantages of planning. (*Chapter 5, pp 53–54*)
C. Manpower planning. (*Chapter 12, p 120*)

Rajasthan University of Health Sciences, Rajasthan
BSc (Nursing) Part IV Examination
Held in August 2008
Old Scheme
Introduction to Principles of Administration and Nursing Services

Q.1. A. Define hospital.
B. Discuss the function of hospital. (*Chapter 10, p 99*)
C. Sketch the organization chart of hospital in district level. (*Chapter 7, p 75*)

Q.2. A. Define administration. (*Chapter 3, p 38*)
B. Explain the principles of administration in detail. (*Chapter 3, pp 39–40*)

Q.3. Discuss the trends in public health administration and nursing education. (*Chapter 24, pp 317–322*)

Q.4. A. Discuss the administrative function of public health nurse (PHN) in district level.
B. What are the job description of different categories of community health workers?

Q.5. A. Define curriculum.
B. As a principal, working in school of nursing, how will you administer the curriculum implementation in relation with practice field and examination. Explain.

Q.6. A. Define evaluation.
B. What are the component and techniques of evaluation? Explain.

Q.7. Define/describe (any eight) of the following:
A. Budget. (*Chapter 19, p 228*)
B. Personnel management. (*Chapter 13, pp 120–138*)
C. Staff counseling. (*see Glossary, p 370*)
D. Records and reports. (*Chapter 21, p 271*)
E. Career development. (*Chapter 28, p 348*)
F. Management. (*Chapter 3, p 40*)
G. Accreditation. (*Chapter 20, p 254*)
H. Client care. (*see Glossary, p 360*)
I. Resources of nursing unit. (*Chapter 22, pp 287–297*)
J. Techniques of supervision. (*Chapter 13, p 35*)
K. Organization. (*Chapter 7, pp 73–74*)

Rajiv Gandhi University of Health Sciences, Karnataka
IV Year BSc Nursing Degree Examination - September 2016

Time: Three Hours **Max. Marks: 75 Marks**

Management of Nursing Services and Education (RS-2)
QP CODE: 1774

Your answers should be specific to the questions asked draw neat, labeled diagrams wherever necessary

ESSAYS TYPE (ANY TWO)

(2 × 10 = 20 Marks)

Q.1. A. Define supervision.
B. What are the objectives of supervision?
C. List the principles of supervision.

Q.2. A. Define personnel management.
B. List the objectives of personnel management.
C. Explain in detail the recruitment process.

Q.3. A. Define staff development.
B. Explain the need for staff development.
C. Describe the staff development programs.

SHORT ESSAYS TYPE (ANY SEVEN)

(7 × 5 = 35 Marks)

Q.4. Explain disaster management.
Q.5. Enumerate the techniques of communication.
Q.6. Describe the Consumer Protection Act.
Q.7. Explain about performance appraisal.
Q.8. Explain about INC code of ethics.
Q.9. Describe about nursing audit.
Q.10. Enumerate the job description of female health assistant.
Q.11. Explain principles of budgeting.
Q.12. Describe leadership styles.

SHORT ANSWERS

(10 × 2 = 20 Marks)

Q.13. Define skill training.
Q.14. Define halo effect.
Q.15. What is graphic rating scale?
Q.16. Define accreditation.
Q.17. What is cost benefit analysis?
Q.18. Define motivation.
Q.19. Define bureaucracy.
Q.20. List the criterias of a good report.
Q.21. What is collective bargaining?
Q.22. What is malpractice?

Rajiv Gandhi University of Health Sciences, Karnataka
IV Year BSc Nursing Degree Examination - May 2016

Time: Three Hours **Max. Marks: 75 Marks**

Management of Nursing Services and Education (RS-2)
QP CODE: 1774

Your answers should be specific to the questions asked draw neat, labeled diagrams wherever necessary

ESSAYS TYPE (ANY TWO)

(2 × 10 = 20 Marks)

Q.1. A. Define material management.
B. Explain the elements of material management.

Q.2. A. Define communication.
B. Explain the communication process.
C. What are the barriers of communication?

Q.3. Define job description.
Describe the job description of a nursing superintendent Grade-I working in 1000 bedded multispecialty hospital.

SHORT ESSAYS TYPE (ANY SEVEN)

(7 × 5 = 35 Marks)

Q.4. Enumerate the qualities of a professional nurse.
Q.5. Describe about nursing assignments.
Q.6. Explain about quality assurance model.
Q.7. Describe the principles of supervision.
Q.8. Enumerate the classification of hospitals.
Q.9. Describe about in-service education for staff nurses.
Q.10. Enumerate various career opportunities for nurses.
Q.11. Explain the management of disciplinary problems.
Q.12. Differentiate between guidance and counseling.

SHORT ANSWERS

(10 × 2 = 20 Marks)

Q.13. Define autocratic leader.
Q.14. What is fixed budget?
Q.15. Define disaster.
Q.16. What is interpersonal relationship?
Q.17. Define negligence.
Q.18. Define curriculum.
Q.19. What is collective bargaining?
Q.20. What is decision-making?
Q.21. Types of reports.
Q.22. Define span of control.

Rajiv Gandhi University of Health Sciences, Karnataka
IV Year BSc Nursing Degree Examination - September 2015

Time: Three Hours **Max. Marks: 75 Marks**

Management of Nursing Services and Education (RS-2)
QP CODE: 1774

Your answers should be specific to the questions asked draw neat, labeled diagrams wherever necessary

ESSAYS TYPE (ANY TWO)

(2 × 10 = 20 Marks)

Q.1. Define management. State the principles of management. Explain the role of nurse as a manager in intensive care units.

Q.2. Explain in detail the role of human resource manager in recruiting, selecting and retaining the staff nurses of a multi speciality hospital.

Q.3. Which are the regulatory bodies for the college of nursing? Explain the physical and clinical facilities for the college of nursing.

SHORT ESSAYS TYPE (ANY SEVEN)

(7 × 5 = 35 Marks)

Q.4. What are the legal aspects in nursing?

Q.5. Describe communication process.

Q.6. Explain Bench marking.

Q.7. Describe the role of nursing service department in emergency and disaster management.

Q.8. Explain the components of staff development programme.

Q.9. Role of ward manager in orienting the newly recruited staff to NICU

Q.10. Explain the principles of adult learning.

Q.11. Write a note on collective bargaining.

Q.12. Explain the job description of principal of nursing educational institution.

SHORT ANSWERS

(10 × 2 = 20 Marks)

Q.13. Define delegation and control.

Q.14. List the objectives of planning.

Q.15. Differentiate between guidance and counselling.

Q.16. List the records maintained in the hospital.

Q.17. Define accreditation.

Q.18. State the characters of professional nurse.

Q.19. What are the different types of patient care assignment?

Q.20. What is curriculum planning?

Q.21. List nursing organizations for the professional membership

Q.22. List the leadership styles.

Rajiv Gandhi University of Health Sciences, Karnataka
IV Year BSc Nursing Degree Examination - April 2015

Time: Three Hours **Max. Marks: 75 Marks**

Management of Nursing Services and Education (RS-2)
QP CODE: 1774

Your answers should be specific to the questions asked draw neat, labeled diagrams wherever necessary

ESSAYS TYPE (ANY TWO)

(2 × 10 = 20 Marks)

Q.1. What is planning? What are the steps of planning? Discuss its advantages and disadvantages.
Q.2. Define motivation. List-down the theories of motivation. Explain any one theory in detail.
Q.3. Define nursing audit. Explain the steps of nursing audit process.

SHORT ESSAYS TYPE (ANY SEVEN)

(7 × 5 = 35 Marks)

Q.4. Types of accreditation.
Q.5. Importance of effective coordination.
Q.6. Factors influencing curriculum development.
Q.7. Key elements of informed consent.
Q.8. Principles of management.
Q.9. Career opportunities for nurses.
Q.10. Activities performed by TNAI.
Q.11. Responsibilities of nursing service administration.
Q.12. Principles of guidance.

SHORT ANSWERS

(10 × 2 = 20 Marks)

Q.13. Incident report.
Q.14. Sources of nursing standards.
Q.15. Four important aspects of educational evaluation.
Q.16. In-service education.
Q.17. Qualities of public relation officer.
Q.18. Type of need.
Q.19. Selection of a student to the college of nursing.
Q.20. Consumer Protection Act.
Q.21. Channels of communication.
Q.22. Negligence.

Rajiv Gandhi University of Health Sciences, Karnataka
IV Year BSc Nursing Degree Examination - September 2014

Time: Three Hours **Max. Marks: 75 Marks**

Management of Nursing Services and Education (RS-2)
QP CODE: 1774

Your answers should be specific to the questions asked draw neat, labeled diagrams wherever necessary

ESSAYS TYPE (ANY TWO)

(2 × 10 = 20 Marks)

Q.1. List the principles of management and explain the role of nurse as a manager.
Q.2. Explain the role of a Principal in curriculum planning for a college of nursing which conducts BSc nursing programme.
Q.3. Discuss the techniques of good leadership.

SHORT ESSAYS TYPE (ANY SEVEN)

(7 × 5 = 35 Marks)

Q.4. Principles of adult learning.
Q.5. Criteria of a profession.
Q.6. Consumer Protection Act.
Q.7. Nurse-patient relationship.
Q.8. PERT.
Q.9. Staff welfare.
Q.10. Patient care unit.
Q.11. Nursing audit.
Q.12. Waste management.

SHORT ANSWERS

(10 × 2 = 20 Marks)

Q.13. Master plan.
Q.14. Define budget.
Q.15. ABC analysis.
Q.16. Critical incidents.
Q.17. Policies.
Q.18. Channels of communication.
Q.19. Define accreditation.
Q.20. Committees in the college.
Q.21. Malpractice.
Q.22. Career opportunities for a nurse

Rajiv Gandhi University of Health Sciences, Karnataka
IV Year BSc Nursing Degree Examination - April 2014

Time: Three Hours **Max. Marks: 75 Marks**

Management of Nursing Services and Education (RS-2)
QP CODE: 1774

Your answers should be specific to the questions asked draw neat, labeled diagrams wherever necessary

ESSAYS TYPE (ANY TWO)

(2 × 10 = 20 Marks)

Q.1. Define Management. Discuss material management in hospital set-up.

Q.2. Define profession. Explain the characteristics of a professional nurse. Describe code of professional conduct.

Q.3. Describe the principles and techniques of supervision in nursing, giving suitable examples from nursing services.

SHORT ESSAYS TYPE (ANY SEVEN)

(7 × 5 = 35 Marks)

Q.4. Principles of adult learning.

Q.5. Public relations in context of nursing.

Q.6. Leadership styles.

Q.7. Malpractice and negligence in nursing.

Q.8. Performance appraisal.

Q.9. Collective bargaining.

Q.10. Job description.

Q.11. Quality assurance model.

Q.12. Program evaluation review technique.

SHORT ANSWERS

(10 × 2 = 20 Marks)

Q.13. Four techniques of supervision.

Q.14. Patient classification system.

Q.15. Nursing rounds.

Q.16. Interpersonal relationships.

Q.17. Affiliation.

Q.18. Scope of in-service education.

Q.19. Philosophy of nursing educational institutions.

Q.20. Indian nursing council act.

Q.21. Continuing nursing education.

Q.22. Principles of budgeting.

Rajiv Gandhi University of Health Sciences, Karnataka
IV Year BSc Nursing Degree Examination - August 2013

Time: Three Hours **Max. Marks: 75 Marks**

Management of Nursing Services and Education (RS-2)
QP CODE: 1774

Your answers should be specific to the questions asked draw neat, labeled diagrams wherever necessary

ESSAYS TYPE (ANY TWO)

(2 × 10 = 20 Marks)

Q.1. Define budget. Enumerate the types and advantages of budget.
Q.2. Define supervision. Explain the principles and techniques of supervision.
Q.3. Discuss nursing as a profession. Explain the characteristics of a professional nurse.

SHORT ESSAYS TYPE (ANY SEVEN)

(7 × 5 = 35 Marks)

Q.4. Performance appraisal.
Q.5. Continuing education.
Q.6. Guidance and counseling.
Q.7. Malpractice and negligence in nursing practice.
Q.8. Equipment and supplies.
Q.9. Principles of audit.
Q.10. Current trends and issues in nursing.
Q.11. Principles of management.
Q.12. Patient classification system.

SHORT ANSWERS

(10 × 2 – 20 Marks)

Q.13. Affiliation.
Q.14. Recruiting.
Q.15. Leadership styles.
Q.16. Essentials of good control.
Q.17. Human relation.
Q.18. Tools for evaluating nursing standards.
Q.19. Delegation of responsibility.
Q.20. Records and reports.
Q.21. Professional organizations.
Q.22. Problems in health administration.

Rajiv Gandhi University of Health Sciences, Karnataka

IV Year BSc Nursing Degree Examination - March 2013

Time: Three Hours **Max. Marks: 75 Marks**

Management of Nursing Services and Education (RS-2)

QP CODE: 1774

Your answers should be specific to the questions asked draw neat, labeled diagrams wherever necessary

ESSAYS TYPE (ANY TWO)

(2 × 10 = 20 Marks)

Q.1. Discuss the points to be kept in mind by nurses regarding legal issues arises in nursing practice.
Q.2. Discuss the nursing as a profession by using standard criteria of a profession.
Q.3. Explain the importance and responsibilities of nursing in maintaining recording and reporting.

SHORT ESSAYS TYPE (ANY SEVEN)

(7 × 5 = 35 Marks)

Q.4. State philosophy and objectives of BSc nursing course.
Q.5. State the principles of adult learning.
Q.6. Describe the elements of material management with references to nursing.
Q.7. Explain the role of nurse manager in emergency and disaster.
Q.8. Describe public relations in the context of nursing.
Q.9. Explain the total quality management in Nursing.
Q.10. List the objectives of staffing in nursing department.
Q.11. State the principles of supervision in nursing.
Q.12. Explain the importance of theories in management.

SHORT ANSWERS

(10 × 2 = 20 Marks)

Q.13. POSDCORB.
Q.14. Accreditation.
Q.15. Continuing education.
Q.16. Interpersonal relationship.
Q.17. Leadership styles.
Q.18. Staff development.
Q.19. Collective bargaining.
Q.20. Indian nursing council.
Q.21. Negligence.
Q.22. Nursing rounds.

Rajiv Gandhi University of Health Sciences, Karnataka
IV Year BSc Nursing Degree Examination - September 2012

Time: Three Hoursr **Max. Marks: 75 Marks**

Management of Nursing Services and Education (RS-2)
QP CODE: 1774

Your answers should be specific to the questions asked draw neat, labeled diagrams wherever necessary

ESSAYS TYPE (ANY TWO)

(2 × 10 = 20 Marks)

Q.1. A. Define quality assurance.
B. Discuss methods adopted to maintain quality in a hospital.
Q.2. Discuss the tools and techniques used in supervision.
Q.3. Explain theories of management.

SHORT ESSAYS TYPE (ANY SEVEN)

(7 × 5 = 35 Marks)

Q.4. Role of nurse manger in maintenance of supplies and equipments in wards.
Q.5. Current trends and issues in nursing.
Q.6. Emergency and disaster management.
Q.7. Philosophy and norms of staffing.
Q.8. Concepts principles and types of budget.
Q.9. Staff development.
Q.10. Performance appraisal.
Q.11. Guidance and counseling.
Q.12. Leadership styles.

SHORT ANSWERS

(10 × 2 = 20 Marks)

Q.13. Inventory.
Q.14. PERT.
Q.15. Records in a school of nursing.
Q.16. Consumer Protection Act.
Q.17. INC code of ethics.
Q.18. Characteristics of a professional nurse.
Q.19. Malpractice.
Q.20. Supervision.
Q.21. Collective bargaining.
Q.22. Cost-benefit analysis.

Rajiv Gandhi University of Health Sciences, Karnataka
IV Year BSc Nursing Degree Examination - Feb/Mar 2012

Time: Three Hours **Max. Marks: 75 Marks**

Management of Nursing Services and Education (RS-2)
QP CODE: 1774

Your answers should be specific to the questions asked draw neat, labeled diagrams wherever necessary

ESSAYS TYPE (ANY TWO)

(2 × 10 = 20 Marks)

Q.1. Define management and discuss the principles of management.
Q.2. Discuss the process of recruitment and selection.
Q.3. A. Discuss the principles of adult learning
B. Explain the steps in organizing in-service education programme.

SHORT ESSAYS TYPE (ANY SEVEN)

(7 × 5 = 35 Marks)

Q.4. PERT
Q.5. Budgeting.
Q.6. Job description.
Q.7. Role of nurse as a manager.
Q.8. Tools and techniques of supervision.
Q.9. Performance appraisal.
Q.10. Staff welfare.
Q.11. INC code of ethics professional conduct.
Q.12. Continuing nursing education.

SHORT ANSWERS

(10 × 2 = 20 Marks)

Q.13. Collective bargaining.
Q.14. Nursing audit.
Q.15. Channels of communication.
Q.16. Nursing rounds.
Q.17. Interpersonal relationship.
Q.18. Accreditation.
Q.19. Records and reports.
Q.20. Quality assurance model.
Q.21. Superanuuation.
Q.22. Malpractice and negligence.

Rajiv Gandhi University of Health Sciences, Karnataka
IV Year BSc Nursing Degree Examination - Aug/Sep 2011

Time: Three Hours **Max. Marks: 75 Marks**

Management of Nursing Services and Education (RS-2)
QP CODE: 1774

Your answers should be specific to the questions asked draw neat, labeled diagrams wherever necessary

ESSAYS TYPE (ANY TWO)

Q.1. What is job description? Prepare a job description for the post of a principal working in a college of nursing.
Q.2. How will you design evaluation program of staff members working in the department of nursing?
Q.3. Discuss the role and responsibilities of an educational administrator for curriculum planning and implementation.

SHORT ESSAYS TYPE (ANY SEVEN)

Q.4. Nursing audit.
Q.5. Institutional records and reports.
Q.6. Professional ethics.
Q.7. Legal aspects in nursing.
Q.8. Current trends and issues in nursing.
Q.9. Functions of management.
Q.10. Principles of material management.
Q.11. Budget for nursing service.
Q.12. Theory of human motivation.

SHORT ANSWERS

Q.13. Purposes of good coordination.
Q.14. Aims of in-service education program.
Q.15. Supervision.
Q.16. Advantages of planning.
Q.17. Staff development program.
Q.18. Division of work.
Q.19. Nursing protocols.
Q.20. Personnel policies.
Q.21. Interpersonal relations in organization.
Q.22. Career opportunities for nurses.

Index

Page numbers followed by *b* refer to box, *f* refer to figure and *t* refer to table, respectively.

C

D

E

F

G

H

I

J

K

L

M

N

O

P

X

Y

Z